# SPORTS INJURIES
## *and their Treatment*

# SPORTS INJURIES
## *and their Treatment*

Edited by

## Basil Helal MCh (Orth), FRCS FRCSE

*Consultant Orthopaedic Surgeon to the London Hospital, The Royal National
   Orthopaedic Hospital and Enfield District Hospital*
*Vice President and Former Chairman, British Association of Sports and
   Medicine*
*Orthopaedic Adviser to the British Olympic Association*

## John King FRCS

*Senior Lecturer, the London Hospital Medical College*
*Consultant Orthopaedic Surgeon to the London Hospital and Newham
   District Hospital*
*Director, the Diploma Course in Sports Medicine, L.H.M.C.*
*Board member, the London Sports Medicine Institute*

and

## William Grange MA, FRCS

*Consultant Orthopaedic Surgeon to the London Hospital*

LONDON
CHAPMAN AND HALL

RD
97
S695
1986

First published in 1986 by Chapman and Hall Ltd
11 New Fetter Lane, London EC4P 4EE

© 1986 Chapman and Hall Ltd

Printed in Great Britain at the
University Press, Cambridge

ISBN 0 412 23950 7

**British Library Cataloguing in Publication Data**

Sports injuries and their treatment.
1. Sports——Accidents and injuries
I. Helal, Basil   II. King, John B.
III. Grange, William J.
617'.1027        RD97

ISBN 0–412–23950–7

# Contents

# Contents

Contents

# Contents

Contents

# Contents

Contents

# Contents

# Contributors

John Blandy MA DM MCh FRCS FACS
Professor of Urology, The London Hospital Medical College and Institute of Urology, London

G. B. Brookes FRCS
Senior Registrar, Department of Otorhinolaryngology, The London Hospital

J. M. Cameron MD PhD FRCS FRCPath DMJ
Professor of Forensic Medicine, The London Hospital Medical College
Honorary Medical Advisor, Amateur Swimming Association

Hugh Cannell MD MSc FDSRCS
Reader and Consultant, The Department of Oral and Maxillo-facial Surgery, The London Hospital

John Challis FRCS
Consultant Orthopaedic Surgeon, The North Middlesex Hospital

Shwing Chong Chen BA (Tech.) FRCS
Consultant Orthopaedic Surgeon, Enfield Group of Hospitals

Margaret E. Ellis FCOT
District Occupational Therapist, The London Hospital

John Emens MD MRCOG
Consultant Gynaecologist, Birmingham Maternity Hospital

John Gleave FRCS
Consultant Neurosurgeon, Addenbrooke's Hospital, Cambridge

Anthony Goode MD FRCS
Assistant Director, Surgical Unit, The London Hospital

Vivian Grisogono MA MCSP
Chartered Physiotherapist, Honorary Lecturer to the London Hospital Medical College (Sports Medicine Course)

xiii

# Contributors

Mark G. Harries MD MRCP
Consultant Physician, Northwick Park Hospital and the Clinical Research Centre, Harrow

Basil Helal MCh (Orth), FRCS, FRCSE
Consultant Orthopaedic Surgeon, The London Hospital, Royal National Orthopaedic Hospital and Enfield District Hospital

John King FRCS
Senior Lecturer, The London Hospital

Ivor S. Levy FRCS
Consultant Ophthalmic Surgeon, The London Hospital, Moorfields Eye Hospital and The Hospital for Sick Children

Terence Lewis FRCS
Consultant Cardiothoracic Surgeon, The London Hospital

Peter McKelvie MD ChM FRCS DLO
Consultant in Otorhinolaryngology, The London Hospital

James Robertson FRCS
Consultant Orthopaedic Surgeon, Southampton General Hospital

Joseph S. Torg MD
Sports Medicine Center, University of Pennsylvania, Philadelphia

Joseph J. Vegso A.T.,C.
Sports Medicine Center, University of Pennsylvania, Philadelphia

Alastair Wilson FRCS
Consultant in Accident and Emergency Medicine, The London Hospital

Maurice Yaffé MSc ABPsS
Senior Clinical Psychologist, Guy's Hospital, Hon. Psychological Adviser to the British Olympic Association

# Foreword

During the past ten years or so many books have been written on 'sports medicine' and 'sports injuries' – probably reflecting the rapid growth of interest in these subjects in an age in which 'sport for all' and increased leisure time for recreation have become matters of social and political concern. And now comes this new book – new in its fresh and stimulating approach to well worn topics and emphasizing the wide scope of preventive measures available, and the over-riding effect of the time element in any consideration of sports injuries. The term, used somewhere in the text that it is dealing with the 'art of interference' is highly relevant.

It is a large book – comprehensive, detailed and yet eminently readable with ample figures, diagrams and tables together with a list of valuable references to each chapter. It is essentially a book for doctors, written by doctors, but that it will have a wider appeal is underlined by the fact that the (excellent) chapter dealing with prevention and prophylaxis (and embodying what might be called the philosophy of sport and sports injuries) is written by a physiotherapist. The editors and most of the contributors stem from that tried and proved sector of sports medicine – The London Hospital – but authors from other centres and from the USA are responsible for some most valuable chapters.

The book would seem to divide naturally into two main parts – general subjects and orthopaedic problems. Both provide a mass of valuable information and practical advice, both prophylactic and therapeutic. It is not easy to select special features from either section as all are of a very high standard. But in the general section, a separate chapter on ENT injuries is surely unusual; the contribution on psychology, linked as it is with consideration of pain and stress and the importance of motivation, underlines the growing significance of non-physical factors in sports injuries; the combination of 'unconsciousness' and 'resuscitation' taken together with the cardiac chapter offers much sound advice, and the article on gynaecological problems is practical and straightforward, including as it does, sensible counsel on the use (and misuse) of the anabolic steroids.

I am sure readers will be intrigued with the information made available

# Foreword

on the relation of weight training to back pain, the high risks of riding (especially for women) in comparison to rugby, soccer and boxing in producing head injuries, the solitary kidney in athletes, and even the esoteric subjects of 'joggers' nipple' and 'groin strain'.

In the orthopaedics section, as one would expect with this editorship, the coverage is detailed, essentially practical and remains closely linked to sports injuries. An interesting feature is the use of the major joints as chapter headings for the various anatomico-geographical areas, although the hand and foot (the special interest of the senior editor) deservedly stand under their own names. Finally, this fascinating book, reverting again to one of its primary objectives, prevention, produces two most valuable chapters on footwear, playing surfaces and protective devices, and on some of the legal problems involved in sports medicine. In the introduction it is stressed that sports injuries are but a part of sports medicine which is itself a part of sports science. It is this all encompassing concept, rigorously adhered to throughout the book, that gives it its wide-ranging appeal. I am sure that for many years it will prove an invaluable book of reference and an essential requisite of all those who have to deal with the complex problems of sports injuries. I wish it well.

PORRITT

# Preface

Sports science embraces very many disciplines: sports medicine is but one of these and a small section of sports medicine is concerned with injury. This is the main subject with which this book is concerned. It is intended for those who have to treat the consequences of the double epidemic of 'sport for all' and the expectation of good health. Cure, especially after severe and complex injury, may be imperfect and may take time to achieve. This is especially important to the athlete at the peak of a career; precaution and prevention are therefore the wisest counsel.

Paracelsius said 'the wound needs nothing so much as to be left alone'. The body's response to injury does not differ whether the individual is a sports person or otherwise. We do not propose that the athlete be given preferential treatment, but hope that the reader of this book may offer more appropriate management for the patient with high sporting aspirations, be they professional or amateur. It must always be remembered that an apparently trivial complaint may make all the difference between success and failure at the highest levels. Awareness of the likely causes of injury, the methods of prevention, the injuries common to a particular sport, combined with accurate history taking and examination will facilitate precise diagnosis and correct management. In the phase of rehabilitation, motivation and physical capacity will influence the speed of return to full fitness. Wolfe's law states that tissues respond to demands made upon them and will strengthen and enlarge accordingly. It is at this stage that the 'art of interference' is applied and protected exercise in mobile splints or cast braces will permit early mobility and allow some stress to be taken without damage.

The possible courses of treatment available have been mentioned, but it must be stressed that expertise is all important and those who are responsible for the care of sports people, whether they be medically qualified or not, must be warned against embarking on diagnosis and treatment beyond their ability, and indeed are liable in law if they make such an attempt at the expense of their patient's well being. Sound advice can always be obtained. The British Olympic Association has a panel of medical practitioners which includes experts in every specialty and doctors from the governing bodies of almost all sports who bring their special knowledge of the sport to bear on the problem in hand.

It has been said that sport is a substitute for job satisfaction and contact sport a substitute for war. Would that this were so. Governments should recognize this and encourage their subjects by putting more financial resource into sport. It is so much cheaper than both war and the outcome of social unrest. Unwarranted displays of dangerous aggression in contact sport seem to be on the increase. The sports person is not immune to a liability in law for wilful injury to a fellow player, nor a doctor for negligence in his or her treatment. Perhaps it is time that those concerned with sports medical care had a say in the revision of the rules of the game.

Medical influence in industry has resulted in more consultation by the manufacturers of sports equipment with those who are concerned with the treatment of injuries. The rewards are seen in the preparation of better playing surfaces, winter sports courses, sports footwear and equipment such as ski bindings, and the better design of helmets, gloves and face, eye and tooth protectors, all of which have substantially reduced the incidence of injuries.

Injuries within the sports context are simply injuries as in any other field and their initial management is much the same. It is important, however, to appreciate the immense pressures placed particularly on top class competitors. The pressures are produced by high motivation, by trainers, teams, clubs or nations and are sometimes overwhelming. It is the responsibility of the medical advisor to protect the individual from him- or herself and from the other pressures whilst restoring him or her to full fitness in the shortest possible time. Much of this book is devoted to these aims and we hope it will not only prove useful to medical practitioners, but that the bulk of its content will be easily understood by other non-medical people who are concerned with the care of sports people.

It is not surprising that many of our contributors have links with The London Hospital since the editors work there and The London Hospital Medical College has pioneered a three term full time course in Sports Medicine. We are grateful to our authors who have given so much of their precious time to the making of this book and to our publishers who have been constantly helpful and sympathetic.

# Acknowledgements

We are grateful to Herr W. Troger, General Secretary of the FDR Olympic Association for permission to use the pictograms and to Dick Palmer, General Secretary of the British Olympic Association for his advice.

The patience and co-operation of our publishers, Chapman and Hall, and their Medical Editor, Dr Peter Altman, is greatly appreciated.

We are most honoured that Lord Porritt has kindly written the Foreword to this book.

Grateful thanks are also due to the British Equestrian Federation, the British Canoe Union, the Amateur Boxing Association of England and the Great Britain Men's Hockey Board for their financial assistance with the cost of the colour illustrations.

Finally we greatly appreciate the tolerance of all at home who share our lives and apologize for robbing them of so many hours of our company.

# 1 *Prevention and prophylaxis*

VIVIAN GRISOGONO

The campaign for fitness and health through exercise has spread world-wide in recent years, despite conflicting opinions among scientists and doctors about its benefits (Holloszy, 1983). It has become axiomatic that the 'sport for all' campaign implies 'sports injuries for all' as its corollary (Sperryn, 1983).

Historically, physical fitness has often been identified with a nation's fitness to fight, and therefore encouraged by governments. Many of the earliest descriptions of injuries related to physical activity were described in soldiers. Devas (1975) cites descriptions by Breithaupt (1855), Aleman (1929) and Nordentoft (1940) of exercise-related bone injuries among soldiers. With the gradual acceptance of sports medicine as an entity, papers on sports injuries have proliferated, both in the old-established orthopaedic and rheumatological journals, and in the more recently founded specialist sports medicine journals. Various factors are making it easier to define the relationship between sport and injuries. Top-level competitors in all countries usually do little other than train for their events, while the growing mass of keep-fit enthusiasts and recreational sportsmen are often relatively inactive in the rest of their working and leisure time. Clinicians' interest in the subject and the provision of sports medicine clinics have led to epidemiological studies (Godshall, 1975; Compton and Tubbs, 1977; Sonne-Holm and Sorensen, 1980; Bedford and Macauley, 1984; Chan, Fu and Leung, 1984; Jorgensen, 1984; Sandelin *et al.*, 1985).

The surveys on sports injuries have naturally stimulated an interest in injury prevention measures. All of the surveys to date present the experience of practitioners working within a particular context, such as with teams, in sports clubs and centres, in casualty departments or in sports medicine units. Many of the surveys simply describe the work within the clinics or centres (Grisogono, 1981; Galasko *et al.*, 1982; Brodie, 1983; Devereux and Lachmann, 1983; Hutson, 1984). Although the surveys therefore differ according to local conditions and individual

1

viewpoints, they serve to provide a broad view of the scope of sports injuries treatment, contrasting with the very narrow definition provided by Williams (1976) when he differentiated between 'injuries occurring in sport' and 'technopathies' which he terms 'true sport-specific injuries'. It is of course important, when discussing injury prevention, to distinguish between injuries incurred during sport, competition and training, and those which happen at other times, even though the injuries may be similar in nature, and rehabilitation for either type has to take into account the patient's needs as a sportsman.

Damage from sports injuries ranges from minor soft-tissue strains to major disruption of vital organs. All the surveys cited show the majority of injuries occurring in the lower limb; most conclude that, probably because of knowledgeable diagnosis and early treatment, the majority of the injuries do not have serious consequences, nor do they cost the patients excessive loss of time from work or sport. Injury prevention measures have arisen largely from practical experience of the dangers in sports. The key factors are recognition of injury types and an understanding of the associated risks. Other factors which need to be considered when advising sportsmen on injury prevention include: levels of participation, including training levels; physiological capacities; and the sportsman's mental attitude to sports participation, to competition where relevant, and to injury (Yaffe, 1983; Sanderson, 1981).

## 1.1 Classification of injuries

Of the various possible methods of categorizing injuries, one of the most logical is according to cause (Williams, 1971). Injuries may occur through extrinsic or intrinsic factors.

An extrinsic cause involves a recognizable abnormal incident which results in damage to body tissues, usually causing pain and loss of function in the affected area. The incident is usually sudden, and may be mild or severe. Examples of extrinsic causes of injury include: a fall; a sheering stress across a joint or bone; a direct blow; or a sudden force exerted across a bone, joint or soft tissue, which causes distortion. There is always a direct relationship between cause and effect in extrinsic injuries, so the sportsman can always identify the event which caused his symptoms.

Intrinsically caused injuries, on the other hand, usually seem to happen without an identifiable cause. Tissues are damaged, causing pain and loss of function, as the result of apparently normal sporting activity. Intrinsic injuries can be subdivided into two categories: overuse and traumatic. Overuse injuries are generally of gradual onset. Characteristi-

2

cally, they occur in the first instance as a slight ache or nagging pain, related to a particular movement pattern, and not noticeable at other times. If the activity is continued, the pain becomes increasingly severe, to the stage where it causes loss of function. Traumatic intrinsic injuries happen suddenly, despite having no obvious cause. The squash player's Achilles tendon rupture is an example of traumatic intrinsic injury; the runner's tight niggling hamstring is an overuse injury. A stress fracture in bone, in its early stages, is an overuse injury, but if it develops to the stage of becoming complete, it is then a traumatic intrinsic injury.

Any injury may have an acute phase, the initial moment of injury, and a chronic phase, when the injury has become established over a period of time. In the acute phase of extrinsic or traumatic intrinsic injuries there may be obvious, gross signs of damage, such as bruising and haematoma formation, joint swelling, muscle spasm, pain on movement and tenderness on palpation. In the chronic phase, the initial signs usually abate, leaving residual functional loss. Overuse intrinsic injuries generally do not have an obvious acute phase, and show no dramatic evidence of damage, other than gradually increasing pain accompanied by decreasing functional efficiency.

## 1.2 Predisposing factors

Intrinsic injuries of both kinds are especially influenced by various underlying causative factors, which, when analysed, may help explain otherwise totally unexpected injuries. Extrinsic injuries happen independently of inherent factors, although these may contribute to the severity of an injury. Commonly recognized predisposing factors include:

(1) Fatigue and overload. Excessive repetition of an activity, or excessive weight loading within an activity, can cause localized fatigue leading to tissue breakdown.
(2) Previous, incompletely rehabilitated injury.
(3) Muscle tightness and soreness, which may be due to fatigue, cold, previous injury, cramp episodes, excessive exercise, tension, viral infection, congenital inflexibility or insufficient flexibility training.
(4) Muscle weakness, which may be due to previous injury or inadequate training.
(5) Muscle imbalance, which may arise through injury or inappropriate training.
(6) Joint limitation.
(7) Poor, inefficient technique.
(8) Inappropriate equipment.

3

(9) Inadequate body preparation, whether for each session, or overall for the sport.

(10) Inappropriate choice of sport.

## 1.3  Hazards in specific sports

It is artificial to assign specific injuries to certain sports, as any human activity can cause musculo-skeletal strains in the widest variety and most unlikely of situations. Academically, one can accept the narrow definition of 'true sport-specific injuries' proposed by Williams (1976), but when dealing with injured sportsmen on a practical level, the practitioner has to take the broadest view of sports injuries. However, it is possible to identify risk factors within sports which lead to an increased likelihood of certain types of injury. Papers have been written reviewing the injuries seen within sports, and highlighting certain injuries in the context of causative sports (for instance Weightman and Browne, 1974; McLatchie, 1976; Williams and McKibbin, 1978; Mack, 1982).

A total of 1740 injuries was seen during a two-year period within the Injuries Unit at the Crystal Palace National Sports Centre in London, in sportsmen from some fifty events. The majority were athletes, the largest group using the centre for training for some level of competition. The other patients were drawn from centre users such as the semi-professional basketball squads, recreational sportsmen, resident school groups and visiting elite squads. Although the Injuries Unit provided facilities for immediate treatment, 59% of the injuries seen over the two years were of the overuse type, totalling 1025. Of these, 94 (9%) were 'growing problems' such as Sever's disease, Osgood-Schlatter's disease, and primary chondromalacia patellae, reflecting the fact that the majority of patients were teenage, between twelve and seventeen years. Overall, the age-span of the patients ranged from eight to sixty-five years.

Extrinsic injuries are a risk in many kinds of sport. In combat sports the principle of controlled assault gives rise to various situations where injuries can occur. The growing medical concern over brain damage and deaths among boxers indicates what serious consequences traumatic injuries may have. Team sports involving direct confrontation between opposing players, such as football, basketball, rugby and water polo, carry the risk of harmful physical contact. The injury risk is increased when the players are also wielding implements, as in hockey and lacrosse. Similarly, in individual sports where the players are in close proximity, like Eton Fives, there is the risk of accidental collision, and the danger is greater when implements are involved, as in rackets, racketball and squash.

4

Speed in sport can increase the severity of accidents, for instance in downhill ski-ing, cycle racing and bobsledding. Some individual sports carry an inherent risk of injury by virtue of their technical difficulty, like gymnastics, sports acrobatics and diving. Environmental hazards can add to the dangers of sports like rock climbing, ski-ing and canoeing.

Overuse intrinsic injuries are particularly associated with sports which involve repetitive movements, like long-distance running, swimming, rowing and cycling. Repetitive patterns of training carry similar risks, for instance extended sessions of hopping and bounding for hurdlers, or service practice for tennis players. The constant gripping action of racket sports makes the wrist and forearm prone to overuse injury.

Traumatic intrinsic injuries are a risk for any sportsman who has to move in varied directions at speed, or has to exert powerful muscle force suddenly, or is subjected to a sudden overload. The lower limbs are vulnerable in sports like football, hockey and sprinting, while racket games also pose a risk to the upper limb. One sport in which the risk of overloading is inherent is competitive weightlifting, where the participant is constantly trying to improve on his best one-repetition-maximum lift.

Figure 1.1 indicates areas of the body commonly affected by intrinsic and extrinsic injuries arising from specific sports.

## 1.4   Preventing extrinsic injuries

Accidents will happen, but risks can be minimized. Foresight and anticipation of possible dangers are prerequisites for this. Risk factors should be identified and understood pertaining to the participant, his sport, his equipment, protective gear, clothing, footwear, and environment.

### 1.4.1   RESPONSIBILITY

Various people can be considered responsible for safety in sports. Firstly, the participants, or where children are concerned, games and physical education teachers and parents; secondly, coaches teaching the sports; thirdly, umpires, markers and referees; fourthly, any medical or paramedical advisers to clubs, centres or teams, or any trained first-aiders; finally, the organizers, and possibly sponsors, of exhibition or competitive events.

### 1.4.2   THE PARTICIPANT

When learning the techniques of a sport, the participant must be made aware of potential dangers to himself, his opponents, and to any other

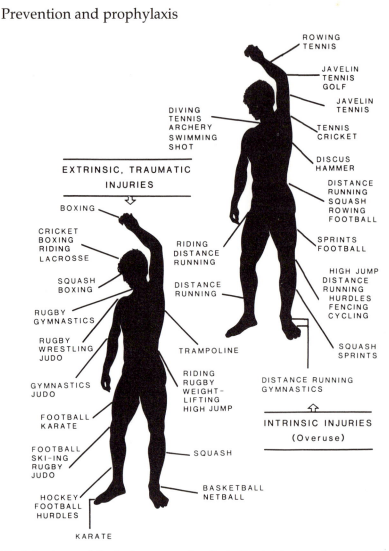

*Fig. 1.1* Areas of the body commonly affected by intrinsic and extrinsic injuries arising from specific sports.

people in the vicinity. In squash, where players are confined in a relatively small space, style must be modified to avoid striking the opponent. In sports involving direct physical confrontation, opponents should be size-matched. Most combat sports incorporate this principle in their rules, but schoolboy rugby is an example of a sport in which it is fairly common to see smaller boys mismatched against physically better developed opponents, who happen to be the same age.

### 1.4.3  THE SPORT

The choice of a sport is sometimes made for more or less logical reasons, like natural aptitude, or appropriate physique, but it is more often arbitrary. A totally unsuitable choice can pose dangers to the participant or others, for instance if someone with poor co-ordination tries to perform gymnastics or throw the hammer.

   Correct and strict application of a sport's rules can be a factor in injury prevention. A boxer has to be passed medically fit before a bout, and it is part of the referee's task to stop a fight if one of the contestants has taken visibly excessive punishment. Foul play is not permissible in any sport, but all too often participants in contact and combat sports are only deterred from it by strict refereeing. In squash, the 'let' and 'point' rules were devised to discourage dangerous and obstructive play. The effectiveness of these protective rules depends on the players' willingness to abide by them, and, more importantly, on the referee's perceptiveness and strict enforcement.

### 1.4.4  EQUIPMENT

Making sure that any equipment is in a fit state for use is fundamental to safety in sport. A squash racket with a cracked shaft may break, allowing the head to fly off. Quick-release safety catches on skis must be working efficiently, in case of a bad fall. The sharp point of a broken fencing foil can penetrate an opponent's protective clothing, so these weapons must be checked for visible signs of fragility or loss of pliability. A rowing boat should not be used without the protective bobble over the sharp end of the bow: the bobble was introduced following the death of a cox who was pierced by a rival boat.

### 1.4.5  PROTECTIVE GEAR

Most sports involving special risks have specifically designed protective gear to reduce risks for participants. In many sports protective clothing is constantly being revised, as new materials become available, or as changes within the sports make different types of protection necessary. Helmets are now routinely used to protect the skull from direct blows in American football, amateur boxing, show jumping, skateboarding, and more recently cricket. Face masks are used by fencers, and by goalkeepers in lacrosse and hockey. These sportsmen also wear padded protective coverings over the chest and abdomen. Mouthguards protect the teeth and gums in contact sports, and they may also help reduce the shock to the skull from direct blows to the chin. Groin boxes shield the genitals.

Many basketball and volleyball players use padded knee boxes against direct trauma to the knees. The shins are protected by thick padded guards in cricket, and by smaller snug-fitting pads in football and hockey.

Where possible, protective gear should be fitted to the individual. Mouthguards, for instance, are best when made up by a dentist, rather than moulded from a shop-bought ready-made plastic shield. Participants should be strongly encouraged to use such protective gear as is available for them. Too often, sportsmen spurn the use of protective items, even when they recognize the need for their use, as Chapman (1985) found in a study on mouthguards for rugby players. Where improvements are being made to existing protective equipment and clothing, information about the developments should be spread as quickly as possible through the sport.

It is the duty of governing bodies in sport to encourage the use of protective equipment, and to promote the development of better versions of available items.

### 1.4.6 CLOTHING

Dress for sport, if it is not specifically designed for protection, should serve not to impede movement. Clothing should be neither too loose nor too tight. Materials should allow for evaporation of sweat. For many sports, there is a dual need for a cooling effect together with insulation against sudden chill. Removable layers of clothing are needed for the warming-up and cooling-down periods of any sports session.

Safety pins, jewellery, or any sharp accessories should not be worn during physical activity, and especially not during combat sports. Fashion often dictates sportswear and the participant's appearance, but common sense should prevail, if fashionable items create potential hazards.

### 1.4.7 FOOTWEAR

Shoes should be protective, but inappropriate or poorly fitting sports shoes can be a source of injuries.

Shock absorption underfoot is an important function of shoes in all sports involving running and jumping. Thick but flexible soles are vital for intensive running training, especially for long distances run on hard surfaces. Competition shoes are usually made as light as possible, but their shock absorption qualities can be greatly increased by the use of the modern resilient polymer insoles.

Grip underfoot is important for sports involving running, twisting and turning, like basketball, football and racketball. In field sports, studs provide for necessary traction, as spikes provide grip for track athletes. They should be correctly sited under the forefoot area, and firmly anchored to prevent protrusion upwards into the wearer's foot. Studs should not be sharpened metal, which would be dangerous for other players. Sole materials should suit the needs of the sport and those of the wearer: some nimble court games players may prefer shoes without a firmly gripping sole, whereas others in the same sport, especially if they have 'weak' ankles or relatively poor balance, may feel unsafe unless they have a sure grip.

Sports shoe uppers have, in general, improved with the new materials available, which combine the useful qualities of resisting external moisture while encouraging the dissipation of internal damp. However, some synthetic modern materials actually increase foot heating, causing sweating and swelling. One obviously harmful innovation has been the raised heel-tab, which causes friction by dragging into the Achilles tendon on plantarflexion, and results in thickening and pain round the tendon in far too many sportsmen.

## 1.4.8 ENVIRONMENT

The ambient temperature may be too cold to allow efficient body movements, increasing the risk of muscle injuries, awkward collisions in contact sports, or falls in sports like rock climbing. Extreme cold can be life-threatening, leading to frostbite and hypothermia. It is a special risk in winter sports, fell walking and orienteering. Extreme heat may also be dangerous if it leads to heat exhaustion, which is a risk especially in endurance events performed in a hot climate. The lesser risk of sport in a hot climate is that of cramp, if the sportsman fails to maintain a good fluid and electrolyte balance. Visibility in outdoor sports can be dangerously reduced by fog, sleet or snow. Sudden dazzling shafts of sunlight or reflected light can temporarily blind a person, causing particular hazards in throwing and shooting events, and contact sports.

Wet and icy conditions underfoot create the risk of sliding, falling, and collisions. Uneven or dirty floors create similar hazards in indoor sports. Mat separation in sports such as judo, gymnastics and high jumping can make the sportsman trip, or deprive him of the expected cushioning on landing from a height.

Adequate space must be allowed for sports. Every court or pitch should have space around it, to allow for player movement beyond the defined area of play. Safe spectator space must be allowed, where appropriate. Any fixed structures in or near a field of play must be covered with protective padding. In an indoor arena, there should be no jutting or overhanging structures to threaten players' safety.

## Prevention and prophylaxis

If there are any visible hazards in the playing conditions, the decision must be taken by any of the people designated as responsible that play should not take place.

## 1.5 Preventing intrinsic injuries

By recognizing the common predisposing factors which may underlie intrinsic injuries, it is possible to formulate practical suggestions for minimizing the risks.

### 1.5.1 BALANCED TRAINING

To avoid fatigue from excessive repetitive training, the sportsman has to learn how to progress his training gradually, allowing recovery days, and preferably varying his muscle work by doing various forms of physical training, rather than a single activity. The stress fracture has become a common injury, through the recent popularity of marathon running (Norfray, Schlachter and Kernahan, 1980; Orava, 1980; Hajek and Nobel, 1982). Typically, the programmes followed by new runners are based on the principle of a weekly total mileage produced by running a certain distance virtually every day. Arguably, it is the lack of recovery days to allow for adaptation which is the major cause of the overuse syndromes.

There is debate as to whether children should be allowed or encouraged to do long-distance running or other endurance events. Children suffer from similar overuse syndromes to adults from repetitive exercise (Walter and Wolf, 1977; Kaltas, 1981). But they also suffer from problems relating to growth areas (Siegel, 1968; Orava and Virtanen, 1982). It is probably to be hoped that the International Amateur Athletics Federation maintains its stand in not allowing children under eighteen years to run in official marathon races. Logistically, it is difficult to set up a viable scientific survey to establish whether the high incidence of Osgood-Schlatter's disease among teenage footballers is due to over-playing, as young footballers of promise are encouraged to play and train intensively, or to inherent dangers in the game related to running, kicking and tackling. In practice, it seems sound sense to encourage children to try various sports, and to discourage them from pursuing a single sport intensively, without at least paying attention to the problems and needs relating to their growth.

### 1.5.2 FULL INJURY RECOVERY

Any injury disrupts normal patterns of movement. If a sportsman is allowed to participate before recovering completely from an injury, he is very likely to suffer re-injury, or a secondary injury elsewhere.

### 1.5.3 MAINTENANCE AND IMPROVEMENT OF MUSCLE FLEXIBILITY

It is commonly held that stretching muscles before strenuous exercise helps reduce the risk of muscle strains, although inevitably there is little scientific proof of this. Static stretching exercises are now the method of choice for improving muscle flexibility (De Vries, 1962), and they are known to play an important part in preventing muscle stiffness after exercise (De Vries, 1961, see also Figs 1.2 and 1.3).

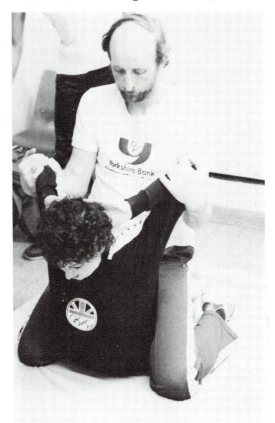

*Fig. 1.2* Passive stretching: physiotherapist Tony Power assisting 1980 Olympic swimming medallist Margaret Kelly.

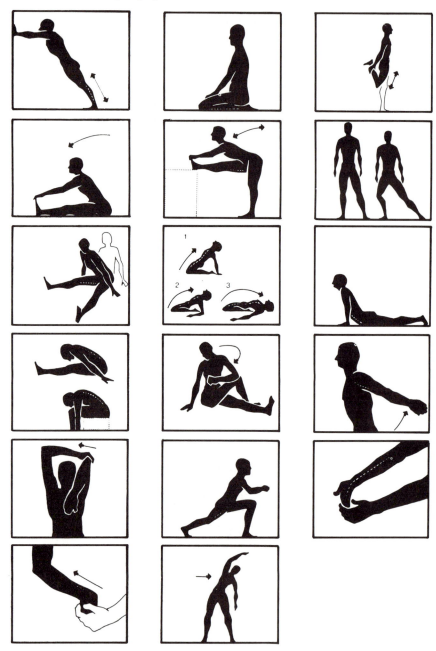

*Fig. 1.3* Passive stretching exercises.

Massage also has a part to play in reducing muscle soreness after strenuous exercise, and therefore improving flexibility in this situation (Whitney, 1980), but it should never be seen as a substitute for stretching exercises.

### 1.5.4 MAINTENANCE AND IMPROVEMENT OF MUSCLE STRENGTH

Strength training can be an important background factor in preparing adequately for a sport. In virtually all top-level sports, some element of weight training is used as part of the conditioning programme (Jensen and Fisher, 1972). In many sports, performance is enhanced by weight training. For instance, runners frequently suffer from soreness in the shoulder and neck muscles, which is reduced by appropriate weight

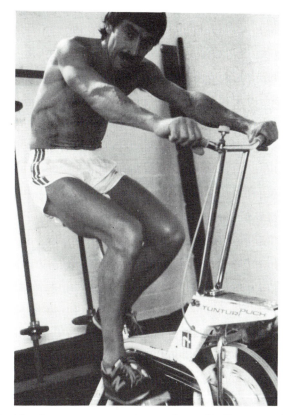

*Fig. 1.4* The bicycle ergometer can be used specifically to regain power and mobility following a knee injury or generally for cardiorespiratory fitness.

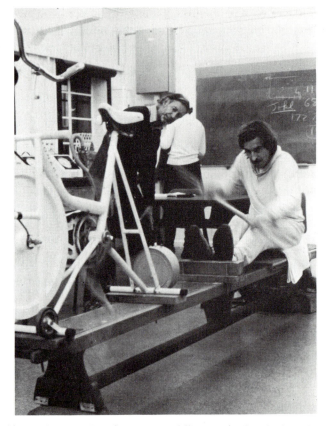

*Fig. 1.5* Alternative exercise: the canoe paddles attached to the bicycle ergometer pedals allow the patient to work at a measurable level, to maintain cardiorespiratory fitness during recovery from a leg injury.

training for these muscles. The increased arm strength provides a more efficient propulsive arm action, improving the runner's ability.

Following an injury, localized strength must be regained in an injured muscle or round a joint, as the first step towards regaining proper co-ordinated movement. Muscle measurement is an invaluable rehabilitation tool (Hyde, Goddard and Scott, 1983). The development of isokinetic measuring devices like the Cybex II and the Kin Kom has been a great advance in sports injury rehabilitation and prevention.

### 1.5.5 BODY BALANCE

Many sports tend to create muscle imbalance in the body. Tennis players and oarsmen may overdevelop the spinal muscles unilaterally; front-

14

crawl swimmers may hypertrophy the anterior shoulder muscles relative to the posterior. This type of imbalance may have an effect on injuries occurring in these sportsmen, like the oarsman's spondylolysis or the swimmer's dislocated shoulder. In the author's opinion, background training, besides being specific to the sport, should also aim to redress this type of imbalance, in favour of developing a more symmetrical musculature, to combat injury.

Chondromalacia patellae is an example of a condition which arises through muscle imbalance, through selective loss of co-ordination involving vastus medialis (Williams and Sperryn, 1976; Kulund, 1982). Protective knee and hip extension exercises as part of background conditioning are invaluable in preventing the condition.

## 1.5.6 JOINT LIMITATION

Joint stiffness can cause problems in related structures, either directly or indirectly. Hip limitation has been found to contribute to hamstring muscle injuries (Liemohn, 1978). Norwegian studies, reported by Sperryn (1982) showed that gymnasts with lower back pain suffered worse pain if they had increased lumbar mobility to compensate for shoulder stiffness.

Joints work in harmony in overall patterns of movement. When a sportsman lands from a jump, each of the lower limb joints gives in turn, to dissipate the shock. If part of this pattern is disrupted, greater shock will be transmitted through the limbs: therefore it seems unwise to reduce a joint's proprioception and mobility through restrictive taping, in order to allow a sportsman to continue activity.

## 1.5.7 GOOD TECHNIQUE

In highly skilled sports, there is often no rigid standard pattern of movement. The basic skill of tennis, striking the ball with the racket, is achievable with innumerable variations of style. Whether single- or double-handed, no two successful tennis players look identical in style.

Defining good technique is almost as difficult as defining good posture. One possible definition might be 'the efficient and comfortable application of body movements to fulfilling the patterns required for the given sport effectively'. Excessive effort is inefficient, and is likely to lead to breakdown.

## 1.5.8 APPROPRIATE EQUIPMENT

Sports equipment usually comes in different sizes, to suit the capacities of the user. There are scaled-down javelins for children to throw, and junior sized rackets for squash and tennis. Sportsmen have to learn to choose equipment objectively, rather than being influenced by marketing pressures or current fashions.

The sportsman should also be aware that any change in individual equipment is likely to cause problems, unless time is allowed for gradual adaptation. A sudden change of racket, coupled with intensive play, can bring on tennis elbow; tenosynovitis in the wrist in oarsmen often results from a change of blade or alteration of the blade handle, without a modification of the training load.

### 1.5.9 BODY PREPARATION

It has been established that a thorough warm-up improves the body's efficiency, and therefore improves sporting performance (Astrand and Rodahl, 1977). The recommended warming-up period varies from a minimum of five minutes, up to thirty minutes. The usual format is a combination of stretching and mobilizing exercises, followed by ballistic or sprinting movements, sufficient to cause sweating.

It has been widely held that warming up may help prevent injuries. It has also been indicated that warming up may help to limit the severity of knee injuries, while not preventing them altogether (Hede, Hejgaard and Jacobsen, 1985).

Overall preparation for a sport involves gradual progression, similar to balancing a training programme for progressive fitness training. With seasonal sports, like outdoor tennis or snow ski-ing, there is always a high risk that the sportsman tries to do too much in the first few days. Pre-season or pre-holiday preparation, with gradual training, is necessary to prevent stiffness and injury. The first sessions should be gentle, with recovery periods or days allowed.

### 1.5.10 CHOICE OF SPORT

If a child is introduced to many sports at the age when skill acquisition is easiest, he will be able to continue to enjoy several sports as he grows up, or he may choose to specialize in one or more sports that he does well, and particularly enjoys. One obvious guideline is that, where possible, the child should learn scaled-down versions of the game. Short tennis and rugby played across the pitch are examples of reduced-size sports which allow children to learn the skills without the physical stresses of the adult game.

For top-level competition, there is no guarantee that the person with the most appropriate build, physiological and psychological profile will be the champion. There have been many studies identifying qualities present in top-level sportsmen and women (Carter, 1984; Khosla, 1983). Self-selection for competitive or professional sport is more commonly based on natural aptitude, enjoyment, and application, than on objective factors.

For the adult, choosing a new sport may be inspired by a desire to get fit, a need for a new physical challenge, or social reasons. More rarely, the adult novice may intend to achieve competitive success. Probably the most important factor in making a sound choice is the ability to take a balanced approach to the new sport, and to accept the physical restraints related to maturity. The adult should be able to set out attainable goals, and to understand the possible good or bad effects which might result from the new activity.

## 1.6  Conclusion

Everyone concerned with sport in any capacity must accept a degree of responsibility for safety. Lay people need to be aware of biomechanical and medical factors underlying sport; medical practitioners have to understand the physical and psychological needs of people involved in sport at recreational or competitive levels. The implications of exercise and movement patterns for growing and mature bodies have to be recognized.

Those directly involved in sport must know the basic first-aid techniques appropriate for major and minor accidents. They must also understand the importance of full recovery from injury before sport can safely be resumed. Minimizing risks in sport depends on an awareness of hazards and the mechanisms of injury. Maximum safety levels in all the different types of sport can be achieved through an interweaving of communication and education between participants, sports coaches, organizers and enthusiasts, and the medical and paramedical professions.

## References

Aleman, O. (1929) Omsk marchschalst (syndesmites metatarsea). *Tidskrift i Militar Halsovard*, **54**, 191.

Astrand, P.-O. and Rodahl, K. (1977) *Textbook of Work Physiology*, McGraw-Hill, p. 562.

Bedford, P. J. and Macauley, D. C. (1984) Attendances at a Casualty Department for sports related injuries. *Brit. J. Sports Med.*, **18**, 116.

Breithaupt (1855) Zur Pathologie des Menschlichen Fusses. *Med. Zeitung, Berlin*, **24**, 169.

## Prevention and prophylaxis

Brodie, D. A. (1983) The University of Liverpool Sports Injury Unit – a practical initiative. *Physiotherapy*, **69(8)**, 277.

Carter, J. E. L. (ed.) (1984) *Physical Structure of Olympic Athletes: Part II Kinanthropometry of Olympic Athletes*, S. Karger, Basel.

Chan, K. M., Fu, F. and Leung, L. (1984) Sports injuries survey on university students in Hong Kong. *Brit. J. Sports Med.*, **18**, 95.

Chapman, P. J. (1985) Orofacial injuries and attitudes to the use of mouthguards by the 1984 Great Britain Rugby League touring team. *Brit. J. Sports Med.*, **19**, 34.

Compton, B. and Tubbs, N. (1977) A survey of sports injuries in Birmingham. *Brit. J. Sports Med.*, **11**, 12.

Devas, M. (1975) *Stress Fractures*. Churchill Livingstone, Edinburgh, London and New York.

Devereux, M. D. and Lachmann, S. (1983) Athletes attending a Sports Injuries Clinic. *Brit. J. Sports Med.*, **17**, 137.

De Vries, H. A. (1961) Prevention of muscular distress after exercise. *Res. Q.*, **32**, 468.

De Vries, H. A. (1962) Evaluation of static stretching procedures for improvement of flexibility. *Res. Q.*, **33**, 222.

Galasko, C. S. B., Menon, T. J., Lemon, G. J., Banks, A. J., Morris, M. A., Bourne, M. S. and Bentley. S. (1982) University of Manchester Sports Injury Clinic. *Brit. J. Sports Med.*, **16**, 23–26.

Godshall, R. W. (1975) The predictability of athletic injuries: an eight-year study. *Amer. J. Sports Med.*, **3**, 50.

Grisogono, V. A. L. (1981) The Injuries Service at Crystal Palace. *Brit. J. Sports Med.*, **15**, 39.

Hajek, M. R. and Nobel, H. B. (1982) Stress fractures of the femoral neck in joggers. *Amer. J. Sports Med.*, **10**, 112.

Hede, A., Hejgaard, N. and Jacobsen, K. (1985) Sports injuries of the knee ligaments – a prospective study. *Brit. J. Sports Med.*, **19**, 8.

Holloszy, J. O. (1983) Exercise, health and aging: a need for more information. *Med. Sci. Sports Exer.*, **15**, 1.

Hutson, M. A. (1984) The Nottingham Sports Injuries Clinic. *Brit. J. Sports Med.*, **18**, 122.

Hyde, S. A., Goddard, C. M. and Scott, O. M. (1983) The Myometer: the development of a clinical tool. *Physiotherapy*, **69**, 424.

Jensen, C. R. and Fisher, A. G. (1972) *Scientific Basis of Athletic Conditioning*, Lea and Febiger, Philadelphia.

Jorgensen, U. (1984) Epidemiology of injuries in typical Scandinavian team sports. *Brit. J. Sports Med.*, **18**, 59.

Kaltas, D. S. (1981) Stress fractures of the femoral neck in young athletes. *J. Bone Joint Surg.*, **63-B**, 33.

Khosla, T. (1983) Sport for all. *Brit. Med. J.*, **287**, 736.

Kulund, D. N. (ed.) (1982) *The Injured Athlete*, J. B. Lippincott, Philadelphia, pp. 361; 378–81.

Liemohn, W. (1978) Factors related to hamstring strains. *J. Sports Med. Phys. Fit.*, **18**, 71.

Mack, R. P. (ed.) (1982) *Symposium on the Foot and Leg in Running Injuries*. American Academy of Orthopaedic Surgeons. C. V. Mosby, St Louis.

# References

McLatchie, G. R. (1976) An analysis of karate injuries sustained in 295 contests. *Injury*, **8(2)**, 132.

Nordentoft, J. M. (1940) Some cases of soldier's fracture. *Acta Radiol.*, **21**, 615.

Norfray, J. F., Schlachter, L. and Kernahan, W. T. (1980) Early confirmation of stress fractures in joggers. *J. Amer. Med. Assoc.*, **243**, 1647.

Orava, S. (1980) Stress fractures. *Brit. J. Sports Med.*, **14**, 40–44.

Orava, S. and Virtanen, K. (1982) Osteochondroses in athletes. *Brit. J. Sports Med.*, **16**, 161.

Sandelin, J., Kiviluoto, O., Santavirta, S. and Honkanen, R. (1985) Outcome of sports injuries treated in a casualty department. *Brit. J. Sports Med.*, **19**, 103.

Sanderson, F. H. (1981) The psychological implications of injury, in *Sports Fitness and Sports Injuries* (ed. T. Reilly), Faber and Faber, London and Boston.

Siegel, I. M. (1968) The osteochondroses. *Amer. J. Orthop. Surg.*, **10**, 246–49; 266.

Sonne-Holm, S. and Sorensen, C. H. (1980) Risk factors with acute sports injuries. *Brit. J. Sports Med.*, **14**, 22.

Sperryn, P. N. (1982) A personal view of the XXII World Congress on Sports Medicine – Vienna 1982. *Brit. J. Sports Med.*, **16**, 260.

Sperryn, P. N. (1983) *Sport and Medicine*, Butterworths, London.

Walter, N. E. and Wolf, M. D. (1977) Stress fractures in young athletes. *Amer. J. Sports Med.*, **5**, 165.

Weightman, D. and Browne, R. C. (1974) Injuries in Rugby and Association Football. *Brit. J. Sports Med.*, **8**, 183.

Whitney, S. (1980) Record recovery. *Physiother. Sport*, **IV**, 16–17.

Williams, J. G. P. (1971) Aetiological classification of injuries in sportsmen. *Brit. J. Sports Med.*, **5**, 228.

Williams, J. G. P. (1976) Injury in sport, in *Sports Medicine* (eds J. G. P. Williams and P. N. Sperryn), Edward Arnold, London, pp. 243–50.

Williams, J. G. P. and Sperryn, P. N. (eds) (1976) *Sports Medicine*, London, Edward Arnold, pp. 460–64.

Williams, J. P. R. and McKibbin, B. (1978) Cervical spine injuries in football. *Brit. Med. J.*, **282**, 747.

Yaffe, M. (1983) Sports injuries: psychological aspects. *Brit. J. Hosp. Med.*, **3**, 224.

# 2  *Psychological aspects*

MAURICE YAFFÉ

Over the past ten years clinical sports psychology has emerged as a distinct specialty within sports medicine (Yaffé, 1979b, 1981a,b; Kincey, 1981; Waitley, May and Martens, 1983) and the study of sports injuries comprises one of its central areas of concern.

According to Williams (1980) most injuries acquired during sports activity are essentially no different from those obtained during other pursuits although demands by the patient regarding rehabilitation and return to physical activity may be significantly greater. However, true sport-specific injuries or *technopathies* in Williams' terms (1976) are probably small in number; they comprise mainly the overuse type but also include others which derive from the specific movements carried out in sport. They are most usefully classified on the basis of their aetiology (Williams, 1971) into those caused by external violence (extrinsic) and those due to stress within the individual (intrinsic); the former are found in sports such as soccer, rugby football and squash, where there is a constantly changing pattern of play and the latter in those involving repetitive action such as running, swimming and rowing. Psychological factors may be relevant to the onset and maintenance of both types of injury.

In terms of incidence it has been estimated that approximately 5% of all cases seen in accident departments of British hospitals are due to a sporting injury and that in the early 1970s two million of those injured had injuries which prevented them from participating in their sport for one week, of whom 10% took time off work. More recent estimates indicate that the size of the problem is increasing, but according to Muckle (1978) serious sports injuries are rare.

As for the incidence of psychological problems within the population of sports participants, athletes of all ages and degrees of participation are subject to the same mental conflicts as non-athletes but may be less likely to seek psychiatric help – at least that was the experience of Carmen, Zerman and Blaine (1968) at Harvard.

# Psychological aspects

## 2.1 Injury prediction

Even though injuries in all sports are increasing (in spite of technological advances in safety equipment, appropriate emphasis on proper physical conditioning and attention to the rules) the variables that serve to protect or predispose sports participants to injury in a given sport remain to be better defined. The aetiological determinants are both complex and multiple, and include: type of sport, experience, equipment used, level of competitive involvement, coaching technique and physical playing conditions. These components interact with the individual's physical characteristics, for example, size, strength, speed, agility, co-ordination, physical fitness, and flexibility, and personality characteristics, such as degree of conscientiousness, tough-mindedness, over-protectiveness and sensitivity (Jackson *et al.*, 1978). These authors report that on the basis of their research on US footballers, using Cattell's 16 Personality Factor Questionnaire, two factors had some potential for predicting injury: Factor A (the dimension that sorts respondents into reserved, detached, critical, cool versus outgoing, warm hearted, easygoing, participating) was predictive of injury *severity*, and Factor I (tough-minded versus tender-minded) differentiated between injured and uninjured players.

Coddington and Troxell (1980) studied the effect of emotional factors on US football injury rates and found their young players who experienced more family instability – especially parental illnesses, separation, divorces and deaths – were more likely to sustain a significant injury. For example, the risk of injury for a boy who actually lost a parent was five times greater than for one who experienced no losses (threatened or real).

Young and Cohen (1981) examined self-concept and injuries among US female high school basketball players using the Tennessee Self Concept Scale and discovered significant differences between injured and non-injured players. Their injured players had more positive scores on total self-concept, and the identity, physical self and personal self subscales, whereas the non-injured players scored more favourably on the self-criticism scale. The authors suggested that their injured players may be more apt to take additional risks in game play and, subsequently, may find themselves in situations which could result in injury. It is interesting that no self-concept differences were found between injured and non-injured basketball players in their previous study (Young and Cohen, 1979).

Pargman (1976) hypothesized that visual perception characteristics, and visual disembedding specifically, may well be related to motor behaviour involving physical trauma in sport. (Visual disembedding is an

22

individual's ability to hold a configuration in mind despite distraction; for example in football: where and when to run, when to leap in attempting to catch the ball.) He compared uninjured, injured but not disabled, and injured/disabled US college football players with regard to their ability to disembed a complex visual field using a group hidden-figures test, and found significant test score differences between athletes in the uninjured and disabled groups. He concluded that higher mean disembedding in a static visual field may relate to physical injury in football. Dahlhauser and Thomas (1979) took this work a stage further with a similar population but added a test of locus of control (a determination of whether an individual focuses on internal or external explanations of phenomena); their data indicate fewer injuries for football players with independent visual perception and internal locus of control.

In this investigation of injured and non-injured competitive male road runners Valliant discovered that those who received injuries appeared less tough-minded and less forthright; injured runners were also heavier, taller, and ran more miles per week than their non-injured counterparts (Valliant, 1981). Bramwell *et al.* (1975) developed a rating scale in order to assess the role of psychosocial factors (life event changes) in athletic injuries, as they felt that acute trauma and injuries may well be associated with an increased perception of stressful events. Their sample comprised US college football players and they found differences over one and two year intervals between the injured and non-injured groups. Football players with low, moderate and high life change scores could be predicted to be at proportionate risk for sustaining injuries.

Nideffer (1981) summarized the relevant factors that influence who becomes injured; apart from personality characteristics, such as hostility and aggression, level of trait anxiety (associated with attentional and physical changes) and the pressure determined by situation and emotional considerations combine with performance demands and attentional abilities to increase or decrease the likelihood of injury. Those athletes who are likely to be stressed in general, by particular situations (like a specific competition or auditorium), and those competitors who have limited attentional control independent of arousal levels, are significantly more likely to be injured.

Overwork, that is working beyond one's endurance and recuperative capacities, may be a hazard in certain personality types engaged in sport, and clusters of symptoms may then develop, some of which may mimic serious physical ailments (Rhoads, 1977). Boredom and monotony, by no means uncommon in training, are generally conceded to be negative factors that can have adverse effects on morale and quality of performance, and could also influence the likelihood of injury (Thackray, 1981). Monotony, coupled with a need to maintain high levels of alertness, may well represent a combination capable of eliciting considerable stress.

## 2.2 Psychological antecedents of injury

Virtually all committed sports participants are injured at some time during their career, which keeps them out of competition for a while. Players can sustain real injury as a result of psychological pressures. In his doctoral study of injury in professional soccer, Reilly found a positive relationship between apprehensiveness (an anxiety trait) and the number of joint injuries per season. This suggests the importance of commitment and assertiveness on the field of play in reducing the likelihood of physical trauma (Reilly, 1975).

## 2.3 Injury proneness

This has emerged over the past few years as an important concept in sports medicine, which may afford a socially acceptable form of retreat from physical activities that are construed as unrewarding or unduly threatening (socially, psychologically, or physically). From a psychological point of view, injury proneness in sport can be divided into three main categories (Ogilvie, 1978): those participants who have actually been injured, those who continually complain of pain but no injury is apparent, and the individual who intentionally fakes injury. According to Sanderson (1977) these reactions are the product of high levels of stress in those who are highly driven, emotionally vulnerable, and negative thinkers. He provides a descriptive account of various kinds of injury-prone athlete, where conflict and anxiety are prominent causal factors, but quantitative assessment is absent in the presentation, which includes:

(1) *Injury resulting from counter-phobia*. This occurs in individuals who find the aggression-loaded atmosphere of competitive sport anxiety-inducing. Anxiety is dealt with directly by overt aggression and fearlessness, and is seen most commonly in boxing, ski-ing and other high-risk sports.
(2) *Injury as a sign of masculinity*. Here injury is a counter-phobic reaction in a person with low self-confidence where the visible signs of physical trauma are used as a testimony to courage and masculinity.
(3) *Injury resulting from masochism (or inward-directed hostility)*. The high risk-taker or sensation seeker has a higher incidence of injury, which is associated with a failure to meet unrealistically high standards or

24

which, as Sanderson claims, may represent atonement for the injury he or she has caused another.

(4) *Injury as a weapon*. Here injury is used to punish others. The example is given of the reluctant, injured athlete who is forced to compete because of an athletically frustrated parent. The undesired competition can be avoided, and the parent's displaced aspirations can be frustrated.

(5) *Injury as an escape*. The 'training-room' athlete is described who is fearful of competing and so becomes injured in practice. The false belief that 'were it not for the injury, I would be an outstanding competitor' is never proved wrong.

(6) *Injury as a concoction*. This player's injuries cannot be substantiated physically; injuries are created for ulterior motives, e.g. to avoid training, or for fear of injury.

(7) *Psychosomatic injury*. This is where no physical basis of an injury can be found, despite the fact that the individual complains of physical trauma. Emotional problems are somaticized, and the *meaning* of the injury requires investigation (for a review of this aspect see Husman, 1970).

This list closely resembles that put forward by Moore (1966) who also describes other possibilities of injury for psychological reasons, which include the sports equivalent of 'accident proneness' – the person with a history of multiple injuries, where the probability of future injury is high, and the next may be more serious. He also discusses athletes who attempt to conceal their injuries so that they will not be removed from competition; this may well render the person vulnerable to some serious injury through reduced co-ordination and stamina.

The opposite extreme is the exaggeration of injuries where every little bruise requires attention. Such a constant preoccupation with injuries may indicate that the person is apprehensive of the contact of the game. Injury can also provide a way out for those who are unable to tolerate failure following early success when the young athlete who was physically mature, ahead of his age group, finds that his peers have now caught up with him. Rosenblum (1979) discusses the emotional conditions that lead to sports injuries, both physical and psychological, highlighting the relevance of depression, fear of success, competitive inhibition and guilt, but makes no suggestion how these can be quantified. However, Sanderson (1977) calls for the establishment of vulnerability to injury profiles on the basis of the known characteristics of injury-prone athletes, as a move to positive injury prevention.

## 2.4  Psychological consequences of injury

A familiar situation occurs where injury following excessive or improper practice produces psychological sequelae. One example is of tendonitis in a professional tennis player, prior to competition, who avoids going to his physician because he knows from experience that he will be told to stop practising. Continued practice leads to an increase in muscle tension and pressure on the joint, anxiety and a narrowing of his attention away from appropriate perceptual cues. Anxiety keeps him away from seeking help and towards possible permanent damage (Nideffer, 1981). Nideffer also points out that there is often considerable concern associated with having to give up practice for even one day, as the committed sportsperson's very life depends upon maintaining and upgrading skills.

An extreme variant of this can present in runners, which Morgan (1979a) calls 'negative addiction'. The person requires daily exercise to cope and believes that he or she cannot live without daily running; but if deprived of exercise for whatever reason, the person manifests various withdrawal symptoms or aberrant behaviour, which may include depression, anxiety, extreme irritability, insomnia, and generalized fatigue. Moreover, interpersonal relations in the home, work and social settings often deteriorate. The hard-core exercise addict with a severe tendonitis, say, or stress fracture, will run even though his or her physician has recommended rest to permit recovery. Such an individual, Morgan explains, continues running by (1) ignoring the pain or dissociating from it, (2) taking analgesics before runs, or (3) locating physicians who will provide cortisone or analgesic injections. Daily runs are given higher priority than job, family or friends, and exercise is taken to the point where overuse injuries have near-crippling effects, the pain becomes unbearable, and yet they search for the perfect shoe, injection, or psychological strategy that will enable them to continue running.

It is known that the psychological impact of injury is less in certain circumstances: if there has been a previous injury to the same part of the body; when the player/athlete is fresh and rested; when repeated success is experienced the sports participant will not tend to believe he or she is seriously hurt; or when winning a person is less likely to succumb to injury. Sanderson (1978) has discussed the psychological implications of injury, which vary according to personality; the stable (versus neurotic) individual does not experience major problems unless the injury is severe and the prognosis is discouraging; the introvert is apprehensive and needs reassurance, whereas the extrovert is generally reckless and impatient and needs to be discouraged from trying to return to competition prematurely.

# Psychological consequences

A fear several injured athletes have is that physicians may not have found and corrected everything – a common reason for requests for second and third medical opinions by the patient and a psychological opinion by the doctor. However, once the fear has been dealt with directly, improvement generally follows.

Psychological reactions to physical disability can be classified into injury-linked reactions, common emotional reactions to disablement, and idiosyncratic reactions (Suinn, 1967). Injury-linked reactions are those directly associated with the organic injury so as to be part of the clinical picture, for example, injury to the brain is associated with impairment of memory, intellect and orientation (Lishman, 1973). In sport, Yarnell and Lynch (1970, 1973) describe progressive retrograde amnesia in US football players, who after concussion had definite post-traumatic confusion but knew the immediate pre-concussive event. They found that the fixation of short-term memory requires more than rehearsal and is interfered with by the continuing effects of a concussive injury in the period following trauma: in other words, they lost this retrograde memory over a period of a few minutes. Regarding longer-term consequences of injury, Corsellis, Bruton and Freeman-Browne (1973) studied the brains of retired boxers and found that some experienced boxers develop a clinical disorder, which essentially has a neuropathological basis. They indicate that the severity of the condition varies greatly, ranging from a mild clumsiness of speech and movement (with or without some loss of memory) to the ataxic, dysarthric, and perhaps Parkinsonian dement.

The common emotional reactions to disablement concern those associated with the state of being disabled, regardless of the origin or return of the disability, and generally include the following sequential stages: shock, implicit denial, emotionality and adaptation. In sport, however, an acute neurotic syndrome has been described by Little (1969, 1979) that occurs primarily out of the shock of a threat in the form of injury or illness to overvalued but waning physical powers, and is most evident in those males around that fifth decade of life who have always been physically active. Symptoms commonly include somatic complaints in the context of hypochondriasis or panic attacks. Little found an incidence of 9% new male psychiatric out-patient referrals, compared to endogenous depression (13%) and schizophrenia (11%).

The idiosyncratic reactions described by Suinn are related to the individual personality; these are the personal reactions (such as withdrawal or crying) which characterize one person and make that person easily identified from another.

## 2.5 The experience of pain

Pain tolerance and threshold: individual variation in pain response has been approached in two main ways, from the standpoint of personality variables, and from that of cultural determinants. Recent controlled studies (Liebeskind and Paul, 1978) indicate the usefulness of distinguishing between a learned component (reflected in *tolerance*), and an unlearned component (*threshold*) of pain perception. Attention to nociceptive stimulation contributes to the intensity of pain experience, and Melzack (1973) makes the familiar observation that boxers, football players and other athletes can sustain severe injuries during the excitement of the sport without being aware that they have been hurt.

Jaremko, Silbert and Mann (1981) go further in asserting that athletes, in general, and female athletes, in particular, should have higher tolerance and threshold owing to the fact that contingencies in their background pay off insensitivity to pain, especially in terms of behaviour, as in not letting the side down by leaving the field of play. In their experimental study, however, they found partial support for their prediction that pain-related complaints would be higher in an athletic group, arguing that treatment is immediately forthcoming to the athlete who reports pain. Their group of women athletes, compared with male athletes and male and female non-athletes were shown to be the most able to tolerate pain produced by the cold pressor test (familiar to athletes as ice-pack treatment) and ischaemia, and used strategies to cope with it better. Jaremko *et al.* explained this on the grounds that women have to struggle for parity between men's and women's athletics, and have disproportionately less personnel to look after them due to smaller numbers.

Clark (in McPherson *et al.*, 1980) reported that in swimming a high pain tolerance is learned as part of mental training, but this may also lead to a reduction of injury reporting. However, injury is less likely to occur in swimming by pushing harder as is the case in other sports, especially those involving contact. For a recent comprehensive review of methods of pain measurement and assessment the reader is referred to Melzack (1983).

## 2.6 Chronic pain

It is useful to make a distinction between *respondent* pain which is closely linked with the occurrence of an injury and does not require any other support for its establishment or maintenance, and *operant* pain which is not directly elicited by the injury but can become associated with it given appropriate conditions of reinforcement (Fordyce, 1976). A pain problem which has existed for a period of time is likely to have been exposed to potent contingency arrangements which may complicate and extend the difficulty. This occurs when pain behaviours receive direct and positive reinforcement, indirect but positive reinforcement by leading to rest or successful avoidance of noxious consequences, such as strenuous exercise routines, or when activity or positive behaviour efforts are punished or not reinforced. Medical attention is, after all, illness contingent, but restricted activity to the sports person may lead to a sense of helplessness or depression.

## 2.7 Psychological approaches to treatment

Nideffer (1981) considers three major areas of psychological intervention: treatment of problems due to overuse, assisting in the psychological recovery from the trauma associated with previous injury, and altering an athlete's tolerance for pain. However, judging from Yaffé (1979a) and Owen (1980), attention also needs to be paid to 'injuries' which have a psychological manifestation. Out of 418 medical complaints by British competitors at the Moscow Olympic Games, 60 (14%) of these appear to be directly related to stress; diagnoses include: insomnia ($N=40$), headache (13), depression (3), anxiety state (3), and hysteria (1), thus supporting the relevance of psychological intervention.

Until the advent of behaviour therapy, psychotherapy was virtually the only approach available for the athlete with problems (e.g. Pierce, 1969). Recent models of comprehensive health care stress the role of a wide variety of psychological factors, including stress, lifestyle habits, abilities and skills, defensive techniques, and motivational factors in maintaining health and coping with illness and injury. Techniques ranging from desensitization and operant conditioning to self-control and problem-solving are used to complement medical treatments for a wide variety of disorders. Seizures, tics, asthma, and insomnia are common targets for the field which has come to be known as behavioural medicine, and by far the most active area of *publication* is the use of biofeedback for muscular tension and migraine headaches for which frontalis EMG or finger temperature biofeedback appear effective in reducing both tension and migraine headaches (Phillips and Bierman, 1981).

Multiple technique packages which teach coping skills as well as relaxation may be more effective for multiply determined problems such as headaches and physical trauma, and a variety of methods have been developed to control pain (e.g. Turk and Genest, 1979). Pre-exposure to

29

medical procedures and participant modelling may reduce stress, and cognitive-imaginal strategies may increase tolerance of pain; stress inno-culation programmes which include relaxation, cognitive skill training and environmental manipulations have already demonstrated their effec-tiveness in helping injured individuals to cope with pain (Weisenberg, 1977) and Kabat–Zinn (1985). Similarly, Faris's (1985) approach empha-sizes the importance of making sure the patient understands their athletic injury and rehabilitation plan, before helping them to work through their feelings in relation to these.

Nideffer (1981) provides the most comprehensive account of the appropriateness of different psychological procedures for the prevention and treatment of injury in sport which include: biofeedback, meditation, progressive relaxation, hypnosis (see also Morgan, 1979b), attention control training, and cognitive rehearsal techniques (comprising mental rehearsal, psycho-cybernetics, positive thinking, discriminant cue analysis, visuomotor behaviour analysis and cognitive behaviour modifi-cation). As no formal comparisons (i.e. controlled trials) of techniques are presented, it is difficult to tease out with accuracy the active ingredients of the therapies described. This remains a fruitful area for future research.

## 2.8 Prevention of injury

Nideffer (1981) calls for an identification of individuals who are likely to be stressed by certain athletic situations (thereby increasing the likelihood of injury) and the situations themselves, for example, learning a difficult and dangerous skill, which are likely to be stressful. He emphasizes the importance of determining the physical and attentional abilities involved with respect to muscle groups and optimal tension levels, as well as appropriate attentional cues (which he divides into broad versus narrow, internal versus external), and recommends cognitive techniques, includ-ing mental rehearsal, to increase mental control, biofeedback to modify autonomic responses, and attentional control training to facilitate task-relevant concentration; he also suggests the sensitization of athletes to appropriate levels of muscle tension and attentional focus to reduce distractability.

Smith (1979) presents a data-based stress management training pro-gramme specifically for athletes which emphasizes the relationship between the athletic situation, cognitive appraisal processes, physiologi-cal arousal, and instrumental behaviours. The strategies described are directed towards the development of an 'integrated coping response' which permits self-regulation of emotional arousal, but requires further validation using heterogeneous groups.

## 2.9 Crisis intervention

As Nideffer (1981) points out, one of the determinants of preventing loss of control (and reducing the likelihood of injury) is the early detection of rising levels of arousal and disturbances in concentration. He lists several signals which need to be monitored:

(1) Any change in the athlete's arousal level, such as significant increase or decrease in activity level.
(2) Increased tension in muscles, especially upper body and neck.
(3) Changes in breathing, particularly hyperventilation.
(4) Presence of small facial twitching movements.
(5) Increase in muscle tension of jaw.
(6) Alterations in ability to shift attention. The analytical individual may become preoccupied with internal events, and the person with an external style of attention becomes highly distractable.
(7) Change in the frequency of natural tension reducers, such as yawning, stretching, coughing.

In order to regain control, Nideffer recommends the following:

(1) Do not overload the athlete with information.
(2) Provide structure and specific direction.
(3) Get feedback.
(4) Establish eye contact and physical contact (to increase kinaesthetic cues).
(5) Direct attention to a couple of task-relevant cues.
(6) Distract those with low self-esteem to neutral or pleasant cues (dissociation with stressful event); for those with high self-esteem distract by getting persons to think about what is going on around them.
(7) Legitimize the response – point out that others feel the same way they do.
(8) Maintain some physical activity, such as running on the spot, as a tension reducer.

## 2.10 Ethical concerns

Sports situations, in general, and injury, in particular, highlight the crucial interaction between psychology and physical factors. As psychologists are not qualified to treat the physical aspects of injury it is important that the athlete is screened medically before referral for a psychological opinion, and reviewed after the completion of any behavioural programme.

## Psychological aspects

Although their value has been demonstrated in general clinical practice, a good deal more empirical evidence is needed to measure the effectiveness of the above approaches in sport. The exciting new specialism of clinical sports psychology should, over the next decade, provide most of the answers, now some of the relevant issues have been debated.

## References

Bramwell, S. T., Masuda, M., Wagner, N. N. and Holmes, T. H. (1975) Psycho-social factors in athletic injuries: Development and application of the social and athletic readjustment rating scale. *J. Hum. Stress*, **1**, 6.

Carmen, L. R., Zerman, J. L. and Blaine, G. B. (1968) *Ment. Hyg.*, **52**, 134.

Coddington, R. D. and Troxell, J. R. (1980) The effect of emotional factors on football injury rates – a pilot study. *J. Hum. Stress*, **6**, 3.

Corsellis, J. A. N., Bruton, C. J. and Freeman-Browne, D. (1973) The aftermath of boxing. *Psychol. Med.*, **3**, 270.

Dahlhauser, M. and Thomas, M. B. (1979) Visual disembedding and locus of control as variables associated with high-school football injuries. *Percept. Motor Skills*, **49**, 254.

Faris, G. J. (1985) Psychologic aspects of athletic rehabilitation. *Clinics in Sports Medicine*, **4**, 545.

Fordyce, W. E. (1976) *Behavioral Methods for Chronic Pain and Illness*, Mosby, New York.

Husman, B. F. (1970) Psychological and psychosomatic problems of athletes. *Maryland State Med. J.*, **19**, 71.

Jackson, D. W. Jarrett, H., Bailey, D., *et al.* (1978) Injury prediction in the young athlete: a preliminary report. *Amer. J. Sports Med.*, **6**, 6.

Jaremko, M. E., Silbert, L. and Mann, T. (1981) The differential ability of athletes and non-athletes to cope with two types of pain: a radical behavioural model. *Psychol. Rec.*, **31**, 265.

Kabat–Zinn, J. (1985) The clinical use of mindfulness meditation for the self-regulation of chronic pain. *J. Behav. Med.*, **8**, 163.

Kincey, J. (1981) Sport psychology and clinical psychology: what value in a closer relationship? *Int. J. Sports Psychol.*, **12**, 216.

Liebeskind, J. C. and Paul, L. A. (1978) Psychological and physiological mechanisms of pain. *Ann. Rev. Psychol.*, **28**, 41.

Lishman, W. A. (1973) The psychiatric sequelae of head injury: a review. *Psychol.*

Little, J. C. (1979) *Psychiat. Ann.*, **9**, 148.

McPherson, B., Marteniuk, R., Tihanyi, J., *et al.* (1980) Age group swimming: a multi-disciplinary review of the literature. *Can. J. Appl. Sport Sci.*, **5**, 109.

Melzack, R. (1973) *The Puzzle of Pain*, Penguin, Harmondsworth, Middlesex.

Melzack, R. (ed.) (1983) *Pain Measurement and Assessment*, Raven Press, New York.

Melzack, R. (1973) *The Puzzle of Pain*, Penguin, Harmondsworth, Middlesex.

Moore, R. A. (1966) *Sports and Mental Health*, Charles C. Thomas, Springfield, Illinois.

Morgan, W. P. (1979a) *Phys. Sports Med.*, **7**, 58.

Morgan, W. P. (1979b) in *Handbook of Hypnosis and Psychosomatic Medicine* (eds G.

Burrows and L. D. Donnerstein), Elsevier/North-Holland Biomedical Press, Amsterdam.

Muckle, D. S. (1978) *Injuries in Sport*, John Wright and Sons, Bristol.

Nideffer, R. (1981) *The Ethics and Practice of Applied Sport Psychology*, Mouvement Publications, Ithaca, New York.

Ogilvie, B. (1978) *Proceedings of 19th Conference on the Medical Aspects of Sports*, American Medical Association, Washington DC.

Owen, R. (1980) *Medical Report: Olympic Games Moscow 1980*, unpublished manuscript, British Olympic Association.

Pargman, D. (1976) Visual disembedding and injury in college football players. *Percept. Motor Skills*, **42**, 762.

Phillips, J. S. and Bierman, K. L. (1981) Clinical psychology: individual methods. *Ann. Rev. Psychol.*, **32**, 405.

Pierce, R. A. (1969) Athletes in psychology: how many, how come? *J. Amer. Coll. Health Assoc.*, **17**,·244.

Reilly, T. (1975) An ergonomic evaluation of occupational stress in professional football, unpublished doctoral thesis, Liverpool Polytechnic.

Rhoads, J. M. (1977) Overwork. *J. Amer. Med. Assoc.*, **237**, 2615.

Rosenblum, S. (1979) Psychologic factors in competitive failures in athletes. *Amer. J. Sports Med.*, **7**, 198.

Sanderson, F. H. (1977) The psychology of the injury-prone athlete. *Brit. J. Sports Med.*, **11**, 56.

Sanderson, F. H. (1978) The psychological implications of injury. *Brit. J. Sports Med.*, **12**, 41.

Smith, R. E. (1979) in *Psychology of Motor Behavior and Sport* (eds C. H. Madeau, W. R. Halliwell, K. M. Newell and G. C. Roberts), Human Kinetics, Champaign, Illinois.

Suinn, R. M. (1967) *J. Assoc. Phys. Mental Rehabil.*, **21**, 13.

Thackray, R. J. (1981) The stress of boredom and monotony: a consideration of the evidence. *Psychosom. Med.*, **43**, 165.

Turk, D. C. and Genest, M. (1979) in *Cognitive-behavioral Interventions: Theory, Research, and Procedures* (eds P. C. Kendall and S. D. Hollon), Academic Press, New York.

Valliant, P. M. (1981) Personality and injury in competitive runners. *Percept. Motor Skills*, **53**, 251.

Waitley, D. E., May, J. R. and Martens, R. (1983) Sports psychology and the elite athlete. *Clin. Sports Med.*, **2**, 87.

Weisenberg, M. (1977) Pain and pain control. *Psychol. Bull.*, **84**, 1008.

Williams, J. G. P. (1971) Aetiological classification of injuries in sportsmen. *Brit. J. Sports Med.*, **5**, 228.

Williams, J. G. P. (1976) in *Sports Medicine* (eds J. G. P. Williams and P. Sperryn), Arnold, London.

Williams, J. G. P. (1980) *A Colour Atlas of Injury in Sport*, Wolfe Medical, London.

Yaffé, M. (1979a) Unpublished report, British Olympic Association.

Yaffé, M. (1979b) The contribution of psychology to sport: an overview. *Medisport*, **1**, 16.

Yaffé, M. (1981a) The contribution of clinical psychology to sports medicine. *Brit. J. Sports Med.* **15**, 16.

## Psychological aspects

Yaffé, M. (1981b) Sport and mental health. *J. Bio-social Sci.*, Supplement 7, 83.

Yarnell, P. R and Lynch, S. (1970) Retrograde memory immediately after concussion. *Lancet*, **i**, 863.

Yarnell, P. R. and Lynch, S. (1973) The 'ding': amnestic states in football trauma. *Neurology*, **23**, 196.

Young, M. L. and Cohen, D. A. (1979) Self-concept and injuries among female college tournament basketball players. *Amer. Correct. Ther. J.*, **33**, 139.

Young, M. L. and Cohen, D. A. (1981) Self-concept and injuries among female high school basketball players. *J. Sports Med. Phys. Fit.*, **21**, 55.

# 3 Management of the unconscious patient

## MARK HARRIES

Soft tissue or bony injuries sustained in sport are a nuisance to the athlete. Training is disrupted and performance diminishes as a result. Injuries such as these usually heal in due course despite treatment, but traumatic injury resulting in unconsciousness is in a different league altogether. Regardless of the dexterity with bandages or the wet sponge, unskilled handling of the unconscious sportsman at the accident site may result in permanent injury or even death.

### 3.1  Assessment of the unconscious patient

The airway, breathing and finally circulation, must be assessed in that order. This is known as the A (airway), B (breathing) and C (circulation) of emergency resuscitation. Ensuring a clear airway is the most important part of the resuscitation procedure without exception. Whether the patient lives or dies is decided at this stage regardless of the excellence of any hospital care which may become available later.

### 3.1.1  THE AIRWAY

The mouth is opened using the triple airway manoeuvre, a term used to describe the three movements required:

(1) Extend the neck (except in those instances where a fracture of the neck is suspected).
(2) Open the mouth.
(3) Support the jaw by pulling forward on the chin.

Without neck extension, the tongue falls back and obstructs the airway. As the neck is extended the airway is opened, but its width is approximately doubled by adding jaw support (Fig. 3.1(a), (b) and (c)). So, both jaw support and neck extension is essential and this method of opening

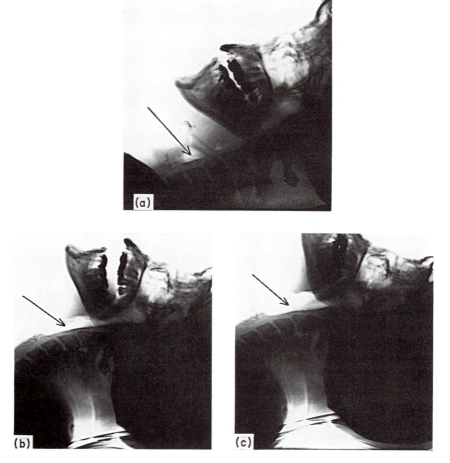

*Fig. 3.1* With the head unextended the tongue obstructs the posterior pharynx (a). With neck extension the airway is clear (b). Addition of jaw support almost doubles the width of the airway (c).

the airway is taught by the American Heart Association (1986), the St John's Ambulance, the International Red Cross and the Resuscitation Council (UK) (1984).

### 3.1.2 BREATHING

Even those people with practical experience of major accidents sometimes find it difficult outside hospital to make clinical decisions

36

which they would ordinarily have made instantly in the hospital setting. The best way to decide whether or not the patient is breathing is to use the look, listen and feel technique. After first opening the airway the operator turns his head to one side and looks down along the patient's chest to see if it moves with respiration. If the chest is not moving the operator then obstructs the patient's mouth gently with his cheek and listens and feels for breathing. If the patient is not breathing his mouth is cleared with the fingers, leaving well fitting dentures in place (performing mouth to mouth resuscitation on edentulous patients is quite difficult). The patient is then given two deep breaths of expired air resuscitation in rapid succession aiming to expand the chest maximally.

### 3.1.3  CIRCULATION

Deciding whether or not the pulse is present is the most difficult and critical of all the decisions to be made. Following cardiac arrest the skin looks ashen or blue and has a mottled appearance especially over the upper chest. The normal pattern of breathing is replaced by irregular deep gasping movements which cease within two to three minutes. This early phase following an accident is horrific and frightening. The pulse is assessed by palpating any large artery which passes close to the skin. Both the carotid and radial pulses are readily accessible even if the patient is clothed. The pupillary reaction to light is notoriously unreliable as a sign of cardiac arrest. The pupils become fixed only after circulation has ceased for three to four minutes. Fiddling with a torch and gazing into the eyes is likely to waste valuable time.

## 3.2  Expired air resuscitation (E.A.R.)

Manual methods of ventilating the lungs by compressing the chest with the patient prone (Holger-Neilson's method) or supine (Silvester-Broche's method) should never be used. Tests performed on paralysed volunteers show that oxygenation of the blood is inadequate when manual methods are used (Nolte, 1968). In contrast expired air resuscitation results in satisfactory arterial oxgyen levels regardless of whether the mouth to mouth or mouth to nose method is used (Fig. 3.2(a) and (b)).

### 3.2.1  THE TECHNIQUE OF E.A.R.

A patient who is not breathing should be given expired air resuscitation using either mouth to mouth or mouth to nose methods, whichever is more convenient. The mouth to nose method may be particularly useful

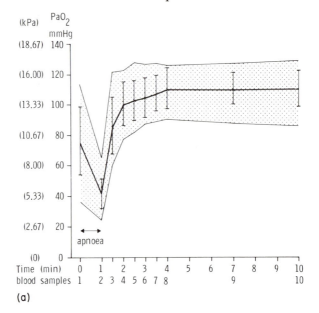

**(a)**

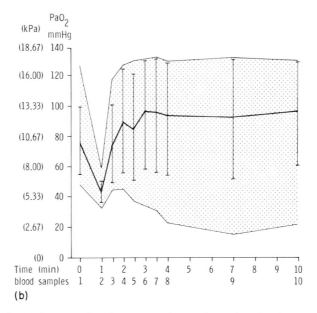

**(b)**

*Fig. 3.2* Arterial oxygen levels in anaesthetized paralysed volunteers after one minute's apnoea. (a) Mouth to mouth ventilation; (b) Silvester-Brosche's method. Note the low arterial oxygen in some given Silvester-Brosche's method. (Reproduced by kind permission of Dr H. Nolte.)

in those with extensive injuries to the mouth or fracture of the jaw or if for any reason jaw support is proving difficult. The rate at which the breaths should be delivered is 12–15 per minute in an adult (more than eight years old), 15–20 per minute for a child (one to eight years old) and 20–30 per minute in an infant (less than one year old). The head of the infant should not be tilted backward but instead held in a neutral position. The reason for this is that the infant's tracheal rings are relatively soft and the trachea will kink if the neck is extended. In children and infants it may be more convenient to cover both mouth and nose during expired air resuscitation, thus combining both mouth to mouth and mouth to nose resuscitation.

## 3.3 External chest compression (E.C.C.)

Following cardiac arrest circulation must be supported artificially by external compression of the chest together with expired air resuscitation. In common with assessment of breathing, feeling for a pulse is much more difficult at the accident site than it is in hospital. For this reason the pulse should be palpated for at least ten seconds after first having cleared the airway and given four to five breaths, before a decision on chest compression is made.

### 3.3.1 THE TECHNIQUE OF E.C.C.

It is now thought that the heart probably plays little part in the pumping mechanism of blood and current evidence suggests rather that the entire rib cage becomes the pump. Blood is made to flow from left to right and from arteries to veins by a rise and fall in pressure within the chest caused by external compression (Chandra et al., 1981) (Fig. 3.3(a) and (b)).

At present it is held that the ideal pace at which to compress the chest in an adult (eight years or older) is about 80 times in each minute (American Heart Association, 1986). The compression technique is critical, squeezing actions with compression and relaxation each occupying about half the cycle allows adequate time for the chest to empty and refill with blood. At compression rates much higher than this there is evidence to suggest that the pumping mechanism becomes less efficient (Taylor et al., 1977).

Correct placement of both hands over the centre of the chest and over the lower third of the sternum is important, the aim being to depress the sternum bone between one and a half and two inches but without breaking ribs. In older people this may be difficult to avoid but in youth the ribs are very springy and it should be possible to avoid damage in most instances.

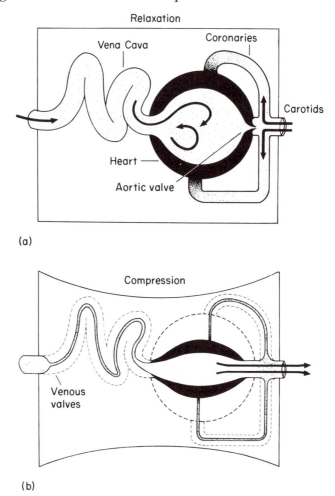

Fig. 3.3 During relaxation (diastole) the vessels of the chest fill. The aortic valve prevents backward flow into the heart and instead blood fills the coronary arteries. During compression (systole) coronary filling is impeded, pressure rises uniformly throughout the chest cavity and the blood is squeezed out of the vena cava, arteries and capillaries rather like water from a sponge. The heart valves move very little, the heart acting as a passive conduit. Backward flow is prevented by venous valves at the thoracic outlet.

In children (one to eight years old) the compression rate needs to be a little higher using one hand to depress the sternum to between one and one and a half inches; while with infants (less than a year old) the rate is 100 compressions per minute using just the finger tips to depress the sternum a half to one inch (see Table 3.1).

*Table 3.1* Recommended timings for expired air resuscitation (E.A.R.) and external chest compression (E.C.C.)

---

*Two man operation*
Adult (eight years or older)
       E.A.R.  12 breaths/minute
       E.C.C.  80 compressions/minute
                (sternal depression $1\frac{1}{2}$ in – 2 in)
       Ratio:  5:1

Child (one to eight years old)
       E.A.R.  15 breaths/minute
       E.C.C.  80 compressions/minute
                (sternal depression 1 in – $1\frac{1}{2}$ in)
       Ratio  5:1

Infant (under one year)
       E.A.R.  20 breaths/minute
       E.C.C.  100 compressions/minute
                (sternal depression $\frac{1}{2}$ in – 1 in)
       Ratio  5:1

*One man operation*
Adult
       E.C.C.  80 compressions/minute
       Ratio:  15:2

Child
       E.C.C.  80 compressions/minute
       Ratio:  5:1

Infant
       E.C.C.  100 compressions/minute
       Ratio:  5:1

---

## 3.4  Timing E.A.R. with E.C.C.

Attempting resuscitation as a solo operator in an adult is vastly less efficient than doing it with a team of two. Wherever possible a solo operator should therefore enlist the help of a bystander. Since chest compression requires less skill than airway management, the most highly trained person should always look after the airway and breathing, allowing the bystander to do the chest compression. It has been agreed internationally that a breath should be interposed between every fifth compression, allowing a short pause in the compression rhythm for the breath.

    A solo operator must interpose two full breaths every 15 compressions allowing no more than five seconds pause in the rhythm to deliver these breaths. The compression rate for adults used by both solo and two operators is the same, 80 compressions per minute (see Table 3.1).

Effective chest compression causes a pulse wave in the carotid artery which is difficult to distinguish from the true pulse. When rechecking the pulse therefore, chest compression should stop briefly, so that the operator performing E.A.R. can check the carotid pulse. This is done every two minutes approximately.

### 3.5   The recovery position

The recovery position is used for a patient who is breathing, whether conscious or unconscious; he may be turned either to the left or to the right side, a position known variously as the coma position, recovery position, or lateral position. It is a good principle to use the recovery position for any seriously injured breathing patient should the severity of the injuries permit it. The airway and carotid pulse should be watched constantly. A patient lying in the recovery position should never be left alone.

### 3.6   Common pitfalls and problems with resuscitation

(1) The novice tends to be in too much of a rush and therefore lacks control. It requires training to slow down, to be cool and to be in command.

(2) Vomiting occurs frequently during the recovery period or actually during resuscitation. If the patient is allowed to inhale vomit he can rarely be revived. The operator must be ready to act promptly and turn the patient to the recovery position in the event of vomiting.

(3) Inexperienced operators tend to breathe too fast, and this causes them to feel dizzy.

(4) Blowing too hard with an improperly extended neck causes air to fill the stomach instead of the lungs and greatly increases the risk of vomiting.

(5) Many operators fail to realize how difficult it is to feel the carotid pulse. Nothing is lost by taking around ten seconds over the carotid pulse decision.

(6) Operators should not be too worried about getting the intricacies of chest compression absolutely right, but should concentrate rather on the airway and breathing.

**3.7 Mouth mask resuscitation**

Use of a mask avoids the unpleasantness of direct contact with the patient's lips, avoids the possible risk of infection and also enables the operator to administer oxygen. Neck extension and jaw support is still essential. The operator kneels at the head of the patient and lifts the jaw forward by using the fingers of both hands hooked around the angles of the jaw. With his thumbs free the operator pushes the mask down on to the patient's face forming a perfect seal. A transparent mask with an inflated or flexible cushion rim is preferred so that the airway is in clear view throughout.

**3.8 Bag/mask resuscitation**

Ventilation is effected via a mask by air squeezed from a hand-held bag. This frees only one hand to hold the mask and considerable practice is required to a achieve a good seal. Bag resuscitators can be adapted to enriching the air supply with oxygen simply by connecting oxygen to the air intake. With the addition of a reservoir bag the inspired oxygen concentration can be raised from 60% to close to 100%.

3.8.1 CONTINUOUS OXYGEN THERAPY

Continuous oxygen via mask should only be offered to a patient who is breathing (conscious or unconscious). The highest concentration which it is possible to deliver in this way is around 60% oxygen. The rate of flow is governed by the design of the oxygen inhalator but is usually fixed at around four to eight litres per minute.

Fully conscious patients often find a mask held or strapped to the face uncomfortable and usually prefer to hold the mask themselves. Giving oxygen in this way is perfectly safe and can also be useful in those who have been injured in other ways, for example following heart attack.

**3.9 Mechanical ventilators**

Mechanical ventilators use the pressure of oxygen delivered from an oxygen cylinder to ventilate the lungs. They should only be used on a patient who is not breathing. The cycle may either be automatic or under manual control (pressure cycled ventilators are unsatisfactory because they cannot be used in conjunction with chest compression). Manually triggered devices are probably preferable to automatic ones because ventilation can then be interposed precisely between compressions. The flow rate of oxygen required to do this is considerably higher than when using continuous oxygen therapy (around sixty litres per minute).

### 3.9.1 PROBLEMS AND PITFALLS USING MECHANICAL VENTILATORS

(1) While E.C.C. is continuing it may be difficult to see the chest rise and fall with ventilation. A good check on this is to listen to the amount of air driven out of the patient's lungs by the compression following each ventilation. If in doubt E.C.C. should be stopped briefly so that the operator can check that the chest really does rise and fall with ventilation. If in doubt still, switch immediately to E.A.R.
(2) Inexperienced operators do not hold the trigger of the ventilator down for long enough, which results in poor ventilation. The trigger should be depressed at the end of the compression down stroke and held down until the next compression empties the lungs.
(3) Ventilating the patient out of phase (i.e. during compression) or maintaining poor neck extension causes oxygen to fill the stomach instead of the lungs. This problem also occurs, though much less often, with E.A.R. A good check on this is to watch the stomach which should rise and fall with ventilation. If the stomach rises but does not fall check the head tilt and the timing of the ventilations.

### 3.9.2 CARE OF THE OXYGEN SUPPLY

If full a D cylinder contains 340 litres of oxygen. The trigger on the ventilator head, if held down, will empty the contents of the cylinder in three and a half minutes. Used properly during resuscitation a full cylinder lasts between ten and fifteen minutes. The operator should instruct a third person to change the cylinder whilst he continues with E.A.R. If a third person is not available then the use of oxygen should be abandoned and E.A.R. continued instead.

### 3.10  Artificial airways

A face mask gives very little control over the airway because the tongue is still able to obstruct the pharynx when neck extension is lost. This is particularly likely to happen when the patient is transported. Artificial airways pass a variable distance into the mouth over the surface of the tongue, thus preventing it from falling back.

The Goudal airway is a simple curved tube which passes over the surface of the tongue distally and fits flush with the lips, thus allowing a mask to be placed over it for bag/mask or mouth to mask resuscitation.

The Brook airway is similar but has a proximal extension from the mouth to facilitate resuscitation. The nose is not covered as it is with a mask and so must be pinched shut during ventilation. Transporting a patient with a Brook airway in place is impractical and a Goudal airway is preferred.

### 3.10.1 ENDOTRACHEAL AND OESOPHAGEAL OBTURATOR AIRWAYS

The greatest hazard faced by the unconscious patient is aspiration of vomit. The endotracheal airway passes down the trachea and the oesophageal obturator obstructs the oesophagus. Both prevent aspiration of vomit. Proficiency with endotracheal intubation requires specific training and regular practice but this is undoubtedly the most satisfactory way of securing an airway in a deeply unconscious patient. It should be pointed out that although the oesophageal obturator has been used with some success in the United States of America (Don Michael, 1981), the trend is towards training in the use of endotracheal tubes.

## 3.11  Management of fractured neck

The same principles of 'airway, breathing and circulation' still apply. However, when opening the airway the operator should allow as little neck movement as is necessary. It may be possible to ventilate adequately without any neck extension by using good jaw support alone. Whilst transporting the patient gentle traction should be applied to the head with hands placed one over each ear trying, if possible, not to change the position of the head with respect to the body. This position, together with traction, should be maintained from ground to stretcher and from stretcher to hospital. Fixing the neck on a spinal board or with a Heinz splint may also be useful.

## 3.12  Intravenous infusion

Intravenous access is essential both for the administration of drugs if immediate action is required, or for support of circulation with rapid fluid replacement. Placement of the intravenous cannula does not take precedence over attempts to re-establish breathing and circulation. With this

45

one proviso, puncture of a large vein as early as possible is important because shock results in peripheral venous collapse and makes entry into a vein later extremely difficult. There is little to choose between the types of fluid replacement available and normal saline seems satisfactory in most instances.

## 3.13  Legal aspects of resuscitation

The Samaritan laws in this country exempt the operator from liability provided he has done his best under the circumstances. The position is less clear if the operator is using mechanical aids. In this instance it is usually sufficient to provide evidence that the operator has been specially trained in the use of mechanical aids. It is for this reason that the administration of oxygen and the use of mechanical aids are reserved for those aged seventeen years or older and who have completed an intensive course of instruction in advanced resuscitation.

## References

American Heart Association (1980) Standards and guidelines for cardiopulmonary resuscitation (CPR) and emergency cardiac care (ECC). *J. Amer. Med. Assoc.*, **255**, 2905.

Chandra, N., Guerchi, A., Weisfeldt, M. L., *et al.* (1981) Contrasts between intrathoracic pressures during external chest compression and cardiac massage. *Crit. Care Med.*, **9**, 789.

Don Michael, T. A. (1981) The oesophageal obturator airway; a critique. *J. Amer. Med. Assoc.*, **246**, 1098.

Nolte, H. (1968) A new evaluation of emergency methods for artificial ventilation. *Acta Anaesthes. Scand.*, Supplement 29, 111.

Taylor G. J., Tucker, M., Greene H. L., *et al.* (1977) Importance of prolonged compression duration during cardiopulmonary resuscitation in man. *New Engl. J. Med.*, **296**, 1515.

The Resuscitation Council (UK) (1984) *Resuscitation for the Citizen*, Department of Anaesthetics, Hammersmith Hospital, London.

# 4 Head injuries

## JOHN GLEAVE

It seems that there is no circumstance free from the risk of head injury, but in general the risk increases with activity. It is therefore not surprising that sport should be responsible for a significant number of head injuries requiring medical care. The fact that head injuries occur in sport has been known for a very long time and the first recorded instances happened on the plains of Troy at the funeral games of Patroclos (Homer). It is of interest to note that the first injury occurred in a horse race due to equipment failure, and the second in a boxing match.

## 4.1 Incidence

The Cambridge Neurosurgical Unit has undertaken the primary care of all head injuries admitted to the hospital from the Cambridge district (population 350 000) since its opening in October 1961. By 1964 this interest in head injury was widely known and there was a stable referral pattern, so that some reliance can be placed on the figures obtained.

During the years 1964 to 1981 inclusive, there were 12 280 patients from the Cambridge district admitted to Addenbrooke's because of head injury. Of these 981 (8%) received their injury whilst pursuing some form of sport. For comparison there were 7328 (60%) admissions as the result of road traffic accidents.

The criteria for admission following head injury were:

(1) Any history of unconsciousness or the inability to remember the concussive incident (retrograde and post-traumatic amnesia).
(2) The development of drowsiness, vomiting, severe headache or severe neurological deficit following the injury.
(3) The presence of a skull fracture assessed clinically or radiologically.

These criteria were designed to embrace all patients with primary brain damage or at risk of the development of brain damage from oncoming

47

## Head injuries

complications. They do not include simple bruises and lacerations of the scalp and almost certainly some linear fractures of the skull were missed, either because the skull was not X-rayed or because the X-ray did not pick up the fracture. Thus the figures given considerably underestimate the frequency of injury to the head because those cases where there was neither injury to the brain nor risk of injury to the brain were not included. Indeed, the incidence of cerebral injury must also be under-estimated to some degree because sportsmen who have sustained a minor degree of concussion do not always report to the hospital. Such concussion may produce only a momentary loss of consciousness or a very short period of amnesia, but it is quite apparent from the findings of Oppenheimer (1968) that diffuse microscopic damage to the brain occurs even in this type of case. This is the pathological basis of the syndrome of post-traumatic encephalopathy (punch drunkenness) seen in those such as boxers and jockeys who receive minor concussive blows.

Cerebral injury may occur in almost any sport as is shown in Table 4.1. The sex incidence is largely a factor of the numbers involved in any particular sport, though male aggression may play a small part. For example, in sports where both sexes might be thought to participate in approximately equal numbers, or indeed there might even be a female predominance, i.e. hockey, swimming, and gymnastics, there is a con-siderably greater incidence of male head injuries.

*Table 4.1*  Head injuries sustained in sport and admitted to hospital, 1964–81

| Sport | Male | Female | Total |
|---|---|---|---|
| Horse riding | 92 | 247 | 339 |
| Rugby football | 217 | – | 217 |
| Association football | 184 | 1 | 185 |
| Cricket | 37 | 1 | 38 |
| Swimming | 15 | 5 | 20 |
| Hockey | 10 | 8 | 18 |
| Athletics | 12 | 5 | 17 |
| Gymnastics | 9 | 6 | 15 |
| Motor cycle racing (including motorcross/speedway) | 13 | – | 13 |
| Roller skating | 5 | 7 | 12 |

Others (less than 10 cases):
   judo, golf, bicycle racing, boxing, netball, trampoline, go-kart, motor car racing, rounders, squash racquets, ice skating, skateboard, parachuting, tobog-gan, rock climbing, hang-gliding, water-skiing, baseball, angling, badminton, table tennis, land yacht racing, American football, basketball, sailing, punting, fives (rugby), gliding, wrestling, karate and clay pigeon shooting

It has not been possible to draw up a table of the comparative risks of different sports because of the seemingly insuperable difficulty of obtaining information about the numbers who participate in each sport and the hours they spend engaged in the sport.

A problem raised by Table 4.1 is the demarcation between sport and recreation. This is a line which is ill-defined and about which some arbitrary decisions have been made. Thus, hacking has been included as a sport, whereas playing on the apparatus in children's playgrounds has been excluded, though some of these activities seem to be very similar to those carried out in the gymnasium under supervision. The chief justification for this is that hacking has been included as a sport in previous surveys (Baker, 1973; Lindsay, McLatchie and Jennett, 1980; Gleave, 1976; Lewin, 1979).

However, the number of head injuries sustained by children at play are considerable, as shown in Table 4.2. Recent improvements in the design of playground equipment are to be welcomed.

*Table 4.2*  Admissions of children to Cambridge Neurosurgical Unit, 1964–81

|  | Male | Female | Total |
| --- | --- | --- | --- |
| Swing | 53 (1 death) | 58 | 111 |
| Climbing frame | 50 | 21 | 71 |
| Slide | 39 | 20 | 59 |
| Seesaw | 2 | 10 | 12 |
| Climbing rope | 10 | 1 | 11 |

In addition 172 injuries occurred in unsupervised play at home, 63 of which were due to falls from trees.

With regard to the ages of those sustaining head injury in sport, this is almost entirely a reflection of the ages of those involved in the sport. However, it does seem possible that an undue proportion of older men sustain head injuries playing cricket and association football. In horse riding the age incidence is set out in Table 4.3. The peak in the second decade may indicate lack of strength, skill, and experience, but it also underlines the remarkable love affair between the adolescent female and her horse.

The different admission criteria do not permit direct comparison of these figures with the Glasgow series of Lindsay *et al.* (1980). However, if allowances are made for this difference, it would seem that the pattern of sports in East Anglia differs considerably from that in south-west Scotland. In East Anglia there is far more horse riding, more rugby football and no mountains. In south-west Scotland there is far more golf, and more association football than rugby football.

Table 4.3 Age incidence of equestrian head injuries requiring admission to hospital

| Ages (decades) | Male (N=92) (%) | Female (N=247) (%) |
|---|---|---|
| 0–9 | 8.9 | 5.3 |
| 10–19 | 35.6 | 58.9 |
| 20–29 | 15.6 | 20.5 |
| 30–39 | 13.3 | 8.1 |
| 40–49 | 11.1 | 6.3 |
| 50–59 | 6.7 | 0.9 |
| 60–69 | 4.4 | – |
| 70+ | 4.4 | – |

## 4.2 Mechanism of cerebral injury in sport

The majority of injuries are caused by the moving head hitting the ground or some other relatively large and relatively stationary object, for example: falls from a horse or motor cycle, being tackled or carrying out a crash tackle at rugby and a collision of heads at soccer. If the velocity of the head is great, or if the ground is rough, deformation of the skull occurs, and this may lead to fracture, but in any event a shock wave is produced which travels through the brain. In all cases the head comes to an abrupt halt, but relative movement of the brain continues with translational and rotational acceleration. This is what concussion means (concutiri – to shake thoroughly) and it is this type of damage which is responsible for loss of consciousness.

A minority of injuries is caused by rapidly moving and relatively small objects striking the head, for example: a hoof, fist, boot, ball, bat, golf club or racquet. If the object is big enough, or the velocity is great enough, this blow will lead to loss of consciousness, but not infrequently a depressed fracture of the skull or local damage to the brain without loss of consciousness is the result.

Different types of injury therefore tend to occur among the players of different sports. Thus in rugby and association football, a closed head injury with concussion from acceleration/deceleration stresses is the most frequent, whereas in golf a depressed fracture from the club and little in the way of concussion is the usual presentation. In horse riding and machine racing, acceleration/deceleration injury is almost invariable, but there may be additional injuries from the head striking irregular objects such as rocks, kerbs or stanchions supporting safety netting.

## 4.3 The causes of head injury in different sports

*(a) Horse riding*

The amateur out hacking provides the greatest number of head injuries (Table 4.4). However, in all categories a fall from the horse was by far the most common cause. In eighteen cases the head was kicked and this proved fatal in one case. Protective headgear of a sort was worn by all except thirty-five of those out hacking. The professionals involved in training used to wear a cloth cap, but this practice seems to be dying out in recent years and the cloth cap has been replaced by a helmet.

*Table 4.4*  Head injuries caused by horse riding

|  | Male | Female | Total |
|---|---|---|---|
| *Amateur* | | | |
| Hacking | 56 | 219 | 275 |
| Hunting | 4 | 2 | 6 |
| Point-to-point | 7 | 7 | 14 |
| Gymkhana | 1 | 2 | 3 |
| Show jumping | 1 | 7 | 8 |
| Cross-country | – | 2 | 2 |
| *Professional* | | | |
| Training | 20 | 5 | 25 |
| Steeplechasing | 2 | – | 2 |
| Flat racing | 4 | – | 4 |
|  | 95 | 244 | 339 |

In spite of increasing publicity about the need for protective headgear there has been no decrease in the number of head injuries (Table 4.5). This is probably an index of the increasing popularity of riding and of sporting

*Table 4.5*  Average annual intake of head injuries in the Cambridge district football

| Quinquennia | All | RTA | All sport | Horse riding | Rugby football | Association football | Other |
|---|---|---|---|---|---|---|---|
| 1966–70 | 670 | 455 | 42 | 12 | 11 | 8 | 11 |
| 1971–75 | 681 | 451 | 49 | 18 | 10 | 11 | 10 |
| 1976–80 | 865 | 528 | 68 | 27 | 13 | 11 | 17 |

# Head injuries

activities in general. The increasing number of road traffic accidents is presumably related to the numbers of vehicles on the road, as crash helmets became compulsory in 1973 and the majority of people now wear safety belts.

## (b)   Rugby and association football

Heavy falls are the most common cause of injury, but collisions, boots and, rarely, fists, make a significant contribution. In two cases, small sub-cortical haematomata were caused in association football by heading a heavy ball incorrectly. In a case not included in this series, bilateral extradural haematomata leading to death were caused by an unskilful crash tackle in rugby football.

## (c)   Cricket

The causes were equally blows from the ball, blows from the bat, collisions with other players and falling over. Depressed fractures have been seen, though not in this series.

## (d)   Swimming

On two occasions, striking the head whilst diving resulted in concussion. In the remainder, slipping on the side of the pool was responsible for the head injury.

## (e)   Hockey

Blows from the stick were the usual cause, and in one case led to a depressed fracture. Blows from the ball were responsible for two head injuries.

## (f)   Athletics

On three occasions the shot and the discus caused head injuries. The remainder were the result of falls in the high jump, the long jump, and sprinting. In an incident not included in this series, death was caused by a javelin.

## (g)   Golf

With one exception, the injury was caused by a blow from the club. The exception was a middle-aged woman who swung at the ball so violently that she overbalanced and concussed herself briefly. She went on to develop a chronic subdural haematoma.

## (h)   Gymnastics

In half the cases, a fall from apparatus was responsible; the remainder were the result of slipping on the floor.

*(i)   Boxing*
It was impossible to decide in the majority of cases whether the blow was directly or indirectly responsible for the cerebral concussion because the recipient was knocked down and struck his head on the floor of the ring.

*(j)   Judo and wrestling*
These were due to heavy falls.

*(k)   Netball, basketball, rounders and baseball*
Collisions and falls were responsible.

*(l)   Squash racquets*
In two cases the injury was due to a blow from the racquet. In one of these, in which the blow was of insufficient severity to knock the player out or even to cause amnesia, an intracerebral haematoma developed over the course of the next hour. On angiography there was no underlying vascular abnormality.

*(m)   Angling and punting*
The injuries were due to bring struck by the weight, the rod, or the pole.

*(n)   Mountaineering and hang-gliding*
These patients lived in the Cambridge district and received part of their treatment here, though their injuries occurred outside the district.

   In the remainder of the sports the causes are self-evident and no comment is required.

### 4.4   Severity of head injury sustained in different sports

The severity of the head injury is considered under four different headings. Where sports are not included in these tables, the reason is that they did not produce an example of this type of injury or deficit.
   Table 4.6 gives the length of the post-traumatic amnesia (P.T.A.). This is the best single index of the severity of cerebral damage following a concussive blow to the head. Only sports in which an injury was sustained producing a post-traumatic amnesia of more than an hour are included in this table. In the remainder of the injuries the length of the post-traumatic amnesia was under 60 minutes. Although the injuries with the relatively short post-traumatic amnesia are often called minor or trivial injuries, as already mentioned, they are associated with diffuse

53

# Head injuries

*Table 4.6*  Severity of brain injury (assessed on length of P.T.A.)

| Sport | Under 60 min | 1–24 h | 1–7 days | 7 days to 1/12 | 1/12 to 3/12 | Permanent coma | Death |
|---|---|---|---|---|---|---|---|
| Horse riding | 264 | 38 | 16 | 10 | 1 | 1 | 9 |
| Rugby football | 179 | 36 | 2 | – | – | – | – |
| Association football | 136 | 45 | 4 | – | – | – | – |
| Swimming | 18 | 1 | 1 | – | – | – | – |
| Gymnastics | 11 | 3 | – | 1 | – | – | – |
| Motor cycling | 9 | 2 | 1 | – | – | – | 1 |
| Roller skating | 9 | 3 | – | – | – | – | – |
| Golf | 7 | 2 | – | – | – | – | – |
| Judo | 8 | 1 | – | – | – | – | – |
| Bicycle racing | 4 | 2 | – | 1 | – | – | – |
| Boxing | 6 | – | 1 | – | – | – | – |
| Rounders | 5 | 1 | – | – | – | – | – |
| Car racing | 1 | 1 | – | 1 | – | 1 | 1 |
| Ice skating | 3 | 1 | – | – | – | – | – |
| Hang-gliding | – | – | – | 2 | – | – | – |
| Badminton | – | 1 | – | – | – | – | – |
| Gliding | – | 1 | – | – | – | – | – |

microscopic damage to the brain, and, if repeated, their effect is cumulative (Oppenheimer, 1968).

Those sports in which players sustained fractures of the skull or face, confirmed radiologically, are shown in Table 4.7. This is therefore almost certainly an underestimate of the true number of fractures of the skull. The presence of a fracture does not necessarily indicate that the brain injury has been severe. Conversely, a lethal injury may be sustained without any skull fracture, particularly if a helmet is worn. However, Mendelow and associates have demonstrated that the risks of intracranial complications is far higher in the presence of a skull fracture (Mendelow *et al.*, 1982).

Table 4.8 is a list of the intracranial complications following head injury sustained in sport. In those sports not listed, no complications have yet been seen.

Permanent deficits occurred in those who returned to 'normal' life following head injuries sustained in sport and are detailed in Table 4.9. It does not include death, which is given in Table 4.6. Some of the patients are included in more than one category of handicap. Focal neurological damage includes such features as hemiparesis, visual defects and cranial nerve palsies (Fig. 4.1).

*Table 4.7* Fractures of the skull or face

| Sport | Skull linear | Skull depressed | Mandible | Facial bones |
|---|---|---|---|---|
| Horse riding | 45 | 16 | 8 | 13 |
| Rugby football | 3 | 3 | 2 | 4 |
| Association football | 8 | 5 | 2 | 10 |
| Cricket | 4 | – | 1 | 1 |
| Hockey | 1 | 1 | – | 2 |
| Gymnastics | 3 | – | – | – |
| Swimming | 2 | – | – | 1 |
| Bicycle racing | 2 | – | – | 1 |
| Motor cycle racing | 1 | – | – | 1 |
| Athletics | – | 1 | – | – |
| Golf | – | 5 | – | – |
| Rounders | – | 1 | – | – |
| Ice hockey | 1 | – | – | – |
| Gliding | 1 | – | – | – |
| Motor car racing | 1 | – | – | – |
| Angling | – | 1 | – | – |

*Table 4.8* Intracranial complications

| Sport | Cerebral damage | | | Cerebral compression | | Meningitis |
|---|---|---|---|---|---|---|
| | Brain laceration | Brain contusion | Intracerebral haematoma | Extradural haematoma | Subdural haematoma | |
| Horse riding | 12 | 20 | 2 | 5 | 8 | 1 |
| Rugby football | 1 | 3 | – | – | – | – |
| Association football | 2 | 3 | 2 | – | 2 | – |
| Cricket | – | – | – | 1 | 1 | – |
| Gymnastics | 1 | – | – | – | 1 | – |
| Motor car racing | – | 2 | – | – | – | 1 |
| Judo | – | – | – | – | 1 | – |
| Rounders | – | – | – | 1 | – | – |
| Baseball | – | 1 | – | – | – | – |
| Golf | 1 | 2 | – | – | 1 | – |
| Hang-gliding | – | 2 | – | – | – | – |
| Boxing | – | 1 | – | – | – | – |
| Angling | 1 | – | – | – | – | – |
| Squash | – | – | 1 | – | – | – |
| Motor cycling | 1 | 1 | – | – | – | – |

# Head injuries

*Table 4.9*  Permanent deficit

| Sport | Impaired mental function | Focal neurological damage | Post-traumatic epilepsy |
|---|---|---|---|
| Horse riding | 10 | 15 | 17 |
| Rugby football | 1 | 1 | 5 |
| Association football | – | – | 6 |
| Cricket | – | – | 1 |
| Hockey | – | 1 | 1 |
| Gymnastics | 1 | 1 | 1 |
| Bicycle racing | – | 1 | 1 |
| Motor cycle racing | – | 1 | – |
| Judo | – | 1 | – |
| Rounders | – | – | 1 |
| Baseball | – | – | 1 |
| Swimming | – | 1 | – |
| Golf | 1 | – | 1 |
| Hang-gliding | 2 | 2 | – |

## 4.5  Management

In any head injury the outcome is determined by two factors: the extent of the primary injury and the development of complications which may be due to intracranial or extracranial factors. Nothing significantly useful can be done about the primary injury although much effort is spent in trying to nurse the patient through the duration of its effects. On the other hand, much can be done to prevent the development of secondary effects and to treat the intracranial complications.

Such management begins at the moment of injury if there is anyone at hand to assist. At race meetings, boxing matches, and major football matches, medical officers are present, but such a provision is impossible during the ordinary Saturday afternoon game or when out hacking. It is not unreasonable to suggest, however, that those in charge of such games and the permanent staff at sports halls, arenas and swimming pools should have some knowledge of first aid to a head injury. The majority will present no problem because they rapidly regain consciousness, but for those who are more seriously injured the most important matter is the care of the airway. The possibility of other injuries, particularly to the neck, should not be forgotten and when the patient has to be moved, care should be taken to prevent further damage occurring. Some simple

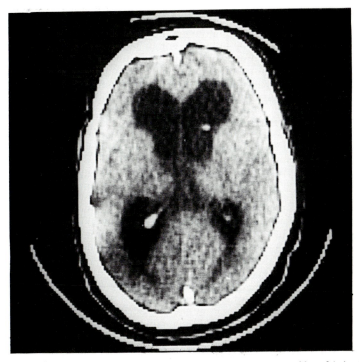

*Fig. 4.1* Ventricular dilatation in a jockey following a series of head injuries. In the right frontal horn the tip of a ventriculoatrial shunt can be seen. This was inserted in case there was an element of obstructive hydrocephalus additional to the post-traumatic encephalopathy. The procedure led to no improvement in his condition.

neurological observations should be noted for the benefit of those who will have the definitive care of the patient.

Many of the so-called minor injuries who regain consciousness within seconds or minutes will wish to play on, but this course of action should not be allowed and medical advice should be sought. Ideally the player should be admitted to hospital for at least twenty-four hours and if he has persistent headache or other symptoms, medical supervision should be continued. The object of admission to hospital of minor head injury is not only the prevention of complications, a point which is generally accepted, but the progressive mobilization of the patient under supervision, which is the most successful method of preventing the so-called post-concussional syndrome with its often prolonged invalidism.

If the concussed player is allowed to continue the game, he is at increased risk of further injury because his speed of reaction will have been diminished and he may be somewhat more reckless due to loss of normal inhibition. Sometimes this leads to him playing above himself, but it is at a risk of further and cumulative damage. It seems that sometimes rugby players are allowed to continue following an injury which would bring an end to a boxing bout (Appendix 1).


## 4.6 Prevention

As even minor blows to the head may be followed by disastrous consequences, all reasonable precautions to prevent them occurring at all should be taken. Obviously in the physical contact sports, head injuries are inevitable but physical fitness, good technique, and the absence of foul play would minimize their incidence. Strong refereeing and the banishing of offenders would also make these games more enjoyable, not only to play in, but also to watch.

Where equipment is used in the pursuance of a sport, this must be of the highest standard and regularly checked. Proper training in its use and supervision while it is being used would again minimize the risk of injury. In the same category is attention to the floor or mat in the combative sports.

Protective headgear should be worn where feasible and must play a significant role in the prevention of injury. Certainly that worn by the racing motorist and motor cyclist seems to be very effective, though nothing yet devised will prevent a serious or fatal injury occurring if the forces involved are sufficiently great. The protective headgear worn by horse riders when not involved in competition seems usually to be inadequate and more part of the general ensemble than a serious attempt to protect the head. There are excellent helmets available and they should be worn by all, and in particular by those in the second decade who either because of inexperience or lack of strength seem most prone to injury. Proper instruction is as important here as in all other sports. There is a limit to the use of helmets, and while they are perhaps justifiable in cricket played as it is today, or apparently as it was in Jardine's tour of Australia, it would seem that there is little place for them in rugby football, for if they were worn they would have to be followed by the whole panoply of protective clothing, and the American experience suggests that the incidence of head injuries in their game is higher than that in the English game (Alley, 1964).

In summary then, it would seem that the best preventive measures are fitness, skill, experience, common sense and adherence to the rules of the game, and, in those sports where it is indicated, the wearing of a properly constructed and fitted helmet.

# References

Alley, R. H. (1964) Head and neck injuries in high school football. *JAMA*, **188**, 418.
418.

Baker, H. M. (1973). Horse play: survey of accidents with horses. *Brit. Med. J.*, **3**, 532.

Gleave, J. R. W. (1976) The impact of sport on a Neurosurgical Unit, Institute of Sports Medicine Symposium, London.

Homer, The funeral games of Patroclos. *Iliad XXIII*, 394–97, 689.

Lewin, W. S. (1979) Head injuries in sport, Institute of Sports Medicine lecture, Cambridge.

Lindsay, K. W., McLatchie, G. and Jennett, B. (1980) Serious head injury in sport. *Brit. Med. J.*, **281**, 789.

Mendelow, A. D., Campbell, D. A., Jeffrey, R. R., Miller, J. D., Hesset, C., Bryden, J. and Jennett, B. (1982) Admission after minor head injury: benefits and costs. *Brit. Med. J.*, **285**, 1530.

Oppenheimer, D. R. (1968) Microscopic lesions in the brain following head injury. *J. Neurol. Neurosurg. Psychiat.*, **31**, 299.

# 5 Eye injuries

IVOR S. LEVY

## 5.1 Introduction

Sports eye injuries are particularly tragic as they often involve children and young adults and should, in most cases, be avoidable. In the USA approximately 100 000 school age children each year have sports related injuries, of which a quarter will suffer serious complications (National Society to Prevent Blindness, 1978). Such injuries may be divided into those involving the eye itself and those involving the lids and orbit, although often the two are combined; these injuries can be penetrating or non-penetrating. Most penetrating injuries occur in sports that involve guns, arrows and darts; others occur from ski sticks, ice skates, fishing hooks and swords. Of equal importance is penetration by broken spectacles; concave lenses used to correct myopia are thinnest at their centre and are particularly prone to shatter. Non-penetrating injuries occur in racket and all contact sports. Orbital injury is a particular hazard in racket sports from both the ball and the racket itself (Fowler, Seelenfreund and Newton, 1980). Injuries to the lids and brow are common in contact sports, especially boxing.

Ideally, all ocular injuries should be referred to an ophthalmologist but where this is impractical, it would be useful for the doctor examining the injured sportsman to have some guidelines to follow so that a decision can be made as to when referral is essential. All serious injuries should be referred. The decision is more difficult in seemingly trivial injuries and when the sportsman has a black eye.

If at all possible the visual acuity should be assessed. A formal test chart is not necessary; the variable print size of a newspaper will enable approximate values to be obtained, particularly when the injured eye is compared with the fellow eye. If there is a black eye or swollen lids, some effort should be made to elevate the lid to obtain a visual acuity. If this is not possible then the patient should be referred to an ophthalmologist. Small differences are of little significance, but if there is a marked

61

reduction in acuity in a previously normal eye, again referral is essential. The movements of the eye should be observed and if diplopia is present the sportsman again should be referred to an ophthalmologist.

Foreign bodies may lodge in the upper or lower fornix. Irrigation with sterile saline may be sufficient to flush them away. If this is not successful they can be wiped away gently with a cotton bud. If a foreign body remains under the upper lid, the lashes should be firmly gripped and the lid everted over a cotton bud to expose the tarsal conjuctiva; any foreign bodies can then be wiped away with another cotton bud. If these simple measures fail to dislodge the foreign body the athlete should be referred. The cornea should be inspected and superficial abrasions, not immediately obvious, may be demonstrated with fluorescein drops which stain the defect green (Plate 1). If an abrasion is detected the eye should be carefully padded, making sure the lids are closed, and the patient referred. The anterior chamber should be inspected particularly for the presence of blood within it (hyphaema); it originates from bleeding vessels at the root of the iris and indicates damage to intraocular structures (Plate 2).

Careful examination of the pupils is most important; their size, shape and reactions should be noted. An enlarged poorly reacting pupil could be due to direct injury to the iris (traumatic mydriasis or iridoplegia) or may indicate damage to the third nerve intracranially. Associated signs of ocular damage would suggest traumatic mydriasis but the differentiation from third nerve palsy becomes particularly difficult when there is diplopia due to orbital injury. A pear-shaped pupil suggests a penetrating injury which may not otherwise be apparent (Plate 3). In such cases expert advice must be sought. The pupillary light reflexes should be tested. The swinging flashlight test is particularly important: a light is shone in the good eye and then swung to the bad eye; dilation of the pupil indicates damage to the optic nerve or retina. A retinal tear should be suspected if the injured sportsman complains of floating black spots in his vision especially when accompanied by flashing lights. If at all possible ophthalmoscopic examination of the fundus should be made; failure to see the fundus clearly may be due to haemorrhage into the vitreous from retinal tears. Tears predispose to retinal detachment and their early detection will facilitate prophylactic treatment and avert this very serious complication. Complete examination of the fundus requires dilation of the pupil though this is not advised at the initial examination as there may be accompanying head injury and dilation of the pupil will destroy one of the most important signs of intracerebral trauma. If the fundus is clearly seen, pallor, especially if associated with haemorrhages, indicates retinal contusion (commotio retinae). At the macula this may produce permanent visual damage. There may also be an accompanying retinal tear so that any such retinal injury requires referral.

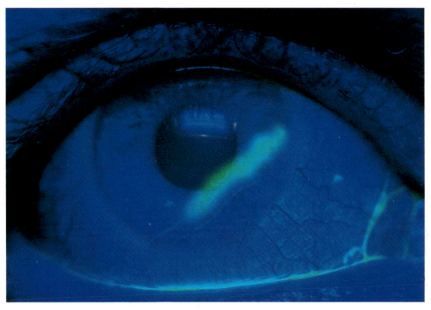

*Plate I*   Corneal abrasion stained with fluorescein.

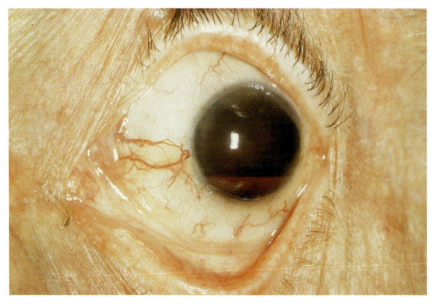

*Plate II*   Blood in anterior chamber (hyphaema).

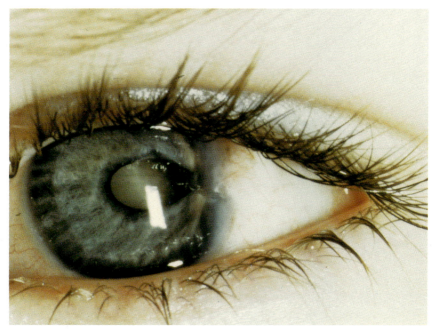

*Plate III*   Penetrating injury showing pear-shaped pupil.

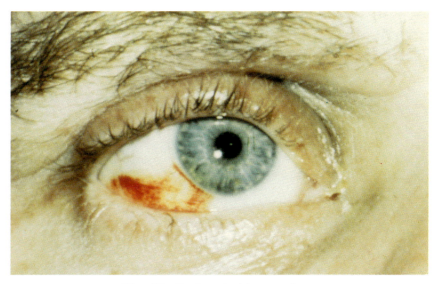

*Plate IV*   Conjunctival haemorrhage.

## 5.2 Penetrating eye injuries

Injuries from BB or pellet guns often produce such damage to the intraocular structures that the eye has to be enucleated, either because surgical repair is not feasible or because, after repair, the eye remains blind and painful. The danger of sympathetic ophthalmia may also contribute to the decision to enucleate the injured eye, although modern techniques of microsurgical repair and the use of steroids lessen this risk. It is now rare to recommend immediate enucleation of a severely injured eye. Even if initially no potential for vision is thought possible, it is still more prudent to attempt primary repair than enucleate. The psychological effect of immediate enucleation can be devastating and the patient may harbour lingering doubts that something could have been done to save the eye. It is easier to accept enucleation of a blind painful eye if some attempt has been made to save it, and on rare occasions, one is surprised at the visual outcome from an eye thought to be unsalvageable. Furthermore, if the eye can be retained even if totally blind, the patient is better off both physically and psychologically. An unsightly but comfortable eye can be made aesthetically quite acceptable with a cosmetic contact lens. Even with the best prosthesis an empty socket, or one containing an implant, can produce many long-term problems.

When repairing penetrating injuries a full assessment of the extent of injury must be made; penetrating wounds to the anterior segment often extend more posteriorly than is immediately obvious and, unless the posterior limits of such wounds are identified, adequate repair cannot be carried out. With eyes filled with blood, assessment of the extent of injury can be aided by the use of ultrasound examination; it is particularly helpful in identifying retinal detachment which would alter the whole surgical approach when attempting to repair such eyes. The detection and localization of retained foreign bodies is crucial. Their presence should be suspected in all penetrating injuries and requires the appropriate radiological and ultrasonographic investigations to be done. Most glass is radio-opaque and detectable by X-rays.

When there are serious intraocular complications of eye injuries such as retinal detachment, lens dislocation or foreign bodies, two approaches can be considered: total primary repair or repair of the wound alone with delayed repair of the intraocular damage. Whilst each approach has its drawbacks, it is often the individual case and circumstances which determine a particular decision. When repairing the only good eye of a young man in a non-specialized unit at night it would be prudent to carry out a simple repair of the wound and transfer the patient to a specialized centre for further surgery. If the patient is initially brought to a large

# Eye injuries

ophthalmic centre with specialized microsurgical vitreo-retinal expertise available, total primary repair may be considered.

## 5.3 Non-penetrating injuries

These occur in racket and contact sports and can be as devastating as penetrating injuries. Damage to the lids and brows is common in contact sports, especially boxing. If there are vertical lid lacerations involving the lid margin or lacrimal drainage system, expert advice should be sought. Inexpert repair can result in a permanently watering eye (Fig. 5.1). Conjunctival haemorrhage is common, it is rarely serious and the athlete can be reassured (Plate 4). If the posterior limit of a conjunctival haemorrhage cannot be seen a more cautious approach should be taken, as such haemorrhages may have tracked forward from an orbital or cranial injury. A hyphaema always suggests intraocular damage and requires referral. Injury to the root of the iris may cause its separation (iridodialysis, Fig. 5.2) or damage the aqueous drainage structures in the angle of the anterior chamber producing a delayed form of glaucoma. Shimmering movements of the iris (iridodenesis) occur after dislocation of the lens. A severe blow to the eye may cause a traumatic cataract, however, this may not develop for months or even years after the injury. Similarly, retinal

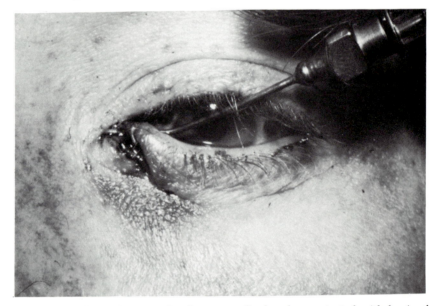

*Fig. 5.1* Lid laceration severing lower canaliculus demonstrated with lacrimal cannula.

64

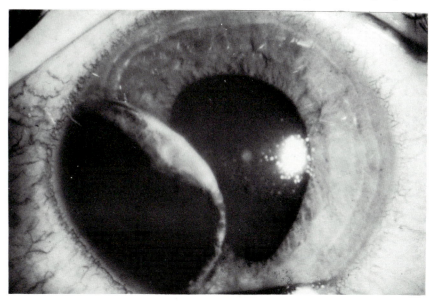

*Fig. 5.2*  Separation of the root of the iris (iridodialysis).

detachment can occur long after the initial injury. When the delay is considerable a direct relationship between the injury and the ocular pathology becomes increasingly questionable.

## 5.4   Orbital injuries

Any structure within the orbit may be injured directly or indirectly by fractured orbital bones. Of particular importance is the so called 'blow-out' fracture. While this is said to occur from small balls it can certainly occur with large ones. If they hit the orbital rim with sufficient velocity the ball is deformed and compresses the globe and orbital contents. Such a rise in intraorbital pressure produces a fracture of the weakest part of the bony orbit, that is, the medial portion of the floor. There is often an associated fracture of the medial wall but this is much less often detected, and produces the dramatic symptom of acute proptosis when the injured sportsman blows his nose, as air from the sinuses pass through the fracture into the orbit. 'Blow-out' fracture produces the classical triad of enophthalmos, diplopia on upgaze and numbness of the cheek (Figs 5.3 and 5.4). The enophthalmos is due to prolapse of orbital fat through the fracture into the antrum, the diplopia on upgaze is caused by tethering of the facial attachments of the inferior rectus muscle and the numbness by damage to the infraorbital nerve.

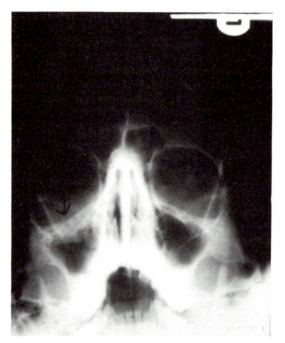

*Fig. 5.3*   Blowout fracture (arrowed).

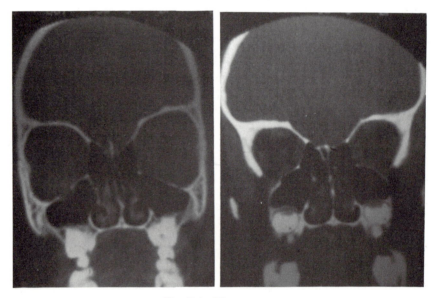

*Fig. 5.4*   Blowout.

If suspected, orbital X-rays using Waters's view may show the fracture but tomography, especially computer assisted tomography, is better as it can not only demonstrate the fracture but reveal its extent (Figs 5.5 and 5.6). The management of these fractures is still controversial. At one extreme some surgeons recommend repair of all demonstrated fractures whilst at the other, surgical intervention is hardly ever recommended. As usual in such a situation the best approach lies somewhere in between with surgery being reserved for patients having diplopia persisting for more than a few days and having significant enophthalmos. Diplopia is also common after other orbital injuries. It may be transient when due to bruising of extraocular muscles or persistent after injury to the trochlea through which the superior oblique muscle passes. Superior oblique paresis also occurs following intracerebral injury to the fourth nerve. This is not uncommon in head injury, particularly from horse riding or motor cycle injuries. It is often bilateral, frequently overlooked and should be suspected if there is double vision on downgaze. Injury to the optic nerve is less common: it can occur anywhere along its course especially where it is tethered, that is, in the optic canal and at its insertion into the globe.

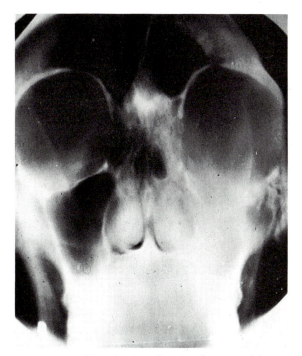

*Fig. 5.5* Blowout fracture: Water's view showing fracture of floor and an opaque antrum.

Eye injuries

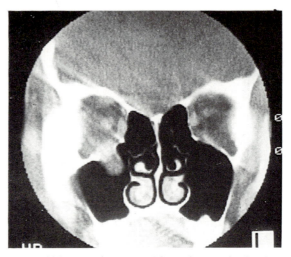

*Fig. 5.6*  C.T. scan of blowout fracture with prolapse of orbital contents in the antrum.

### 5.5  Prevention

Even more important to doctors concerned with sports eye injuries is involvement in their prevention. This entails not only advice about forms of eye protection but ensuring that such advice is adhered to. Many eye injuries occur because advice is ignored, or through careless neglect of the rules of a particular sport. They should encourage their stricter enforcement and, where necessary, suggest changes in the rules to make the sport safer.

Ice hockey in North America produced an epidemic of eye injuries both from the hard rubber puck which reached speeds of over 100 miles per hour and from the sticks, which were too often wielded in a dangerous manner (Pashby *et al.*, 1975). In Canada a Committee on Protective Equipment was set up by the Canadian Standards Association. This finally recommended a face protector made from heavy wire that was meshed tightly enough to prevent the penetration of the smallest hockey stick. The alternative clear plastic polycarbonate shield was rejected by the Canadians because of fogging and scratching. The rules of the game were also changed and strictly enforced; sticks had to be kept below shoulder height. Adequate protection and rule enforcement have almost eliminated trauma to the eye and face which previously had accounted for two-thirds of all injuries in ice hockey.

Unfortunately eye injuries in squash and racquetball continue to increase and will only be reduced when the wearing of eye-guards is mandatory (Vinger, 1980; Easterbrook, 1981a). Open eye-guards allow penetration by the ball and are not recommended. Those not requiring a prescription should wear wrap-around eye-guards giving good lateral protection. If prescription lenses are needed these should be in a nylon sports frame with a steep posterior lip; this allows the lens to project forward instead of being driven into the eye if the frame is struck. Ideally, all lenses should be made of polycarbonate plastic as this is the strongest material. Unfortunately as yet the range of prescriptions available is limited. Industrial plastic lenses which are 3 mm thick at their centre are available in a wider prescription range (Easterbook, 1981b). As fishing-hook injuries often result in loss of an eye, fishermen should be strongly encouraged to wear glasses with either prescription or plane lenses.

Many athletes now prefer to wear contact lenses to avoid the disadvantages of spectacles. However, hard lenses can break and seriously damage the eye (O'Rourke, 1971); soft lenses are more comfortable, and though they can split rarely cause damage. It is still important to wear eye protection in all racket sports, irrespective of whether contact lenses are worn or not. When swimming with contact lenses the head should be kept out of the water or goggles worn. Ultraviolet light can produce an extremely painful form of keratitis. Goggles to filter out the harmful ultraviolet rays should be worn not only by snow-skiers, but also by water-skiers and yachtsmen when weather conditions produce strong light reflection from the surface of the water. Such goggles should be sturdy and of approved safety standard to avoid shattering with subsequent ocular damage.

Finally, athletes at particular risk should be warned of the dangers they run. High myopes have a much higher incidence of detachment. Eyes which have had previous intraocular surgery or injury are more vulnerable. Athletes with an amblyopic (lazy) eye, whilst not at greater risk, would be much more devastated if they injured their good eye. In all such cases the doctor involved should inform the athlete clearly of the risks, stress the need for adequate protection, but leave the final decision whether to retire from a particular sport to the individual, or in some cases, to the appropriate controlling body. The British Boxing Board of Control is very stringent with regard to eye injuries; whether an injured eye which has been surgically successfully repaired is at greater risk than a previously uninjured eye is unproven. Nevertheless it may be prudent to ban such boxers from the ring. Such decisions are particularly difficult in professional sports where the individual's livelihood is at stake.

# Eye injuries

## References

Easterbrook, W. M. (1981a) Eye injuries in racquet sports: a continuing problem. *Phys. Sports Med.*, **9**, 91.

Easterbrook, M. (1981b) Eye protection for squash and racquet players. *Phys. Sports Med.*, **9**(2), 79.

Fowler, B. J., Seelenfreund, M. and Newton, J. C. (1980) Ocular hazards sustained playing squash. *Amer. J. Sports Med.*, **8**, 126.

National Society to Prevent Blindness (1978) Fact sheet, 79 Madison Avenue, New York, NY 10016.

O'Rourke, P. J. (1971) Traumatic fracture of contact lens with corneal injury. *Brit. J. Ophthalmol.*, **55**, 125.

Pashby, T. J., Pashby, R. C., Chisholm, L. D. J. and Crawford, J. S. (1975) Eye injuries in Canadian hockey. *Can. Med. Assoc. J.*, **113**, 663.

Vinger, P. F. (1980) Sports related eye injury. A preventable problem. *Surv. Ophthalmol.*, **25**(1), 47.


## Further reading

Duke-Elder, Sir S. and MacFaul, P. A. (1972) *System of Ophthalmology*. Vol. XIV. Part I *Mechanical Injuries*, Henry Kimpton, London.

Freeman, H. MacKenzie (ed.) (1979) *Ocular Trauma*, Appleton-Century-Crofts, New York.

Vinger, P. F. (ed.) (1981) Ocular sports injuries, in *International Ophthalmology Clinics*, Vol. 21, No. 4, Little, Brown and Company, Boston.

Walsh, F. B. and Hoyt, W. F. (1969) *Clinical Neuro-ophthalmology*. Vol. III. Williams and Wilkins Company, Baltimore.

# 6 Oral, dental and maxillo-facial injuries

HUGH CANNELL

## 6.1 Introduction

The sports most frequently associated with injuries to the face, mouth and teeth are rugby football (Upson, 1982; de Wet, 1981; Davies *et al.*, 1977; Morton and Burton, 1979;), ice hockey (Motyčka and Vašina, 1982; Jarvinen, 1980), horse riding (Lie and Lucht, 1977), competitive bicycling (Jarvinen, 1980), and hockey (Dennis and Parker, 1972).

Surveys of all sports taken together have shown a frequency of injury to the teeth in sportsmen which ranges from 16% in England (Lees and Gaskell, 1976), 18.5% in Poland (Krzychalska-Karwan, 1975), 30–40% in West Germany (Bollman and Wanneumacher, 1974) and up to 50% in the USA (Cathcart, 1968; Heintz, 1968). Teenagers have high frequencies of injury (Jarvinen, 1980; Roberts, 1970).

Comparison of the numbers of cases amongst rugby players in New Zealand (Morton and Burton, 1979) shows that protection apparatus in the form of mouthguards can reduce dental injuries (Nicholas, 1976) by nearly 43%. In the USA, football players wearing face and mouthguards now have fewer dental injuries than boxers, basketball players or hockey players (Roberts, 1970; Fitzner, 1979; Jones, 1979). The incidence of fractures of the bones in the middle and lower thirds of the face in sportsmen is between 5.6–17% of all facial fractures treated by specialist maxillo-facial units (Worrall, 1980; Moos, 1982; Rowe and Killey, 1968; Guise, 1982; Eade, 1969; Schultz, 1970; de Wet, 1981; Bollman and Wanneumacher, 1974; Motyčka and Vašina, 1982 and Fortunato, Fieding and Guernsey, 1982).

The absolute incidence of facial bone fractures in a population of 1.5 million at risk in New Zealand has been estimated to be 0.1% (Guise, 1982). Since most sports, if competitive, are played by cohorts of the population from the second and third decades of life, the true incidence is likely to be much higher. Non-organized but competitive sports must involve large numbers of players, hence it is impossible to determine

71

# Oral, dental and maxillo-facial injuries

frequencies of injury per player-hours. Figures for facial bone injuries recorded as being associated with the playing of sports do give an indication of total numbers of patients (Table 6.1).

Table 6.1 shows that the overwhelming majority of fractures were to the zygomatic (malar) bone complex. Table 6.2 shows that the left side of

Table 6.1  Sites of 193 fractures* of the facial bones recorded as associated with sports, over a five-year period, Canniesburn Hospital, Scotland, UK (Moos, 1982)

| Site | Number | % Sports fractures |
|------|--------|--------------------|
| Mandible | 34 | 17.5 |
| Nasal | 15 | 7.8 |
| Central maxillary | 11 | 5.7 |
| Malar | 133 | 69 |

*193 fractures were 7.2% of total facial fractures surveyed ($n = 2695$)

Table 6.2  Fractures of the zygomatic (malar) bone complex associated with sports in several areas of the UK

| Area | % All fractures | Side | | Reference |
|------|-----------------|------|-------|-----------|
| | | Left | Right | |
| London Hospital | 5.7 | 6.2 | 4.5 | Worral (1980) |
| E. Scotland | 9.2 | 11.8 | 6.4 | Hitchin and Shuker (1973) |
| S.E. Scotland | 12 | | | Haidar (1978) |
| S. England | 3.6 | L | > R | Rowe and Killey (1968) |

Table 6.3  Aetiology of fractures of the mandible (alone) by sport, in three areas of the UK expressed as percentages of all mandibular fractures

| Total of all | Sports sample | Soccer | Rugby | Cricket | Hockey | Boxing | Golf or athletics |
|--------------|---------------|--------|-------|---------|--------|--------|-------------------|
| 465* | 38 | 6.8 | 4.8 | 2.0 | 7.3 | 0.8 | 0.4 |
| 1500† | 127 | 4.13 | 1.6 | 1.94 | | 0.6 | 0.2 |
| 108‡ | 13 | 10.2 | 1.9 | | | | |

* Halazonetis (1968) Bristol area
† Rowe and Killey (1968) Rooksdown and Queen Mary's Hospitals
‡ Haidar (1978) S.E. Scotland

the face was injured more frequently than the right side. Blow-out fractures of the orbital floor through sports comprised nearly 30% of a total of 90 cases over six years in Poland (Bartowski and Krzyskowa, 1982).

Soccer and rugby players had more injuries to the mandible than other sportsmen (Table 6.3) but the numbers playing each sport were not available.

## 6.2 Mechanisms of injury

Trauma to the face, teeth or jaws is responsible for almost all injuries associated with sports activities to the region. Injuries to teeth are particularly common. Damage can take place not only to the crown of the tooth but also to the structures beneath the surface of the gingiva. Fractures of the teeth and of the supporting bone are at their maximum after low velocity injuries such as falls after collisions (Andreasen, 1981). Higher velocity injuries tend to produce horizontal fractures of the crowns of the teeth but the distribution of some of the force may be cushioned by the lips or cheeks. Implements used in sport may, by their shape and size, produce patterns of injury to the teeth.

In general it is the fast moving team games that lead to collisions and produce dental injuries. Where apparatus in the forms of sticks and hard balls or pucks is used, the frequency of dental injury is particularly high. Ice hockey skating speeds may attain 25 m.p.h. and a puck may travel at up to 90 m.p.h. (Wood, 1972). The incidence of dental injury is greater in ice hockey forwards than in defence men (Wood, 1972) but less information appears to be available for injury frequency.

The bony skeleton into which the teeth are inserted is in two parts: the dento-alveolar components which approximate to the length of the tooth roots and the basal bone of the jaws. The upper jaw and its adjacent region is of complex structure as the forces of chewing have to be distributed to the base of the skull. At the same time the weight of the upper jaw and parts of the skull are weakened by the accommodation of the nasal airway, the orbits and the air sinuses. The structure of the middle third of the facial skeleton is therefore a series of thicker struts of bones that buttress the weaker areas against chewing forces from below (Killey, 1971). A fracture of bones in the middle third therefore possibly involves not only the buttress bone, but the very thin walls of the air sinuses or orbits.

The mandible, although a much stronger bone than the maxilla, is weakened at the thin condylar neck and by the length of the roots of some teeth, the common sites for fracture being the neck of the condyle, the

73

# Oral, dental and maxillo-facial injuries

lower wisdom and lower canine regions. Indirect trauma may lead to concussion. This most important result of trauma to the area of the chin may be overlooked unless the mechanism is understood. A blow to the chin is transmitted along this curved bone to the angle of the mandible. The force is then changed in direction up the ascending ramus and is transmitted to the base of the skull via the head of the condyles impacting into the glenoid fossae. The contre-coup effect then produces concussion.

In team games players it has been postulated that since 90 to 95% of the population are right-handed, the precision of motor control through hemispheric dominance may allow better protection of the right side of the face against injury than of the left (Hitchin and Shuker, 1973). Certainly it is true that more left-sided zygomatic complex injuries are encountered (Table 6.3) in sports injuries. Further research with a control group of left-sided players would help investigation of this aspect.

In any episode of trauma, the extent of the injury when vision is present is lessened by an avoiding reaction. In this way the force of a blow is taken on the main buttress bones and high points of the face. Potential injuries to the soft parts of the eye region are prevented by the supraorbital ridges, the nose, the zygomatico-frontal buttress and the prominence of the buttress of the zygoma itself. It would appear that an avoiding reaction also tends to rotate the head about the neck and hence displace a frontal blow laterally.

The facial bones will withstand considerable forces if the load is applied for a short time via a padded surface (Swearingen, 1965). Blows from hard objects impacting over a small area of bone will fracture the bone with much smaller loading forces. Injuries associated with sports implements, such as bats or sticks, may be expected to lacerate soft tissues and lead to displaced comminuted type fractures. Collision injuries from head contacts, elbow or arm blows or from kicks, in general produce less soft tissue damage but the forces impacting against a small area of bone may lead to displacement of fractures.

Blow-out fractures occur (Rowe, 1981) when an impacting object compresses the globe of the eye within its bony socket. The periorbital fat that surrounds the globe and the ocular muscles is virtually incompressible and behaves like liquid. The transmitted force after impact bursts the bony walls of the orbit at one or more of its weakest areas. Since the floor of the orbit is in places only about 0.5 mm thick it is usual for this partition between the orbit and the maxillary antrum to be fractured and displaced (Fig. 6.1). Less frequently the partition at the medial wall of the orbit to the ethmoid air cells may be fractured in a similar way.

Herniation of the periorbital fat through the burst bony wall produces an enophthalmos. Since the cubic capacity of the orbit is effectively increased by the loss of integrity of its restraining walls, the degree of

74

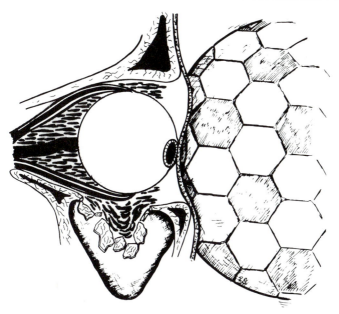

*Fig. 6.1* The mechanism of a blowout fracture of the orbital floor. Note the herniation of periorbital fat into the maxillary sinus.

enophthalmos produced may be considerable. Later if some of the herniated fat undergoes necrosis a degree of enophthalmos may become permanent. Unprotected ball players are most at risk from blow-out injuries. Hard balls such as those used in hockey are an obvious danger. Less obviously dangerous are tennis balls. These may be travelling at up to 100 m.p.h. and their size is such that although the prominent bony ridges that ring the eye must be hit, so also must the globe itself receive part of the force of the blow. Deformation on impact of the soft ball may reduce but not avoid a compressive force to the globe. Smaller balls such as squash balls may fit the size of the external orbital rim and produce severe compression of the globe (Barrel *et al.*, 1981).

Fights on or off the sporting arena are, apart from road traffic accidents, the most frequent cause of blow-out fractures (Converse *et al.*, 1962). The human fist is often the vehicle by which a compressive force is applied to the globe of the eye.

## 6.3 Diagnosis

The history of injury through sport to the face and jaws will be that of direct or indirect trauma. Concussion may complicate the history and pre-

# Oral, dental and maxillo-facial injuries

traumatic and post-traumatic amnesia may be present. Witnesses should be sought to confirm the extent and the probable severity of the traumatic episode.

### 6.3.1 EXAMINATION

Extraoral examination for facial injuries is carried out by careful palpation of the main bony contours. It is best to commence with the mandible by following the lower border then checking for painful movement of the temporo-mandibular joints when opening the jaw. Even undisplaced crack fractures at the condylar neck can be suspected if pain occurs on gentle depression of the mental prominence against resistance. Gentle squeezing of the two bodies of the mandible between forefinger and thumb of the outstretched hand will in the same way give an indication of the site of any fracture.

Dislocation rarely occurs in sports injuries without fracture, but may be recognized by an inability to close the front teeth together. The high points of the rest of the face are then carefully examined. Flattening of the contour of the zygomatico-maxillary complex, including the arch, is recognized more easily by examining the patient, from above and from below, and comparing one side with the other. Oedema may occur rapidly after injuries to the face and tends to mask any flattening of bony contours. Palpation for step defects in the lateral and inferior orbital rims is carried out and may assist preliminary diagnosis despite oedema.

A summary of the physical signs of fractures of the zygomatic complex is given in Table 6.4.

Fractures of the maxilla with displacement are rarely associated with sports injuries but gross bilateral oedema of the face, lengthening of the face and an altered occlusion of the teeth with an anterior open bite should alert the clinician to this possibility.

Intra-oral examination of all cases of injuries to the facial bones is mandatory. Mandibular fractures (Table 6.5) of the angle, body and mid-line usually involve the tooth-bearing regions. Damaged and loose teeth should be sought and a gentle tilting movement of the alveolus between the fingers may reveal fractures of the bone beneath.

Investigations of the injured face should include:

(1) Observation of eye signs, pulse and blood pressure for possible head injury.
(2) Intraoral examination for lacerations and for broken or lost teeth.
(3) Radiographs (*see below*)
(4) Later specialist dental examination, including intraoral radiographs.

76

*Table 6.4*  Summary of signs of fractured zygomatico-maxillary complex

| (1) | Cheek | Oedema of cheek perhaps masking flattening of cheek bone<br>Loss of or diminished sensation of anterior aspect of cheek |
|---|---|---|
| (2) | Eye | Bruising around the orbit<br>Subconjunctival haemorrhage<br>Diplopia especially on upward gaze<br>Enophthalmos<br>Restriction of ocular movement |
| (3) | Orbit | Step defects of rims<br>Obvious distortion of bony contours and width between eyes |
| (4) | Nose | Unilateral epistaxis on side of injury |
| (5) | Mandible | Limitation of full opening<br>Restriction of lateral movement to injured side |
| (6) | Mouth | Anaesthesia of upper teeth and gum<br>Bruising of buccal sulcus<br>Tenderness of zygomatic buttress<br>Loosened teeth<br>Malocclusion |
| (7) | Radiographic | Step defects in bony contours (occipitomental views)<br>Notches in or apparent change in arc of zygomatic arch (sub-mento vertex view)<br>Opaque antrum (blood)<br>'Tear drop' or soft tissue outline at orbital floor (blow-out fracture) |

Extraoral radiographs are necessary before the full extent of any facial bone fractures can be determined. The views that best demonstrate the middle third of the face are difficult to take well and the radiographer should not be asked to attempt them until the patient's condition permits. The standard views are shown in Fig. 6.2. For the mandible, the oblique lateral for each side and also the rotary tomogram are added to this list of extraoral views. Intraoral views of fractured teeth, teeth adjacent to fractures of the jaws and of any suspected midline mandibular fracture are taken using a dental X-ray machine.

# Oral, dental and maxillo-facial injuries

*Table 6.5*  Summary of signs of fractured mandible

| | | |
|---|---|---|
| (1) | Unilateral condylar neck | Tenderness over jaw joint on movement<br>Pain on pressure to mental prominence<br>Possibly slight bleeding at external auditory meatus<br>Deviation of jaw on opening towards injured side |
| (2) | Bilateral condylar neck | Tenderness and pain as above<br>Anterior open bite at attempted closure of jaw<br>Possible associated fracture at mid-line of mandible |
| (3) | Coronoid process | Mild oedema above anterior end of zygomatic arch<br>Pain on closure against resistance<br>Limitation of movement of mandible<br>Exclude condylar fracture |
| (4) | Ascending ramus | Slight swelling over region<br>Pain on movement of jaw |
| (5) | Angle<br>Body | Swelling over fracture site<br>Tenderness<br>Step defect at lower border<br>Pain on movement<br>Anaesthesia of lower lip on injured side<br>Bruising of lingual or buccal sulcus<br>Tender, displaced teeth<br>Derangement of occlusion |
| (6) | Mid-line region | Bruising, tenderness<br>Laceration under chin<br>Loose teeth<br>Possible associated fractures of condyles |
| (7) | Radiographic | Single or branching or double line radiolucencies, often with contour outline defects or obvious displacement<br>Radio-opaque (white) line in cases where bone ends have overlapped |

## 6.4  Treatment

### 6.4.1  SOFT TISSUE LACERATIONS

Lacerations may be to skin or to oral mucosa. Those involving the skin may be irregular in shape and depth following trauma over the bony

78

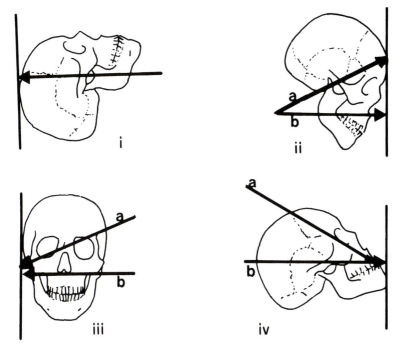

*Fig. 6.2* Standard radiographic views for suspected fractures of the facial bones and lower jaw. (i) Submentovertical view to show zygomatic arches. (ii) (a) Reverse Townes (occipitofrontal) to show head and neck of mandibular condyles. (b) Posterior-anterior view (PA) to show displaced mandibular fractures, displacement of large alveolar fractures and of middle third of face fractures. (iii) (a) Temporomandibular joint views, usually taken in both open and closed positions of the jaw. (b) Lateral view of facial bones and base of skull; demonstrates posterior displacements of maxilla and available airway. (iv) (a) 30° occipitomental view (OM); to show maxillary sinuses and facial bones and orbits. (b) 10° or less occipitomental view, to show lower parts of the facial bones. (Diagrams courtesy of Mrs R. Mason.)

prominences of the face, shelving in collision type injuries or compound to bone in severe trauma. Intraoral lacerations are due to teeth cutting the cheeks or tongue or even penetrating the lips. Partial degloving of the mental prominence may occur with collisions or falls involving a rotational effect about the chin or due to direct downward blows. The apparently superficially torn mucosa of the lower anterior buccal sulcus may conceal the extent of the separation of the soft tissues of the chin from the bone unless the full depth of the wound is explored.

First aid treatment is to control any bleeding by simple pressure. Lacerations more than ¼ cm long should be considered for suture or taping

# Oral, dental and maxillo-facial injuries

if on the facial skin. In sports injuries, lacerations may be contaminated with mud or dirt. Any obvious foreign body should be removed at once at the time of first aid. The preparation of a laceration for suturing should be undertaken as soon as possible after the injury has occurred. Infiltration of local anaesthetic, a solution such as 2% lignocaine hydrochloride containing 1 in 80 000 adrenaline as small vessel vasoconstrictor, confers the advantages of analgesia and a near bloodless field. It is important to note that bottles or cartridges of local anaesthetic solutions containing vasoconstrictors should be carefully marked 'for facial and oral wounds only'. On no account should it be possible for a non-professional first-aider to inject such solutions by mistake into the limbs or digits.

Contaminated wounds should be explored and lightly scrubbed with a sponge or a soft nylon brush and with copious use of sterile normal saline or an electrolytically stable 2% hypochlorite solution diluted 1 part in 40 with sterile water. Pieces of devitalized skin or very ragged edges are resected conservatively. Suturing is in layers using a careful technique whereby sub-epidermal tissues are brought together with catgut to eliminate dead space and so as to form a firm, even base for subsequent skin or mucosal closure. Skin edges on facial lacerations should be handled with non-toothed dissecting forceps and skin hooks. Thin monofilament thread on atraumatic needles should be used. For mucosal closure it is preferable to use a thicker gauge black silk thread on a curved half round eyeless needle. Skin wound edges should be slightly everted at closure and sutures removed and replaced if necessary by tapes after three days. Superficial shelving skin flaps should be gently explored and then taped back into place rather than sutured.

Lacerations that involve the eyebrows should be sutured without removal of the hair. Eyelid lacerations are best repaired by an expert. Lacerations over obvious fractures should be loosely sutured and referred for specialist treatment. All athletes with contaminated wounds should be given a short course of antibiotics and tetanus prophylaxis. Lacerations involving the vermilion border of the lip should be carefully sewn so that the first surface suture precisely brings together the two edges of the mucosa to skin junction. Ragged contaminated wounds of the lip may be excised by a small wedge resection.

## 6.4.2 INJURIES TO TEETH

Every coach, physiotherapist, dental surgeon or doctor responsible for first aid for injured sportsmen should be able to offer appropriate on-the-spot care for injuries to the mouth and teeth. The detailed management and definitive treatment plan is thereafter within the remit of the experienced dental surgeon. The frequency of injuries to the teeth has

80

suggested to many amateur and professional sports associations that a dental surgeon should be present or on call during all competitions (de Wet, 1981).

Table 6.6 summarizes the first aid treatments. For a full description of

*Table 6.6*  First aid treatment of injuries to the teeth. This table is intended as a first aid reference for club doctors, physiotherapists or trainers. In all cases of tooth injury an experienced dental surgeon's advice should be sought as soon as circumstances permit

| *Diagnosis of trauma* | *First aid treatment (Scheer, 1982)* |
|---|---|
| In all cases, check carefully for signs of concussion. If head injury is suspected the athlete must be referred for hospital advice. | |
| Fractures of crown of tooth | |
|    enamel only | Remove tooth fragments. Check for foreign bodies in lip wounds |
|    + dentine | Fit celluloid crown former filled with calcium hydroxide paste |
|    + pulp | Fit celluloid crown former filled with calcium hydroxide paste |
| Fracture with subluxation (Fig. 6.3(a) and (b)) | Use calcium hydroxide paste and a length of tin or lead foil so as to splint to adjacent teeth |
| Root fracture alone | Splint as above<br>If fracture at gum margin, remove, and retain loose piece<br>Calcium hydroxide paste |
| Complete avulsion | Clean tooth with saline<br>Attempt to replace and use tin foil splint<br>If replant attempt fails place tooth in athlete's blood, or in saline or milk and refer within one hour |
| Alveolar bone fracture | Reposition by squeezing together<br>Stop bleeding<br>Check for other tooth or jaw fractures<br>Tin-foil splint |
| Jaw and facial bone fractures | Remove mouthguard, dentures, tooth fragments<br>Maintain airway<br>Control bleeding<br>Concussion probable<br>If unconscious, transport in prone position |

the details of definitive dental techniques the reader is referred to Andreasen's (1981) excellent text *Traumatic Injuries to the Teeth*.

The minimum first aid set for dental purposes should consist of:

- Calcium hydroxide (medicinal quality); this can be purchased as a paste which sets on exposure to air.
- Tin foil as strips of about $10 \times 3.5$ cm (4 in $\times 1\frac{1}{2}$ in) or lead foil from used dental X-ray packets.
- Scissors.
- Celluloid crown formers, for front upper teeth, to act as a temporary cover.
- 3/0 silk suture on cutting 22 mm half curved needle.
- Curved Mosquito artery forceps.
- Plastic or rubber oral airway.
- Cold cure acrylic powder and liquid – useful for splinting several loose teeth.
- Local anaesthetic cartridges and dental syringe and needles.

The kit should include the name, telephone number and address of the dental surgeon who is usually responsible to that club or sports association. It is important to note that in a severe accident from a games implement or a collision, more than one type of injury to the teeth, facial and head region may occur.

The technique of replacement of an avulsed anterior, single rooted tooth, is a useful first aid measure (Fig. 6.3(a)–(c)). Officials in charge of children's sports may find that this injury is common. The tooth should first be washed with normal saline or even tap water, so as to remove any articles of dirt. By comparing the face of the tooth with adjacent teeth, it should then be possible to push the tooth correctly into place into its socket. If an appropriate local anaesthetic is available, a small amount should first be injected into the buccal sulcus above the socket and a very small amount into the adjacent palatal gum. The avulsed tooth should be pushed firmly into place so that its length and angle aligns with adjacent teeth. The gum overlying the bone of the socket is then squeezed together with finger and thumb. Tin foil moulded by finger pressure is used as a temporary splint over the replanted tooth and several adjacent teeth. If the attempt to replant the tooth fails, then the tooth should be kept moist (see Table 6.6), bleeding controlled by pressure and the patient referred for expert dental treatment within one hour.

The problem of whether a player in a team game ought to withdraw following tooth injury is an insoluble one. If the injury is slight and the game an important one the athlete will in most cases prefer to go on playing. On completion of the game, a dental opinion and treatment must be obtained as soon as possible. More severe injuries in general produce more pain. Cold air on exposed dentine or pulp tissue may be acutely painful and limit the concentration of the athlete. Teeth which have been partially dislodged from their sockets or are loose due to crown or root fractures are uncomfortable and will prevent a mouthguard being worn. They are also more liable to further injury. Unfortunately it is common for a professional sportsman playing in a competition to prefer to lose the tooth rather than abandon his efforts.

The question of whether to prescribe expensive and sophisticated dental treatment to save the upper front teeth of injured professional athletes is a vexed one. It it were certain that dental fitness was important to that individual and that mouth protection apparatus were to be worn during sports, then every effort to retain teeth should be made. Children need to have especially careful advice given to them and to their parents. More often, as the references previously referred to show, many athletes accept dental disfigurement as an occupational risk. The restoration or replacement of a tooth for the athlete is therefore a matter for decision after discussions with his dental surgeon. Influencing that decision will be whether previous episodes of trauma had occurred and whether, as in rugby players, trauma is likely to occur again.

## 6.5 First aid for fractures of the jaws and facial bones

An athlete suspected of having sustained a fracture of the jaws or facial bones may occasionally be at risk from an obstruction to his airway. An unconscious patient is even more at risk. The sportsman with a facial injury who has been knocked out should be positioned with his head to one side or preferably face downwards on the ground. Blood and saliva can then trickle out of the corner of the mouth. The tongue should be pulled forward with the finger and any loose teeth, fragments, dentures or mouthguards removed by sweeping movements.

A frontal blow to the chin from a games implement or a boot could result in a bilateral anterior mandibular fracture. The anterior insertions of the genioglossus muscles may be on this loose anterior fragment. The tongue having lost its anterior support may then fall backwards and completely obstruct the oral airway. In these circumstances the position of the athlete's head is crucial and if conscious he must hold his head downwards and forwards. A suture inserted deeply into the midline of the dorsum of the tongue and held by a pair of artery forceps will help hold the tongue forward. Emergency stabilization by wires or even by thread so as to tie the teeth on the loose mandibular fragment to adjacent firm lower teeth may then be carried out.

The injured sportsman with facial bone fractures must be transported

# Oral, dental and maxillo-facial injuries

to hospital as soon as possible. If unconscious, the prone position should be maintained and the mouth sucked out at intervals. If a neck injury is suspected the athlete should have been moved as little as possible and his neck stabilized by a pneumatic temporary collar.

Temporary immobilization of the jaw by bandages or supports, except as described above, is not generally useful. The athlete with a fracture of

*Fig. 6.3* Examples of tooth injuries through sport. (a) A young athlete fell and fractured the upper left central incisor (enamel only) but subluxed the upper right central. (b) Emergency treatment. Splinting the loose tooth to others by means of metal foil, in this case as lead foil obtained from small X-ray films. (c) Boxing injury. This upper tooth was avulsed; no mouthguard was worn. (d) The tooth being reimplanted. (e) Splinted into position. (Photographs courtesy of Mr B. Scheer.)

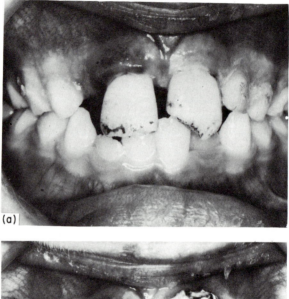

(a)

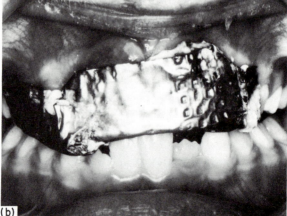

(b)

84

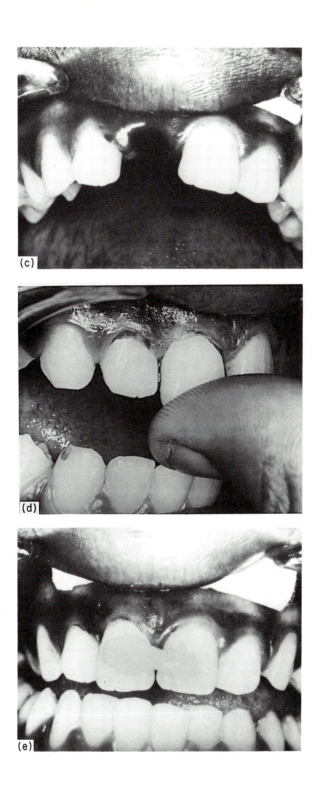

the mandible will not move the part voluntarily and may obtain relief from pain by support from his hand placed under the jaw. No drink or food should be given and if the patient has been unconscious, even for a short time, it is good practice not to give any drug or injection.

Fracture and displacement of the maxilla is rare in sports-associated injuries, except in car and motorcycle racing. If it has occurred or is suspected, the upper jaw displacement may have partially obstructed the airway. This obstruction occurs because the maxilla has been separated from the cranial base. The force of the blow pushes it downwards and posteriorly as it slides down the inclined base of the skull. The palate then rests on the tongue and occludes the oral airway. The nasal airway is often obstructed at the same time due to fractures or blood. The first aid treatment in these circumstances is to insert two fingers in the mouth until the back of the hard palate is felt. The maxilla should be pulled gently forward and the airway maintained as necessary by positioning the patient to lie face downwards and by insertion of a nasopharyngeal or oral tube.

Fractures of the zygomatic complex rarely need emergency first aid except to control bleeding by pressure on any lacerations and by forbidding the athlete to blow his nose. Removal of any caked blood from the nostrils can be performed later. Allowing the athlete to blow his nose in an attempt to remove it may produce air emphysema of the face and around the orbit. It is again emphasized that the athlete who has lost consciousness or who has been dazed should be referred to hospital for observations for possible head injury.

## 6.6   Definitive treatment of maxillo-facial fractures

When observation or treatment for head injury allows, the treatment of facial bone fractures is by accurate reduction and fixation and immobilization.

### 6.6.1   THE ZYGOMATICO-MAXILLARY COMPLEX

Clean breaks of the zygomatic arch or minor displacements of the zygomatic buttress are treated by open operation via the classic temporal approach. After reduction the fracture is usually stable provided that the athlete is not allowed to apply pressure to the part, particularly when asleep, for the next few days. Bony union in a fit athlete should be complete by three weeks after an uncomplicated injury (Fig. 6.4(a), (b) and (c)).

Blows of greater force may produce comminution about the zygomatic complex and tend to result in unstable reductions after operation. Of particular concern are injuries in which the thin bone supporting the heavier buttresses of the face has been fractured at the lateral and anterior walls of the maxillary sinus or about the orbit. Comminuted or unstable fractures are treated by direct fixation techniques at open operation. Injuries of these types take between three and six weeks to heal sufficiently well for sport to be resumed.

Fractures of the zygomatico-maxillary complex may be complicated by damage to the soft parts of the eye. In order to reduce the chance of complications due to oedema producing pressure on retinal vessels (Varley, Holt-Wilson and Watson, 1968), it is advisable to postpone open or closed reductions until the majority of the swelling due to the trauma has subsided. This delay before operation may be as long as three to five days.

Blow-out fractures of the orbit are treated by open operation and repair. Complications possibly following severe zygomatico-maxillary and orbital bony injuries (Rowe, 1981) apart from direct damage to the globe at the time of trauma, may include diplopia, enophthalmos, intraorbital haemorrhage, post-traumatic iridoplegia, optic nerve damage, oculomotor nerve palsy, superior orbital fissure syndrome and the orbital apex syndrome.

6.6.2   FRACTURES OF THE MANDIBLE

Fractures of the jaws inevitably involve the tooth bearing areas. Definitive treatment of the fractures is by reduction by accurate localization of the occlusion of the teeth, one arch of the jaw against the other. Once the natural bite (occluded) position of the teeth has been obtained the vertical height of the jaw is also probably corrected. In the majority of cases fixation and immobilization of the teeth to one another is enough to reduce the fracture and ensure healing after three to six weeks. Lacerations or tears of the mucosa or skin may indicate displaced fractures and invite open reduction and fixation.

In the UK a fracture of one condyle of the dentate mandible is treated by immobilization only if it is necessary to do so to control pain. Early movement is preferred so that chewing maintains the vertical height of the affected side. In other countries, such as the USA or France, open reductions of displaced condylar fractures are often undertaken. Satisfactory post-treatment results are obtainable by either conservative treatment or open reduction but it seems preferable to avoid operative interference where possible. Complications subsequent to fractures of the condyle are uncommon (Rowe and Killey, 1968).

# Oral, dental and maxillo-facial injuries

*Fig. 6.4* Injury during a football game. (a) This 45° occipitomental view shows the right zygomatic arch is depressed. (b) This rotated submentovertical view (SMV) displays the comminuted arch well by avoiding superimposition of the bones of the skull. (c) Occipitomental view, post-operative, shows that the zygomatic arch form has been restored.

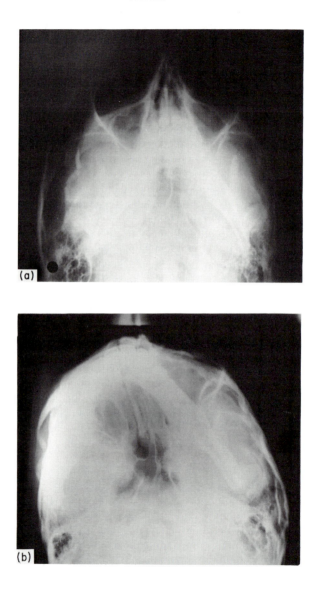

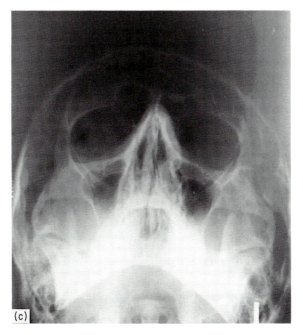

(c)

Figure 6.5 shows the commonly used method of eyelet wiring and intermaxillary fixation for immobilization of simple fractures of the mandible. The tie wires run through the eyelets from one jaw to the other. It is useful for doctors or dental surgeons to be able to use this form of treatment, especially in countries without specialized care facilities for maxillo-facial injuries. The period of immobilization for fractures of the mandible in young healthy adults should be a minimum of three weeks. At four weeks it is usual for bony union to have been obtained. Unusually, infection or displacement of fragments may occur. A liquid diet (high

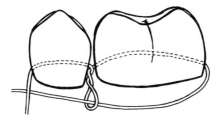

*Fig. 6.5* Eyelet wiring for immobilization of the jaws via the teeth. The wires, when pulled tight, should disappear beneath the gum margin. The eyelet remains visible and is linked to other eyelets in the upper jaw by wire loops. The teeth should be in occlusion before final tightening of the intermaxillary wire loops.

calorie) is necessary for feeding during the period of immobilization by intermaxillary fixation.

### 6.6.3 MAXILLARY FRACTURES

The principle of treatment of fractures involving the upper jaw is to control any displacement by using an intact lower jaw to close against it. The lower jaw is then fixed to the cranium by means of external pins. Alternatively, rods are fastened to splints on the teeth and then linked to a cranial halo frame. Since maxillary fractures with displacement are rarely encountered in sports injuries the reader is referred to specialist text books for further reading.

### 6.6.4 TEMPORO-MANDIBULAR JOINT INCLUDING THE MENISCUS

Trauma to the temporo-mandibular joint may produce a variety of injuries, some overt and some occult, but leading to later complications. Dislocation can be produced if the mandible is hit in a collision or fight whilst the mouth is in the open position. In those circumstances the condyle becomes locked in in the forward position anterior to the articular eminence. Rarely, dislocations may be posterior and associated with fracture of the bony part of the auditory canal or superior (after high speed road traffic accidents) when the head of the condyle is forced in the middle cerebral fossa. Reduction of anterior dislocations is best achieved at once by downward and backward pressure with the thumbs placed in the mouth to the lateral side of the lower back teeth. Longer standing dislocations should be referred to an oral surgeon. Direct blows to the chin result in the force being transmitted through the head of the condyle to the joint and the base of the skull leading to concussion. A haemarthrosis within the joint capsule may also result, producing restriction of movement and pain. The meniscus which separates the upper and lower compartments of the joint may become oedematous or even torn from its attachment to the capsule and lateral pterygoid muscle.

Intracapsular fractures of the head of the condyle in any age group may result in an ankylosis later. Post-traumatic osteo-arthritis occurred in 38.3% of a group of 165 patients presenting with temporo-mandibular joint disorders (Norman, 1982). The same author found that trauma was the aetiological agent in about two-thirds of cases of recurrent mandibular dislocation and in about two-thirds the causes of ankylosis of the joint. Trauma may also precipitate temporo-mandibular pain and dysfunction in susceptible patients.

The definitive treatment of temporo-mandibular joint injuries is a specialized task not within the remit of this chapter. It must be noted, however, that all injuries to the joints of children must be followed up long-term lest complications with disfigurement occur later. In adults it is imperative that the occlusion of restored and intact dental arches is checked by an expert. Rehabilitation of sportsmen with closed injuries to the joints, including unilateral fractures, should rarely exceed three weeks. Treatment is based on early movement but in a few cases continuing pain may force the athlete to discontinue competitive sport for up to six weeks. Boxers should not attempt to resume sparring for at least this time.

## 6.7 Prevention of injuries to the teeth

Regular dental advice and treatment should become a matter of habit for all full-time and occasional sportsmen. Yet in athletes, dental and oral neglect is common. For a while such neglect may be unnoticed. Unfortunately the stress of a major competition may be the time at which dental pain jeopardizes the ability of an athlete to take part (Forrest, 1969). For example, stress is a well known precursor of acute ulcerative gingivitis and also of inflammation around erupting wisdom teeth. Some forms of dental disease are more common in sportsmen. Due to mouth breathing at rigorous training schedules, athletes have been found to suffer from resorption of alveolar supporting bone following gum disease (Bodenham, 1970; Lamendin and Davidovici, 1981). Decay of the anterior teeth has been reported in athletes due to their habit of frequent consumption of glucose and fruit drinks (Finidori and Lamendin, 1981).

Loss of teeth and their effects upon function and appearance is compounded by the need to accept dentures or bridges for life. In the long term, teeth adjacent or opposite to those damaged, as well as the originally damaged teeth, may lose their vitality and become infected. Boxers may present, many years after ceasing their sporting activity, with a discharge from a sinus on the chin subsequent to death of a lower incisor tooth. Pulp canal obliteration, necrosis of the pulp and either external root resorption or, more rarely, internal root resorption may occur in teeth which have been traumatized. Disturbances in the eruption and development of permanent teeth after trauma to deciduous teeth in young children may be as high as 58% (Andreasen and Rava, 1973).

Appliances worn in the mouth, such as orthodontic bands or plates may contribute to patterns of injury. Mouthguards can be constructed so as to fit over such appliances.

Children or adults with prominent upper anterior teeth are especially likely to sustain injury to them through trauma (McEwen, McHugh and

Oral, dental and maxillo-facial injuries

Hitchin, 1967). Where there is a dento-alveolar or skeletal base disproportion, the position of one jaw may be markedly anterior to the other. Injuries are even more common in these groups of patients. USA football players with grossly maligned bites due to crowding of the teeth or due to disproportion of the jaws (Fig. 6.6), tend to give up the sport as adequate comfort and protection from mouthguards prove impossible (Smith, 1982).

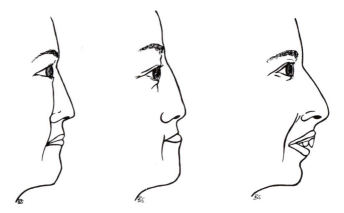

*Fig. 6.6* Profiles of facial types. Left to right: normal contour, slight mandibular prognathism and the type most at risk from injury to the teeth – maxillary prominence with a receding lower jaw.

The presence and position of unerupted teeth in the mandible have been shown to be associated with sites of mandibular fractures. The angle of the mandible is the weakest site for single fractures (Halazonetis, 1968) and this liability to fracture may be associated with the presence of impacted lower third molar teeth. Schwimmer, Stern and Kritchman (1983) quoted that 17% of patients over twenty years of age have at least one impacted third molar and advocated removal of such teeth in athletes engaged in collision sports. Eleven athletes out of thirty-four had impacted lower third molars (Randell, 1983) and these were players of American football.

Cysts of the jaws are symptomless until they reach a large size or become infected. The weakening of tooth support and of basal bone makes injury more likely after mild trauma. Dental screening including radiographs could eliminate this problem. Regular dental advice and treatment should be part of the overall care offered to all athletes. The more so if it is accepted that dedication to a sport often hides a lack of interest even in basic oral hygiene (Lamendin and Davidovici, 1981).

## 6.8 Facial and oral protection for sportsmen and women

In the author's view even one maimed person or one death through sports is one too many. Some sports are inescapably dangerous. Boxers, horse riders and rugby players seem particularly at risk from at least injury and occasionally from death.

Protective apparatus for use in high speed sports, collision sports and contact sports is available and in some cases (e.g. American football) has proved its worth. It is most unfortunate that adequate protection for all players at risk is not mandatory. Professional sportsmen are opinion formers as regards the acceptability of wearing protective apparatus during sports. In the UK it is now commonplace for cricketers to bat against fast bowlers only when a protective helmet with facial shield is being worn. A few years ago such apparatus would have been regarded as less than manly and possibly as not quite fair. The amateur team coaches, selectors and club officials should adopt the professional view, that the wearing of some protective apparatus does indeed save sportsmen from injury or worse. Failure to offer appropriate advice points to a lack of concern for their athletes.

The design of helmets with face bars for USA footballers has received much attention. Loft (1981) pointed out that movement of the helmet about the head should be prevented by careful fit, maximum coverage and by a balanced point of attachment for the retention strap at the chin. Schneider (1982) suggested that the helmet must have a resilient shell capable of withstanding many impacts and two separate inflatable crowns in order to minimize the risk of a closed head injury. It is important to note that helmets must be individually fitted for each athlete.

Helmets as worn by USA footballers, cricketers, motor cyclists, ice hockey players and hockey goal keepers undoubtedly reduce maxillofacial injuries. Nevertheless the helmet must be well fitting (Kendrick, 1981) and of proper design (Wood, 1972) so that concussive effects of blows are minimized and it should be worn with a mouthguard when appropriate to the sport. Unfortunately the standards applied to the thickness and to the design features of helmets vary between countries. Sports with international regulations, such as motor cycling or formula car racing, have higher standards for helmet regulations than is common for non-sporting use. Designs to offer maximum facial protection vary between branches of sports and yet not every part of the helmet possibly subject to loading forces is necessarily tested and subject to rigorous quality control (Cannell, King and Winch, 1982). Failure to insist upon adequate head, facial and dental protection for fast moving collision sports or in sports where falls are commonplace (Lie and Lucht, 1977) contributes to the extent and complexity of injuries.

Where inadequate refereeing of the game allows the rules to be broken, so the frequency of injuries increases. The high frequency of facial injuries (Wilson *et al.*, 1977) and particularly of eye injuries (Pashby *et al.*, 1975) in North American ice-hockey players resulted in the drafting of regulations for the sport. All players in official games are now wearing facial protection. The material and the design of the apparatus is distinctive for goal-minders, whilst outfield players have more varied forms of facial protection.

Although helmets and face guards undoubtedly reduce injuries to players they also have been used as offensive weapons. The helmeted head has been used as a battering ram in American style football. Leverage on face guards has been used to hyperextend the neck of an opponent. Only adequate discipline within the sport can hope to eliminate these non-accidental type of sports injuries.

### 6.8.1 MOUTHGUARDS

Mouthguards could be used by the majority of sportsmen. Professional boxers are required to wear so-called gum shields (in fact mouthguards) over the upper teeth and amateurs in the UK are the subject of present legislation (Blonstein, Cutler and Mason, 1977). Hockey, ice-hockey and USA style footballers are accustomed to their use. Rugby footballers of all ages (de Wet, 1981; de Wet *et al.*, 1980a, b) have been encouraged to wear mouthguards but compliance remains a definite problem (Upson, 1982).

Protection of the upper teeth is obtained by their coverage with a resilient material that can absorb the energy of an impact. The lower teeth are also protected against damage through forced closure against the upper jaw by the cushioning effect of biting against the material. Dissipation of the energy of a blow from below to the chin is also achieved and the well constructed mouthguard absorbs much of the force which would otherwise be transmitted through the heads of the condyles to the base of the skull.

The design of mouthguards may differ slightly according to intended use. Squash players may prefer a semi-rigid material covering the anterior upper teeth with padding or resilient material labially (Blonstein *et al.*, 1977). Boxers require fuller coverage of the upper teeth, thinned, shaped buccal flanges and slight imprints in the lower occlusal surface into which the lower teeth can fit. All other sportsmen seem to prefer mouthguards of the minimum size and shape necessary to protect their maxillary teeth (Turner, 1977).

The material from which mouthguards should be constructed is of great importance (Fig. 6.7). Durability, protectivity and water absorption have been tested for 57 different products by Going, Loehman and Chan (1974). Silicone has a high bounce recovery factor (Blonstein *et al.*, 1977) and is especially suitable for players of contact sports. Thermoplastic sheets of polyvinyl acetate–polyethylene copolymer are widely used and can be made in various overall thicknesses.

Whatever material is used it is of the utmost importance that the dedicated sportsman has his mouthguard made for him by a dental

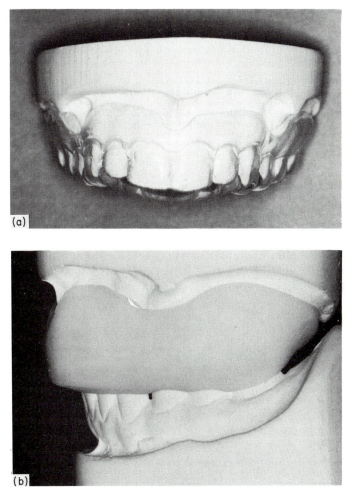

(a)

(b)

*Fig. 6.7* Pressure formed (a) and heat treated (b) individually fitted mouth-guards. Pressure formed mouthguards are cheaper to produce but costly in laboratory equipment. Heat treated mouthguards are even more costly due to the large amount of labour involved in making them.

surgeon. The guard should vary in design and thickness according to the degree of protection needed. It should cover his upper teeth at least as far posteriorly as the second premolar but leave as much of the palate uncovered as is compatible with adequate strength. It should be of sufficient size to minimize the risk of accidental inhalation. Latex rubber mouthguards, whilst expensive to produce, seem to repay financial outlay by satisfactory use under all conditions. Mouthguards bought as stock sizes, or adapted to the shape of the teeth by self-curing materials, give some protection against impacts. They are, however, likely to be uncomfortable to wear and less efficient than individually designed and fitted mouthguards. Crudely fitting mouthguards may be placed in the same category as grandad's old set of dentures for chewing or as high heels on football boots.

Since the cost of even one porcelain crown to restore a fractured incisor is about 95% more expensive than one mouthguard (Kendrick, 1981), the sports doctor should advise all team sportsmen, contact sportsmen and horse riders to obtain and wear individually constructed mouthguards.

When these requirements of a mouthguard for a particular sport are met, compliance in wearing them is high (de Wet et al., 1980a, b). Mouthguards should be lightly scrubbed with soap and water after use, kept in a box or preferably on a model of the athlete's teeth and kept slightly damp. They should be renewed every season. Growing children participating in collision sports should have the fit of their mouthguards checked every six months, or as made necessary by erupting teeth. If, despite use of a mouthguard, fracture or dislocation of a tooth occurs, then the appliance can be used as a temporary splint.

## 6.8.2  KINESIOLOGY

Mandibular orthopaedic repositioning devices (M.O.R.A.) made of acrylic or urethane have been put forward as increasing the strength and stamina of athletes as well as providing mouthguard type protection. These devices are similar in construction to mouthguards but include a well fitting surface into which the cusps of all the lower teeth can fit. The theory behind their use is that the device helps correct any previously existing proprioceptive dysfunction of the ligaments of the muscles of the jaws (Jakesh, 1982). Many normal athletes, as many normal non-athletes, without symptoms of temporo-mandibular joint dysfunction must have premature contacts of their teeth when occluding.

Careful adjustment of the bite may improve the standard of comfort when clenching the teeth hard together. Athletes, for example weight lifters, seem to need to grimace and to clench their teeth with effort. A M.O.R.A. may help them to do so with a degree of greater comfort and with less stress on an individual slightly malaligned tooth. Whether athletic performance is improved is debatable, but further research is needed. Perhaps the placebo effect of a cushioned bite (Jakesh, 1982) is helpful as indeed it would be to a sufferer from jaw joint dysfunction (Kerr, 1983).

## References

Andreasen, J. O. (1981) Classification, etiology and epidemiology. *Traumatic Injuries to the Teeth*, 2nd edn, Munksgaard, Copenhagen, pp. 19–45.

Andreasen, J. O. and Rava, J. J. (1983) Enamel changes in permanent teeth after trauma to their primary predecessors. *Scand. J. Dent. Res.*, **81**, 203.

Barrel, V. U., Cooper, P. J., Elkington, A. R., *et al.* (1981) Squash ball to eye ball: the likelihood of squash players incurring an eye injury. *Brit. Med. J.*, **283**, 893.

Bartowski, S. B. and Krzyskowa, K. M. (1982) Blow-out fracture of the orbit. Diagnostic and therapeutic considerations and results in 90 patients treated. *J. Maxillo-facial Surg.*, **10**, 155.

Blonstein , J. L., Cutler, R. and Mason, M. (1977) Mouth and jaw protection in contact sports. *Brit. J. Sports Med.*, **11**, 75.

Bodenham, R. S. (1970) A biteguard for athletic training. Case report. *Brit. Dent. J.*, **129**, 85.

Bollmann, F. and Wanneumacher, M. (1974) Individual functional mouth guard for contact sports. *Quintessence Int.*, **5(1)**, 34.

Cannell, H., King, J. B. and Winch, R. B. (1982) Head and facial injuries after low speed motor-cycle accidents. *Brit. J. Oral Surg.*, **20**, 183.

Cathcart, J. F. (1968) Practical preventive dentistry: the use of mouth protectors for contact sports. *Dental Digest*, **58**, 348.

Converse, J. M., Smith, B., Obear, M. F. and Wood-Smith, D. (1962) Orbital blowout fractures: a ten year study. *Plast. Reconstr. Surg.*, **39**, 20.

Davies, R. M., Bradley, D., Hale, R. W., *et al.* (1977) The prevalence of dental injuries in rugby players and their attitude to mouthguards. *Brit. J. Sports Med.*, **11**, 72.

Dennis, C. G. and Parker, D. A. S. (1972) Mouthguards in Australian sport. *Austral. Dent. J.*, **17**, 228.

de Wet, F. A. (1981) The prevention of orofacial sports injuries in the adolescent. *Int. Dent. J.*, **31**, 313.

de Wet, F. A., Potgeiter, P. J. and Rossouw, L. M. (1980a) Mouthguards for sports participation. *J. Dent. Assoc. S. Afr.*, **35**, 417.

de Wet, F. A., Badenhorst, M. and Rossouw, L. M. (1980b) Mouthguards for rugby players at primary school level. *J. Dent Assoc. S. Afr.*, **36**, 249.

Eade, G. G. (1969) Emergency care of facial injuries. *Northwest Med.*, **68**, 729.

Finidori, C. and Lamendin, H. (1981) Les boissons des sportifs: dietetique et hygiene bucco-dentaire. *Inform. Dent.*, **1.26.**, 2493.

Fitzner, R. (1979) North Dakota High School Activities Association, in *Traumatic Injuries to the Teeth* (ed. J. O. Andreasen), 2nd edn, Munksgaard, Copenhagen, p. 442.

Forrest, J. O. (1969) The dental condition of Olympic games contestants – a pilot study, 1968. *Dent. Practit.*, **20**, 98.

# Oral, dental and maxillo-facial injuries

Fortunato, M. A., Fieding, A. F. and Guernsey, L. H. (1982) Facial bone fractures in children. *Oral Surg., Oral Med., Oral Pathol.*, **53(3)**, 225.

Going, R. E., Loehman, R. E. and Chan, M. S. (1974) Mouthguard materials: their physical and mechanical properties. *J. Amer. Dent. Assoc.*, **89**, 132.

Guise, R. B. (1982) Personal communication. Wellington region, New Zealand. Accident Compensation Corporation.

Haidar, Z. (1978) Aetiology of zygomatic complex fractures. *Brit. J. Oral Surg.*, **15**, 265.

Halazonetis, J. A. (1968) The weak regions of the mandible. *Brit. J. Oral Surg.*, **6**, 37.

Heintz, W. D. (1968) Mouth protectors – a progress report. Bureau of Dental Health Education. *J. Amer. Dent. Assoc.*, **77**, 632.

Hitchin, A. D. and Shuker, S. T. (1973) Some observations on zygomatic fractures in the Eastern Region of Scotland. *Brit. J. Oral Surg.*, **11**, 114.

Jakesh, J. (1982) Can dental therapy enhance athletes' performance? *J. Amer. Dent. Assoc.*, **104**, 292.

Jarvinen, S. (1980) On the causes of traumatic dental injuries with special reference to sports accidents in a sample of Finnish children. *Acta Odontol. Scand.*, **38**, 151.

Jones, J. J. (1979) Wisconsin interscholastic athletic association, in *Traumatic Injuries to the Teeth* (ed. J. O. Andreasen), 2nd ed, Munksgaard, Copenhagen, p. 442.

Kendrick, R. W. (1981) Some 'sporting' injuries. *Int. J. Oral Surg.*, **10**, Supplement 1, 245.

Kerr, L. (1983) Dental problems in athletes, in *Clinics in Sports Medicine*, **2. 1.**, W. B. Saunders, Philadephia, pp. 115–121.

Killey, H. C. (1971) Surgical anatomy. *Fractures of the Middle Third of the Facial Skeleton*, 2nd edn, J. Wright and Sons Ltd, Bristol, pp. 11–15.

Krzychalska-Karwan, Z. (1975) Trauma to the anterior teeth of sportsmen in the light of statistics. *Czasopisma stomatol.*, **28(5)**, 479.

Lamendin, H. and Davidovici, M. (1981) Practique sportif de haut niveau et alveolysen precoces. *Rev. d'Onto-Stomatol. (Paris)*, **10**, 305.

Lees, G. H. and Gaskell, P. H. F. (1976) Injuries to the mouth and teeth in an undergraduate population. *Brit. Dent. J.*, **140**, 107.

Lie, L. H. and Lucht, U. (1977) Ridesportsulykker. I. Undersogelse af en rylterpopulation med saerligt henblik pa ulykkesfrekvensen. *Ugeskrift Fur Laeger (Copenhagen)*, **139**, 1687.

Loft, B. I. (1981) Injuries and their prevalence in American football, in *Sports Fitness and Sports Injuries* (ed. T. Reilly), Faber and Faber, London, p. 94.

Mason, R. (1977) *A Guide to Dental Radiography*, J. Wright and Sons Ltd, Bristol, pp. 108–15.

McEwen, J. D., McHugh, W. D. and Hitchin, A. D. (1967) Fractured maxillary central incisors and incisal relationship. *J. Dent. Res.*, **46**, 1290.

Moos, K. F. (1982) Personal communication. Oral and maxillo-facial surgery service, Canniesburn Hospital, Glasgow, Scotland.

Morton, J. G. and Burton, J. F. (1979). An evaluation of the effectiveness of mouthguards in high-school rugby players. *New Zeal. Dent. J.*, **75**, 151.

Motyčka, A. and Vašina, A. (1982) Injuries of the head and face in ice hockey players. *Ceskoslovenska stomatol.*, **1**, 46.

# References

Nicholas, N. K. (1976) Mouthguards in sport. *New Zeal. Med. J.*, **84**, 31.

Norman, J. E. (1982) Post traumatic disorders of the jaw joints. *Ann. Roy. Coll. Surg. Engl.*, **64**, 27.

Pashby, T. J., Pashby, R. C., Chisholm, L. J. and Crawford, J. S. (1975) Eye injuries in Canadian hockey. *Can. Med. Assoc. J.*, **113**, 663.

Randell, S. (1983) Dental trauma and disease in 34 professional athletes. *Phys. Sports Med.*, **11(6)**, 85.

Roberts, J. E. (1970) *Wisconsin Interscholastic Athletic Association*, 1970 Supplement to the 47th Official Handbook, 1.

Rowe, N. L. (1981) The surgical anatomy of the orbit, in *Anatomy of the Orbit, Salivary Glands and Neck. Proceedings of the Consultant Study Day, 1980* (ed. H. Cannell), British Association of Oral Surgeons, pp. 13–36.

Rowe, N. L. and Killey, H. C. (1968) *Fractures of the Facial Skeleton*, 2nd edn. E. and S. Livingstone, London and Edinburgh, Appendix.

Scheer, B. (1982) Traumatic injuries to the teeth, in *General Dental Practice* (ed. J. Manning), Instalment 13, Kluwer, London, pp. 901–9.

Schneider, R. C. (1982) The incidence of head injuries – the potential for protection, in *Head Protection, the State of the Art* (eds J. S. Pedder and N. Mills), Proceedings of a Symposium, 1982, University of Birmingham, pp. 5–14.

Schultz, R. C. (1970) *Facial Injuries*, Yearbook Medical Publishers, Chicago.

Schwimmer, A., Stern, R. and Kritchman, D. (1983) Impacted third molar: a contributing factor in mandibular fracture in contact sports. *Amer. J. Sports Med.*, **11(4)**, 262–68.

Smith, S. D. (1982) Adjusting mouthguards kinesiologically in professional football players. *New York State Dent. J.*, **48**, 298.

Swearingen, J. J. (1965) *Tolerance of the Human Face to Crash Impact*, Federal Aviation Agency, Oklahoma City.

Turner, C. H. (1977) Mouth protectors. *Brit. Dent. J.*, **143**, 82.

Upson, N. (1982) Dental injuries and the attitudes of rugby players to mouthguards. *Brit. J. Sports Med.*, **16(4)**, 241.

Varley, E. W. B., Holt-Wilson, A. D. and Watson, P. G. (1968) Acute retinal arterial occlusion following reduction of a fractured zygoma and its successful treatment. *Brit. J. Oral Surg.*, **6**, 31.

Wilson, K., Cram, B., Rontal, E. and Rontal, M. (1977) Facial injuries in hockey players. *Minnesota Med.*, **1**, 13.

Wood, A. W. S. (1972) Head protection – cranial facial and dental in contact sports. *Oral Health (USA)*, **62**, 23.

Worrall, S. F. (1980) Personal communication. Department of Oral and Maxillo-Facial Surgery, The London Hospital, London.

# 7  Otorhinolaryngology

## G. B. BROOKES and PETER McKELVIE

The growing popularity of sporting leisure activities in recent years has resulted in a significant increase in the incidence of sports related injuries. The true incidence of injuries involving the ear, nose and throat is impossible to define because many are relatively minor, and are not seen in hospital practice nor result in loss of time from work.

The range of possible injuries is as varied as the spectrum of the sporting activities themselves. All types of otorhinolaryngological trauma may be encountered, from the common haematomas and minor lacerations, to the effects of blunt head injury on the inner ear with possible vestibular disability and deafness, and major laryngeal trauma with possible compromise of the airway. Fortunately, as in most other sites, such severe injuries are rare. Body contact games, such as rugby football, soccer, hockey and boxing account for the majority of injuries. Some disorders may occur, albeit occasionally, as a recognized risk in certain other sports such as diving and flying, when differential rapid ambient pressure changes may lead to sinus and otitic barotrauma. It need hardly be stated that the management of sports conditions affecting the ear, nose and throat is as diverse as their anatomical and functional differences. Each of these sites is therefore considered separately.

## 7.1  Otology

Trauma may affect the external, middle and inner parts of the ear either individually or in combination. The middle and inner ear are also susceptible to damage resulting from sudden local pressure changes.

### 7.1.1  TRAUMA

*(a)  External ear*

*(i) Haematoma*  A blow to the auricle may cause haematoma formation due to rupture of vessels in the perichondrium, especially on the outer aspect.

# Otorhinolaryngology

The diagnosis is obvious from the history and the presence of a tender swollen pinna (Fig. 7.1). It is wise to exclude the possibility of concurrent damage to the other parts of the ear by clinically testing the ability to hear the whispered voice with occlusion of the contralateral ear.

It treatment is delayed, fibrous organization of the haematoma occurs with permanent thickening of the auricle, and an unsightly swelling. Figure 7.2 shows the prominent 'cauliflower' ear of an ex-professional wrestler, for which there is no effective treatment. In the early stages the accumulated blood can usually be aspirated as a sterile procedure through a wide bore needle if it has not organized. Alternatively, incision and drainage is necessary. The application of a firm pressure dressing is essential. Cotton wool is carefully placed into the contours of the auricle, and a larger pad packed over the posterior aspect, so that firm and even pressure is applied when a crepe bandage is wrapped over the ear and around the head. This should be left in place undisturbed for one week to prevent the reaccumulation of haematoma which is otherwise likely to occur.

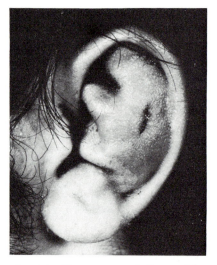 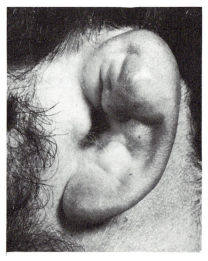

*Fig. 7.1* Haematoma of the auricle which has been inadequately treated.

*Fig. 7.2* 'Cauliflower ear' due to repetitive trauma in professional wrestling.

Figure 7.1 shows the ear of a rugby player injured eight days previously. The acute haematoma had been incised and evacuated by the casualty officer, but an adequate pressure dressing had not been applied. At this stage the swelling was fairly well organized with an associated perichondritis, and inevitable cosmetic deformity.

102

*(ii) Lacerations* All degrees of laceration are encountered, including complete avulsion of the auricle, and are probably most common on the rugby field, where boot studs and teeth are frequently the offending 'weapons'. Shearing injuries of the auricle may cause laceration of the external auditory canal at the bony-cartilaginous junction.

Standard principles of wound cleansing and debridement are employed. In the primary repair, sutures should not pass through the cartilage as they invoke painful irritative perichondritis. Partial or even total avulsion of the auricle is best managed by immediate primary suture if the torn piece can be recovered. The excellent local vascularity will often allow successful healing to occur, and produce a cosmetic result which would be difficult to emulate with delayed plastic surgical reconstruction. Broad spectrum antibiotic cover is required in all these cases. Delayed canal stenosis often follows lacerations of the external auditory meatus. These may require repair with the introduction of a local rotation flap.

Outer ear injuries can be effectively reduced in certain sports by the wearing of protective headgear such as rugby scrum and cycling caps or protective helmets in cricket, motor sports and American football.

## (b) Middle ear

Traumatic rupture of the tympanic membrane may result from sudden air or fluid compression in the external auditory canal. It can be caused by a slap or boxing punch, or the sudden impact of a ball over the meatus, which may be filled with water as in water polo.

The degree of pain is variable but may be severe at the moment of rupture, when a blood-stained discharge may be evident in the meatus. The degree of conductive deafness depends on the size of the perforation, and is often only mild. Temporary tinnitus may be reported. The ear drum does not need to be examined immediately, and in any case the deep meatus is often obscured by blood clot. A perforation can usually be assumed from the history.

The patient is instructed to keep the ear dry. If there is no reason to suspect contamination, antibiotics are not necessary. Most traumatic perforations heal spontaneously, but this process often takes longer than four weeks. Residual perforations after three months, or any conductive deafness due to damage of the ossicular chain, may require elective surgical intervention.

## (c) Inner ear

*(i) Acoustic trauma* Noise is a well recognized cause of sensorineural deafness in the industrial setting, and in a number of sports the participants may also be exposed to high sound pressure levels which will produce inner ear damage. The basal turn of the cochlea which subserves

the higher frequencies, and particularly around the 4 kilohertz level, bears the main brunt of the physical impact of loud noise. Permanent deafness and tinnitus may result, or with less severe and shorter noise exposure this may be temporary, with some degree of recovery being possible.

Firearms are a major threat to hearing. Twelve-bore shotguns, for example, cause a significant deafness in about 10% of individuals (Coles and Rice, 1966). Very high sound levels are also produced by model aeroplanes, motorcycles, racing cars and snowmobiles. The snowmobile, and the rapidly developing interest in racing it in North America and Canada, constitutes a particular hazard. It is run by a usually inadequately silenced motorcycle engine, and Bess and Poynor (1974) found that the majority of regular drivers had marked evidence of high tone deafness.

This type of traumatic deafness is unlikely to be recognized by the patient until the hearing loss is considerable. This is because the sound frequencies required for the discrimination of speech are not affected in the early stages. Tinnitus may be the presenting complaint, which is intermittent at first, but later becomes constant with continued noise exposure. The high tone hearing loss may be asymmetrical, as for example in shooting, because the leading ear is exposed to higher sound levels. Examination usually reveals normal tympanic membranes and normal tuning fork tests of hearing. Pure tone audiometry is necessary to establish the high tone hearing loss.

Avoidance of excessive exposure to loud noise and the use of effective ear protectors are the important preventative aspects of management. Thus Fletcher and Gross (1977), using high frequency audiometric testing, found that motor cycling produced more inner ear damage than shooting, largely because of the fairly routine use of ear defenders among American sports shooters. There is no specific treatment for this type of deafness though the fitting of a hearing aid may reduce the disability in the more severe cases.

*(ii) Temporal bone fracture* Transverse fractures of the petrous temporal bone due to blunt head trauma may involve the inner ear or the internal auditory canal. If the fracture involves the otic capsule the sudden release of inner ear fluids will lead to sudden deafness and acute vertigo. Haemorrhage occurs into the cochlea, vestibule or internal canal, and disruption of the membranous cochlea is frequent.

The tympanic membrane is usually intact but there may be a haemotympanum. Clinical tests will show a severe sensorineural deafness which can be confirmed audiometrically, and marked spontaneous nystagmus is often present. Skull radiology does not always demonstrate the fracture site. If the VIIth nerve is damaged, a lower motor neurone facial palsy will result.

The deafness is usually permanent and severe. The patient is treated with vestibular sedatives and bed rest. Sufficient vestibular compensation occurs in about ten to fourteen days. Total facial palsy at the time of the injury often indicates that the nerve has been severed, and immediate surgical exploration is necessary. A facial paresis or delayed onset palsy usually recovers spontaneously. Systemic steroids may help this recovery.

*(iii) Blunt head trauma* Whilst much attention has been given in recent years to the progressive degenerative central neurological effects of boxing, it is not so widely appreciated that repetitive closed head trauma often causes cochleovestibular symptoms. Labyrinthine concussion results from a blow to the fixed head. Pressure waves passing through the skull base cause a symmetrical high tone deafness similar to that caused by loud noise. Rapid acceleration or deceleration of the mobile head after a blow, in contrast, causes shearing effects of the brain inside the skull, and may tear the auditory nerve. Post-traumatic positional vertigo due to degenerative changes in the ampulla of the semicircular canals sometimes occurs.

Any deafness is commonly only mild to moderate and may be reversible to some degree. Positional vertigo, when present, is characteristically momentary, lasting seconds only, and is precipitated by certain head positions, such as looking up to a high shelf or turning over in bed at night. Typically a fatiguable spontaneous nystagmus is induced during Hallpike positional testing. Other vestibular tests including caloric and electronystagmography are usually normal.

The cochleovestibular symptoms are reversible in the early stages, although tinnitus frequently persists. Repetitive trauma is, however, likely to produce more permanent sequelae. Some degree of recovery occurs in the majority of cases of positional vertigo, whilst the individual also adjusts by learning to avoid head positions which precipitate symptoms. Drugs are rarely of value. The only sensible advice is to retire from the sport at the onset of symptoms.

### 7.1.2 INJURIES DUE TO SUDDEN PRESSURE CHANGES

During the last two decades increasing attention has been directed towards the potentially damaging effects of sudden environmental pressure changes on middle and inner ear function. These effects may occur during ascent or descent in both pressurized or non-pressurized aircraft, and possibly during hot-air ballooning, a rapidly growing sport in North

# Otorhinolaryngology

America. However, they are more and more frequently found among divers, mainly because underwater pressure changes are more rapid due to the density of water. Thus at 10 metres below the water surface, the pressure is twice atmospheric pressure; in contrast, an aviator must ascend some 5480 m (18 000 feet) to experience a comparable pressure change. Boyle's law states that the volume of an enclosed fixed mass of gas is inversely proportional to its pressure. If the openings of the external ear canal and the middle ear space are not readily patent, the rapid equalization of their pressure relative to the external ambient pressure is not possible and may result in otitic barotrauma. This can affect either the middle or inner ear.

*(i) Otitic barotrauma of the middle ear* Middle ear otitic barotrauma is an inflammatory reaction produced in the lining of the middle ear cleft by an excessive negative pressure. This differential pressure gradient occurs as a result of 'locking' of the Eustachian tube which cannot open to allow equalization of the pressure across the tympanic membrane. The mechanism is illustrated in Fig. 7.3. 'Locking' may occur during rapid descent in an aircraft, especially if the flight cabin is not pressurized, or during the descent phase of diving to as shallow a depth as 4.8 m (16 feet). It is more likely to occur in subjects with underlying impaired Eustachian tube function due to obstructive nasal conditions, such as rhinitis, nasal polyps or a deviated nasal septum or with a current upper respiratory tract infection. McNicoll (1982) has found from the analysis of more than

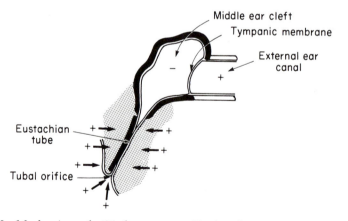

*Fig. 7.3* Mechanism of otitic barotrauma. During descent, increasing ambient pressure forces the tympanic membrane inwards, and unless there is pressure equalization through the Eustachian tube barotrauma will occur (after Head, 1979, reproduced by kind permission of Butterworths Publishing Company).

106

2000 recruits for diving duties that relatively mild degrees of deformity at the mid bony nasal septum can cause Eustachian tube problems in response to increases in the ambient pressure, which are not apparent under normal atmospheric pressure conditions.

The tympanic membrane retracts inwards with the negative middle ear pressure. Oedema of the lining mucous membrane and an effusion follow, with pressure, pain and deafness. Transient vertigo is a rare feature. On examination the eardrum is dull and congested, and bubbles may be visible in the middle ear fluid. Occasionally perforation of the tympanic membrane occurs.

The condition can be prevented by not flying or diving with an upper respiratory tract infection. Frequent autoinflation of the middle ear by Valsalva's manoeuvre as soon as mild pressure discomfort is experienced should avoid Eustachian tube 'locking'. Oral antihistamine or nasal decongestants may also help to improve Eustachian tube function and are essential in the face of nasal airway impairment. Nasal surgery to resolve any obstructive pathology is strongly recommended for individuals regularly pursuing these types of sport. McNicoll (1981) found that submucous resection of an underlying septal deformity in diving recruits with evidence of functional tubal dysfunction resulted in 95% of cases achieving normal tubal function six weeks following surgery. A history of chronic Eustachian tube dysfunction or established chronic seromucinous otitis media, however, should be a definite contraindication.

An established effusion is treated with analgesics and decongestants. Antibiotics have no useful role. If the effusion persists for more than ten days a myringotomy can be performed under local anaesthetic to evacuate the fluid and restore the middle ear pressure to normal. If the condition has become chronic, a grommet, or ventilation tube, may need to be inserted through the tympanic membrane to allow complete resolution.

Changes in the ambient pressure can also cause transient vestibular disturbances by the direct effect of abnormally high or low middle ear pressures on the intracochlear fluid pressure. This condition is termed 'alternobaric' or 'pressure' vertigo, and is quite common, occurring during either ascent or descent in air or water. An incidence of 10–17% has been reported in Royal Air Force pilots (Melville-Jones, 1957; Lundgren and Malm, 1966). Lundgren (1965) found that this phenomenon was even more common (23%) among divers. The condition is not serious, and most subjects are able to learn physiological tricks to reduce the degree and frequency of symptoms.

*(ii) Otitic barotrauma of the inner ear* Sudden middle ear barotrauma or attempts at equilibrating the differential pressure gradient by a forceful

Valsalva manoeuvre may, however, produce actual inner ear damage involving either the cochlea or the vestibular labyrinth. Such inner ear injuries are more often sustained during diving than flying. The sudden pressure changes may induce turbulence in the perilymph and disrupt the intracochlear membranes in the basal turn causing permanent high frequency sensorineural deafness, and tinnitus, and vertigo. The raised intracranial pressure by performing a Valsalva manoeuvre, or by physical exertion during hyperbaric diving, may be transmitted to the perilymph via a wide cochlear aqueduct or the internal auditory canal. Rupture of the membranes in the oval and round windows may follow with leaking of perilymph leading to sudden or progressive sensorineural deafness, with tinnitus or vertigo, depending on the size of the fistula. Five cases of inner ear barotrauma in experienced divers were described by Freeman and Edmonds in 1972, while Farmer has given a full account of the problems of diving barotrauma in his 1977 monograph.

Perilymph fistula may cause sudden and severe deafness, or a fluctuating hearing loss with tinnitus and vertigo which can closely mimic the symptoms of Ménière's disease. Positional vertigo and imbalance can also occur. Inner ear barotrauma is always accompanied by pain from the concomitant middle ear barotrauma. The hearing loss affects the lower frequencies early on, whilst labyrinthine dysfunction may be reflected by abnormalities on caloric and electronystagmographic testing.

Any diver who develops persisting giddiness or sensorineural deafness during or after a dive, in which 'decompression sickness' (see later) is unlikely, has most likely suffered labyrinthine window rupture and must be treated appropriately. Some perilymph fistulas undoubtedly close spontaneously with bed rest, head elevation and avoidance of factors which would raise the CSF pressure, such as blowing the nose or straining at defaecation. If there is no improvement in the hearing loss or vestibular features within forty-eight hours, surgical exploration of the middle ear is indicated for closure of a possible fistula with a fat or fascial plug (Goodhill, 1972). This course of management allows the best opportunity for restoring the hearing. In some cases there may be concurrent intracochlear membrane trauma, or this may be the sole cause of the symptoms. Some degree of permanent deafness therefore often remains. Of course, preventive aspects of middle ear barotrauma are also important for inner ear protection.

*(iii) Decompression sickness of the inner ear* In water the environmental pressure acts on gases in the blood vessel system and Boyle's law also applies. As a diver increases his depth the respired gases are absorbed into the circulation and distributed through the body tissues. Decompression sickness (Caisson disease), or 'the bends', follows a too rapid

decompression during ascent, and usually only occurs following deep diving. Bubbles of nitrogen come out of solution and are released suddenly as emboli in the labyrinthine fluids to cause haemorrhage, and intracellular disruption and also forming in parts of the central nervous system. Bubbles of gas may also block the end-arterial supply to the cochlea.

The main clinical features are sudden severe deafness, tinnitus and vertigo accompanied by vomiting. There is often bleeding into the middle ear, and sometimes general neurological symptoms.

The diagnosis is obvious from the history. Treatment involves recompression followed by slow decompression in a pressurized chamber. Farmer (1977) studied twenty-three cases and found that the earlier recompression was instigated the better was the chance of full recovery.

## 7.2 Rhinology

The nose is the site of the face most frequently injured because of its prominence. Such injuries are quite common in body contact sports such as soccer and rugby football, and are almost universal in boxing. A recent review of a large series of facial fractures showed that overall about 20% of all nasal fractures occurred in sports activities (Starkhammar and Olofsson, 1982).

### 7.2.1  NASAL TRAUMA

Injury to the nose may result in one or a combination of the following:

(a)  Fractures of the nasal bones.
(b)  Fracture or dislocation of the septum.
(c)  Septal haematoma.
(d)  Epistaxis.

*(a)   Fractures of the nasal bones*

Direct injuries to the nose often fracture the bones of the nasal vault. A direct blow on one side of the nose tends to produce a depressed fracture of the bone on the side of the injury. A blow on the front may fracture both nasal bones with depression of the tip, or may cause splaying of the bridge.

If there is displacement the injury can be recognized immediately by distortion and asymmetry, though this quickly becomes obscured by soft tissue swelling which develops in the overlying subcutaneous tissues. Associated injuries to other parts of the face, particularly the zygomatico-

109

maxillary complex, must be excluded. This injury gives rise to symptoms such as anaesthesia of the cheek, diplopia and subconjunctival haemorrhage. Careful palpation of the bony orbital margin is necessary to elicit a step deformity sign. X-rays are important medicolegally but of little clinical value.

Only displaced nasal fractures require surgical reduction. It is most unwise to attempt immediate reduction 'on the field' since the procedure is painful and the sharp bone fragment may tear arterial vessels causing severe acute haemorrhage. By the time the patient arrives at hospital assessment will be difficult due to the soft tissue swelling. Such overlying swelling usually takes five days or so to settle and it is usual practice for the ENT surgeon to carry out review at seven days. If necessary, the nasal bones can be straightened under a short general anaesthetic the following week. A plaster splint may be required if the bones are unstable following reduction, and this is removed at one week. The nasal bones will become set firmly about three to four weeks after the injury, so there is a time limit for this simple management. If the patient presents late and the deformed nasal bones are firmly united, rhinoplasty surgery will be necessary.

Epistaxis is a frequent feature of nasal fractures, but usually settles quickly with appropriate first aid measures (see later). However, when the fracture line extends along the lateral ethmoid wall it may breach the anterior ethmoidal artery causing torrential haemorrhage and requiring surgical ligation.

Rare sequelae, when the fracture involves the roof of the ethmoid labyrinth, are CSF rhinorrhoea and total or partial loss of the sense of smell. A CSF leak will usually require neurosurgical repair, or may later result in recurrent meningitis. About 10% of all cases of post-traumatic anosmia occur following nasal injuries (Zusha, 1982). The mechanism is due to tearing of the tiny olfactory nerve fibres as they pass through the cribriform plate. It is more commonly associated with the general head injuries which are a recognized risk in boxing, horse riding and motor sports, when the mechanism is believed to be due to contusion of these olfactory fibres when the brain rapidly accelerates and decelerates inside the skull. There is no specific treatment, but Zusha (1982) reports that improvement may occur in up to 14% of cases, though on occasions it may take several years.

Fractures of the thin lamina papyracea may open up a communication between the nasal cavity and orbit. Patients are often very alarmed when blowing the nose leads to swelling of the periorbital skin with surgical emphysema and the characteristic crepitus on palpation. If this practice is avoided for several days, however, healing of this false communication occurs without complication.

## (b) Fracture or dislocation of the septum

Fracture or displacement of the nasal septum may occur with or without disruption of the nasal skeleton. The patient reports unilateral nasal obstruction or sometimes general stuffiness. In more longstanding cases headaches over the frontal region or cheek may be present. The septal deviation is readily apparent on examination with a headlight when the head is tilted backwards. Occasionally the septum is snapped out of its bony groove anteriorly in the floor of the nose producing a caudal dislocation.

These septal deformities can rarely be corrected satisfactorily at the same time as the bony nasal fracture. If the condition remains symptomatic the piece of distorted septum can be excised surgically by an intranasal approach several months later (submucous resection), or a septoplasty may be performed for repositioning a caudal dislocation. If the individual is likely to sustain further nasal trauma, such as in boxing or as a rugby forward, it is best to defer any definitive surgical treatment until the player retires from his sport, as in some instances the support of the nose will be weaker.

## (c) Septal haematoma

Septal haematoma occurs uncommonly after a nasal injury, but is nonetheless an important condition to recognize. It causes total nasal obstruction, and gross swelling of both sides of the nasal septum. Such swelling is clearly visible when the head is titled back, and the septum is seen to be touching both lateral walls of the nasal cavity (Fig. 7.4). If secondary infection supervenes, soft tissue swelling of the face and

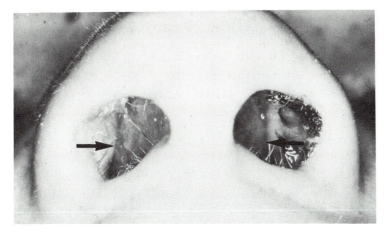

*Fig. 7.4* Septal haematoma following nasal injury; arrows indicate lateral limits of swollen septum.

111

cellulitis may develop (Fig. 7.5). This infective focus is also in the drainage area of the cavernous sinus, so that there is a real risk of life-threatening sinus thrombosis in the absence of prompt treatment.

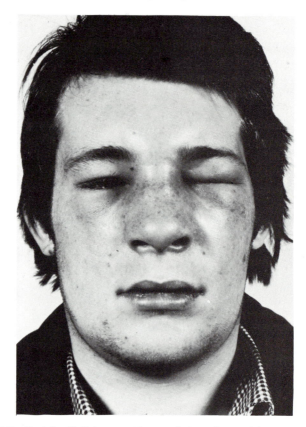

*Fig. 7.5*   Facial cellulitis secondary to infected septal haematoma.

The blood clot should be evacuated under local anaesthetic using either a wide bore needle or through a small incision. The nose is firmly packed for forty-eight hours to prevent recurrent haematoma formation, and broad spectrum antibiotic cover given. If the haematoma is left and becomes infected to form a septal abscess, necrosis of the septal cartilage may ensue followed by collapse of the nose and the ugly 'saddle shape' deformity (Fig. 7.6). This is almost a trademark of the boxing fraternity, and a legacy of repeated trauma and soft tissue haematoma. Surgical correction of the saddle nose requires an implant, usually of costal cartilage or iliac bone, and a good cosmetic result is a difficult surgical challenge.

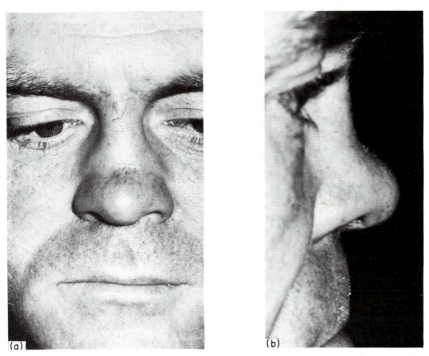

*Fig. 7.6* (a) and (b) 'Saddle nose' deformity following necrosis of supporting nasal cartilage by repetitive trauma.

### (d) Epistaxis

Epistaxis is a frequent concomitant feature of nasal injuries. The amount of blood loss may be trivial or may be severe enough to require blood transfusion in hospital. In most cases the bleeding arises from ruptured blood vessels in Little's area of the caudal septum and usually responds to simple first aid measures. Occasionally sharp bone edges may penetrate arteries; for example, the anterior ethmoidal artery is susceptible to laceration from fractures involving the ethmoid complex. Recently the authors managed the severe epistaxis of an international professional footballer who suffered a nasal injury during the course of a game. Transfusion of eighteen units of whole blood and three operations were necessary during a fourteen day period before control of the bleeding was achieved.

The general management of epistaxis has been well summarized by McKelvie (1972). First aid measures consist of pressure to the caudal septum, the common site of the bleeding, by pinching the anterior cartilaginous part of the external nose between finger and thumb for a minimum period of five minutes. Local ice-packs held to the nasal bridge

113

promote local vasoconstriction, and seating the patient upright may also be useful by lowering the venous pressure. If the bleeding continues despite these measures it is probably best to transfer the patient to hospital.

It is important for the casualty doctor to assess the extent of blood loss, which will be reflected in the pulse and blood pressure measurements. If bleeding has been severe blood should be cross-matched and an intravenous infusion with a plasma expander commenced. Examination may reveal the bleeding point which can be cauterized, following the application of 10% cocaine local anaesthetic by a red hot galvano cautery wire. Chemical methods, such as silver nitrate application, can also be used but are probably less effective. If the bleeding is excessive insertion of a firm anterior nasal pack is necessary to apply pressure to the walls of the nasal cavity. Insertion of a pack is an unpleasant procedure even following adequate local anaesthesia. Gauze (2.5 cm) impregnated with bismuth iodoform paraffin paste (BIPP) is packed in layers using Tilley's dressing forceps. If the epistaxis is controlled the patient may be allowed home providing the general condition is satisfactory. The pack should be left in place for a minimum of forty-eight hours. Bed rest and mild sedation are also of confirmed value. Inflatable devices such as Simpson's and the Brighton balloon, whose modus operandi is that of the Foley bladder catheter, have been specifically designed as an alternative method of nasal packing. They can be positioned without anaesthesia in an emergency, and are probably easier to manage by the non-specialist. In the authors' experience, however, the results are probably less satisfactory than using conventional ribbon gauze.

Bleeding may infrequently persist despite these measures from more posterior sites, when a post-nasal pack may be required, or from damaged arteries. The susceptibility of the anterior ethmoidal artery has been mentioned above. It can be occluded directly by clipping or coagulation through a medial canthal incision to gain access to the medial orbital wall. Rarely ligation of the maxillary arteries in the retromaxillary pterygo-palatine fossa, or one or both external carotid arteries may be indicated. More recently carotid angiography and selective embolization has been found useful in these situations (Kingsley and O'Connor, 1982).

## 7.2.2 SINUS BAROTRAUMA

Pathological changes in the sinus mucosa may result from the sudden lowering of pressure within the sinus compared to the surrounding atmosphere. This condition occurs in similar sports to those predisposing to otitic barotrauma, namely flying and diving. Dickson and King (1954) described 328 patients suffering from barotrauma; 100 had a sinus barotrauma and 250 an otitic barotrauma, with a combination of both lesions present in a further 22. Of 100 cases of sinus barotrauma, King (1965) found that the frontal sinus was involved in 70, the maxillary sinus in 19, and the ethmoid in only one case, the rest developing a combination. Normally the paranasal sinuses contain air, which in the case of the frontal and maxillary sinuses enters through ostia in the middle meatus. Interference with normal aeration can be due to chronic obstructive nasal pathology or the presence of an acute upper respiratory tract infection. In these instances vulvular blockage of the ostia may allow a differential pressure gradient to occur across the sinus walls. Congestion of the lining mucous membrane with mucosal haemorrhages, oedema and effusion may all be induced.

The main clinical symptom is pain felt in either the frontal region or cheek, and usually occurs during descent in an aircraft. On occasions it is severe. Underlying chronic nasal conditions may be found on examination, but there are not often obvious signs of the superadded barotraumatic sinusitis. Occasionally serious nasal discharge occurs or epistaxis. There may be tenderness over the affected sinus, and X-rays frequently show a fluid level.

As with otitic barotrauma, flying should be avoided with a concurrent upper respiratory tract infection or significant chronic nasal obstruction. Decongestant vasoconstrictor nasal drops, such as xylometazoline (Otrovine) or oxymetazoline (Afrazine) possibly with an antihistamine decongestant, help to free the blocked ostium. Definitive treatment of chronic local pathology is advised as an early elective procedure.

## 7.3 Laryngology

Serious laryngeal injuries are rare in sporting activities. This is mainly because the larynx is well protected by the more prominent mandible and sternum, but also because it is composed of pliable cartilage which is relatively resistant to all but the most severe degrees of trauma. In addition it is mobile and tends to slide out of the way when struck. This type of injury is occasionally encountered in sports such as karate, golf and basketball, where players are often looking upwards leaving a large area of the neck unprotected, and also in cricket and ice-hockey. When it occurs in motor sports and snowmobiling high impact injury is likely to cause more severe laryngeal damage.

### 7.3.1 TRAUMA TO THE HYOID BONE

Because most participants in sports are young and their cricoid and hyoid cartilages are not ossified, the type of injury most likely sustained

115

following blunt neck trauma is a fracture of the more rigid hyoid bone, when it is compressed against the unyielding bodies of the cervical vertebrae.

This injury produces the characteristic symptom of severe pain on swallowing. There is usually superficial haematoma and subcutaneous swelling in the upper neck, with acute tenderness of the hyoid bone on palpation. Examination of the internal larynx using a mirror is often unremarkable.

If the symptom persists, it can be readily treated surgically by exposing the fracture site and removing a piece of the body of the hyoid bone on each side following detachment of the muscles. This central bony gap does not cause any longstanding functional problems.

### 7.3.2 TRAUMA TO THE LARYNX

A blow to the larynx itself may cause soft tissue damage to the interior of the larynx as well as the overlying skin and subcutaneous tissues, and a fracture of the major cartilages with disruption of the vocal cords. Once again the larynx is compressed against the posterior vertebrae. The laminae of the thyroid cartilage are spread outwards, and commonly fracture vertically down the anterior prominence (Fig. 7.7). The vocal cords and epiglottis are both attached on the fracture line and may be avulsed. The detached epiglottis may fall into the laryngeal lumen causing respiratory obstruction. The arytenoid cartilages can also be dislocated from the cricoid, and the vocal cords detached posteriorly. An

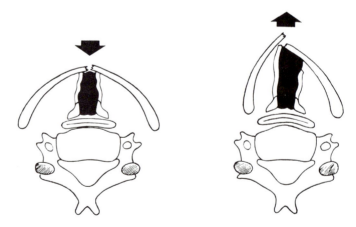

*Fig. 7.7* Laryngeal damage following blunt trauma usually leads to a linear fracture of the thyroid cartilage and detachment of the vocal cords (Maran, 1979, reproduced by kind permission of William Heinemann Medical Books Ltd).

injury at the C6 level may fracture the cricoid cartilage itself. Subsequently if the diagnosis is missed, adhesions may develop between opposing surfaces of lacerated mucosa perhaps eventually leading to chronic stenosis with airway impairment and hoarseness.

The symptoms vary with extent of the injury. Mild degrees of external trauma will only cause internal soft tissue damage with bruising, haemorrhage and secondary laryngeal oedema. More severe degrees of injury can easily be missed because the external signs of trauma may be minimal. In addition, in high-speed accidents which occur in the motor sports (motor car, motor cycle and speedway racing) associated multiple life-threatening injuries, particularly of the head, tend to divert attention away from the larynx.

The most important symptom is respiratory obstruction which may necessitate urgent medical intervention. Dyspnoea secondary to laryngeal haemorrhage and oedema can be marked and occur suddenly, or take several hours to develop. Other features may include haemoptysis, hoarseness, and pain on swallowing. The presence of stridor indicates upper respiratory obstruction, but the loudness bears little relation to its severity. However, two-way stridor that is present on both inspiration and expiration does reflect significant airway limitation, and tracheostomy rather than endotracheal intubation is invariably necessary under these circumstances. External swelling may result from haematoma or from surgical emphysema due to a tear in the perichondrium or the cricothyroid or thyrohyoid membranes. Crepitus will be present on palpation in the latter case, and the emphysema may extend down to involve the mediastinum. Local tenderness may be found on palpation of the larynx, and linear fractures of the thyroid cartilage can sometimes be felt. Internal submucosal haemorrhage and tears or vocal cord disruption may be detected by indirect laryngoscopy.

Cervical spine X-rays should be obtained to exclude fractures of the vertebrae. Plain and tomogram X-rays of the larynx may demonstrate displaced cartilage fragments, avulsion injuries, e.g. the epiglottis, and emphysema in the fascial planes of the neck.

Airway protection is the most important aspect in the management of acute laryngeal injury. Fortunately, most cases of blunt laryngeal sporting injuries can be managed conservatively and there is an excellent prognosis in respect of vocal and airway function. The standard conservative measures include voice rest, humidification and bed rest. The long-term functional results or more severe types of trauma, which are sustained for example in motorized sports, are distinctly less favourable, and only about 50% of these patients are likely to achieve a 'good result' (Maran, et al., 1981).

All cases with significant neck injuries should be transported to hospital immediately by ambulance, as airway problems can develop rapidly. If there is clinical evidence of disruption of the laryngeal cartilages or vocal cords, surgical emphysema and significant airway obstruction, open surgical reduction and mucosal repair is necessary with a temporary elective tracheostomy. Prophylactic broad-spectrum antibiotics are given to prevent possible infective perichondritis. Where the injury is confined to the soft tissues close clinical observation regarding airway adequacy is essential. Endotracheal intubation or, less commonly, tracheostomy may be required in these cases. Systemic steroids may aid resolution of the associated oedema (Olson and Miles, 1971).

## 7.4 Comment

The full philosophy of 'sports medicine' has yet to penetrate the discipline of otolaryngology. The immediacy of much of it falls well within the scope of the day to day work of an ENT department. However, the rapid rehabilitation and expedition of many of these 'cold' procedures and the priorities accredited to the sportsmen are likely to meet with competition. Sportsmen, anxious to return to the fray, still find themselves in company with those afflicted by similar injuries acquired from domestic, road traffic, industrial, criminal and other origins.

## References

Bess, F. H. and Poynor, R. E. (1974) Noise induced hearing loss and snowmobiles. *Arch. Otolaryngol.*, **99**, 45.

Coles, R. R. A. and Rice, C. G. (1966) Auditory hazards of sports guns. *Laryngoscope*, **76**, 1728.

Dickson, E. D. D. and King, P. F. (1954) The incidence of barotrauma in present day service flying. *Flying Personnel Research Committee Report No. 881*, Air Ministry, London.

Farmer, J. C. (1977) Diving injuries to the inner ear. *Ann. Otol., Rhinol. Laryngol.*, **86**, Supplement 36.

Fletcher, J. L. and Gross, C. W. (1977) Noise induced deafness in motor sports and shooting. *Sound and Vibration*, **11**, 26.

Freeman, P. and Edmonds, C. (1972) Inner ear barotrauma. *Arch. Otolaryngol.*, **95**, 556.

Goodhill, V. (1972) Inner ear barotrauma. *Arch. Otolaryngol.*, **95**, 588.

Head, P. W. (1979) Physiological considerations of pressure effects on the ear and sinuses in deep water diving, Chapter 7 in *Scott Brown's Diseases of the Ear, Nose and Throat* (eds J. Ballantyne and J. Groves), 4th edn, Butterworths, London.

King, P. F. (1965) Sinus barotrauma, in *A Textbook of Aviation Physiology* (ed. J. A. Gillies), Pergamon Press, Oxford, p. 112.

# References

Kingsley D. and O'Connor, A. F. F. (1982) Embolisation in otolaryngology. *J. Laryngol. Otol.*, **96**, 439.

Lundgren, C. E. G. (1965) Alternobaric vertigo – a diving hazard. *Brit. Med. J.*, **ii**, 511.

Lundgren, C. E. G. and Malm, L. U. (1966) Alternobaric vertigo among pilots. *Aerospace Med.*, **66**, 178.

Maran, A. G. D. (1979) Trauma and stenosis of the larynx and cervical trachea, in *Head and Neck Surgery* (eds P. M. Stell and A. G. D. Maran) 2nd edn, pp. 205–211, William Heinemann Medical Books Limited, London.

Maran, A. D. G., Murray, J. A., Stell, P. M. and Tucker, A. (1981) Early management of laryngeal injuries. *J. Roy. Soc. Med.*, **74**, 656.

McKelvie, P. (1972) Epistaxis. *Brit. J. Hosp. Med.*, **18**, 339.

McNicholl, W. D. (1982) Eustachian tube dysfunction in submariners and divers. *Arch. Otolaryngol.*, **108**, 279.

Melville-Jones, G. (1957) A study of current problems associated with disorientation in man-controlled flight. *Flying Personnel Research Committee Report No. 1006*, Air Ministry, London.

Olson, N. R. and Miles, W. K. (1971) Treatment of acute blunt laryngeal injuries. *Ann. Otol., Rhinol. Laryngol.*, **80**, 704.

Starkhammer, H. and Olofsson, J. (1982) Facial fractures: a review of 922 cases with special reference to aetiology and incidence. *Clin. Otolaryngol.*, **7**, 405.

Zusha, H. (1982) Post-traumatic anosmia. *Arch. Otolaryngol.*, **108**, 90.

# 8 Injuries to the cervical spine

JOSEPH S. TORG and JOSEPH J. VEGSO

[This chapter is taken from *Athletic Injuries to the Head, Neck and Face* (ed. J. S. Torg), Lea and Febiger, Philadelphia, 1982 by courtesy of the publishers.]

Of the variety of injuries that can occur to the athlete, those involving the head and neck are the most difficult to evaluate and manage on the field. Risks can be high, because of the actual or potential involvement of the nervous system, and consequently the margin for error is low. The initial clinical picture frequently may be misleading. Patients with significant intracranial hemorrhage may at first present with minimal symptoms only to follow a precipitous downhill course. On the other hand, short-lived problems such as neuropraxia of the brachial plexus may at first present with paraesthesia and paralysis, raising the question of a significant spinal injury, only to resolve within minutes with the individual returning to his activity. Fortunately, the more severe injuries that can occur to the neck are infrequent. As a consequence, most team physicians and trainers have little, if any, experience in dealing with them.

There are several principles that should be considered by individuals responsible for athletes who may sustain neck injuries.

(1) The team physician or trainer should be designated as the person responsible for supervising on-the-field management of the potentially serious injury. This person is the 'captain of the medical team'.
(2) Prior planning must ensure the availability of all necessary emergency equipment at the site of potential injury. At a minimum, this should include a spineboard, stretcher, and equipment necessary for the initiation and maintenance of cardiopulmonary resuscitation.
(3) Prior planning ensures the availability of a properly equipped ambulance, as well as a hospital equipped and staffed to handle emergency neurological problems.
(4) Prior planning ensures immediate availability of a telephone for

121

communicating with the hospital emergency room, ambulance, and other responsible individuals in case of an emergency.

Athletic injuries to the cervical spine may involve the bony vertebrae, intervertebral discs, ligamentous supporting structures, the spinal cord, roots, and peripheral nerves, or any combination of these structures. The panorama of injuries observed runs the spectrum from the 'cervical sprain syndrome' to fracture-dislocations with permanent quadriplegia. Those responsible for the emergency and subsequent care of the athlete with a cervical spine injury should possess a basic understanding of the variety of problems that can occur.

## 8.1 Functional anatomy

With the neck in the anatomic position, the cervical spine is extended due to normal cervical lordosis. When the neck is flexed to 30°, the cervical spine straightens. In axial-loading injuries, the neck is slightly flexed and normal cervical lordosis is eliminated, thereby converting the spine into a straight segmented column. Assuming the head, neck, and trunk components to be in motion, rapid deceleration of the head occurs when it strikes another object, such as another player. This results in the cervical spine being compressed between the abruptly deaccelerated head and the force of the oncoming trunk. When maximum vertical compression is reached, the straightened cervical spine fails in a flexion mode, and fracture, subluxation, or unilateral or bilateral facet dislocation can occur.

## 8.2 Nerve root-brachial plexus neurapraxia

The most common and most poorly understood cervical injuries are the pinch-stretch neurapraxias of the nerve root and brachial plexus (Clancy, Brand and Bergfeld, 1977). Typically following contact with head, neck, or shoulder, a sharp burning pain is experienced in the neck on the involved side that may radiate into the shoulder and down the arm to the hand. There may be associated weakness and paraesthesia in the involved extremity lasting from several seconds to several minutes. The key to the nature of this lesion is its short duration and the presence of a full, pain-free range of neck motion. Although the majority of these injuries are short-lived, they are worrying because of the occasional plexus axonotmesis that occurs. However, the youngster whose paraesthesia completely abates, who demonstrates full muscle strength in the intrinsic muscles of the shoulder and upper extremities, and who most importantly has a full, pain-free range of cervical motion, may return to his activity.

Persistence of paraesthesia, weakness, or limitation of cervical motion requires that the individual be protected from further exposure and that he undergo neurological and radiological evaluation.

## 8.3  Acute cervical sprain syndrome

An acute cervical sprain is a collision injury frequently seen in contact sports. The patient complains of having 'jammed' his neck with subsequent pain localized to the cervical area. Characteristically, the patient presents with limitation of cervical spine motion and without radiation of pain or paraesthesia. Neurological examination and radiographs are normal.

Stable cervical sprains and strains eventually resolve with or without treatment. Initially, on the field the presence of a serious injury should be ruled out by a thorough neurological examination and determination of the range of cervical motion. Range of motion is evaluated by asking the athlete to actively nod his head, touch his chin onto his chest, touch his chin onto his left shoulder, touch his chin onto his right shoulder, touch his left ear onto his left shoulder, and touch his right ear onto his right shoulder. The athlete with less than a full, pain-free range of cervical motion, persistent paraesthesia, or weakness should be protected and excluded from further activity. Subsequent evaluation should include appropriate radiological studies, including flexion and extension views to demonstrate fractures or instability. If the patient has pain and muscle spasm of the cervical spine, hospitalization and head-halter traction may be indicated.

In general, treatment of athletes with 'cervical sprains' should be tailored to the degree of severity. Immobilizing the neck in a soft collar and using analgesics and anti-inflammatory agents until there is a full, spasm-free range of neck motion is appropriate. It should be emphasized that individuals with a history of collision injury, pain and limited cervical motion should have routine cervical spine X-rays. Also, lateral flexion and extension radiographs are indicated after the acute symptoms subside.

It should be noted here that many older people are becoming involved in sports such as power boat racing where the cervical spine may be at risk. A hyperextension injury in association with cervical spondylosis can lead to the development of a central spinal cord syndrome. The treatment of this is conservative.

## 8.4 Intervertebral disc injuries

Roaf has provided insight into the sequences of events involved during compressive loading of the vertebra in trauma (Roaf, 1960). The disc is less compressible than the vertebra, which is the first structure to fracture. Initial deformation occurs by vertebral end-plate bulging, and the process eventually continues to end-plate failure. Cortical shell fracture and cancellous bone compression occur as deformation proceeds. Roaf further recognized that there can be asymmetric compression and that the pressure thus transmitted to the annulus results in tearing of the annulus or a general collapse of the vertebra due to buckling at its side. His study included determining the resistance of the annulus fibrosus with and without the presence of a fluid nucleus pulposus. After removal of the nucleus pulposus, compressive loading produced the type of typical annulus prolapse seen in disc protrusion. Thus, Roaf suggested that compressive loading results in vertebral end-plate fracture with extrusion of nucleus pulposus into the vertebral body.

Albright studied 75 University of Iowa freshman football recruits who had radiographs of their cervical spines after having played in high school, but before playing in college (Albright et al., 1976). Of the group, 32% had one or more of the following: 'occult' fractures, vertebral body compression fractures, intervertebral disc-space narrowing, or other degenerative changes. Of this group, only 13% admitted to a positive history of neck symptoms. The development of early degenerative changes or intervertebral disc-space narrowing in this group was attributed to repetitive impact on the cervical spine as a result of head impact in blocking and tackling.

Although not documented completely, the findings of Roaf and Albright suggest the occurrence of intervertebral disc injury without herniation of the nucleus pulposes resulting from axial compression of the cervical spine (Roaf, 1960; Albright et al., 1976). More careful clinical and radiographic examinations determine whether 'occult' injury to the intervertebral disc space occurs more frequently than is currently appreciated.

Acute herniation of the nucleus pulposus as an isolated entity resulting from athletic injuries is rare. However, acute onset of quadriplegia in an athlete who has sustained head impact with negative cervical spine radiographs suggests acute rupture of a cervical intervertebral disc. The syndrome of acute anterior spinal cord injury, as described by Schneider, may be observed.

'The acute anterior cervical spinal cord injury syndrome may be characterized as an immediate acute paralysis of all four extremities with a loss of pain and temperature to the level of the lesion, but with preservation of posterior column sensation of motion, position, vibration and part of touch' (Schneider, 1951; Schneider, Cherr and Pantek, 1954).

The pressure of the disc is on the anterior and lateral columns, while the posterior columns are protected by the denticulate ligaments. Myelography should be performed to substantiate the diagnosis. Anterior discectomy and interbody fusion for a patient with neurological involvement or persistent disability due to pain should be considered.

## 8.5 Emergency management of severe injuries

Managing the unconscious athlete or one suspected of having a significant injury to the cervical spine is a process that should not be done hastily or haphazardly. Being prepared to handle this situation is the best way to prevent actions that could convert a reparable injury into a catastrophe (Fig. 8.1).

Thus, the single most important point to remember is: *prevent further injury*. Be sure that whatever action is taken does not cause further harm. Being well prepared helps to alleviate indecisiveness and second-guessing. Immediately immobilize the head and neck by holding them in the neutral position. Check first for breathing, then for pulse, and then for level of consciousness.

If the victim is breathing, simply remove the mouthguard, if present, and maintain the airway. It is necessary to remove a facemask only if the respiratory situation is threatened or unstable, or if the athlete remains unconscious for a prolonged period. Leave the chinstrap on.

Once it is established that the athlete is breathing and has a pulse, evaluate the neurological status. The level of consciousness, response to pain, pupillary response, and unusual posturing, flaccidity, rigidity, or weakness should be noted.

At this point, simply maintain the situation until transportation is available, or until the athlete regains consciousness. If the athlete is face down when the ambulance arrives, change his position to face up by logrolling him onto a spineboard (Fig. 8.2(a),(b)). Make no attempt to move him except to transport him or to perform CPR if it becomes necessary.

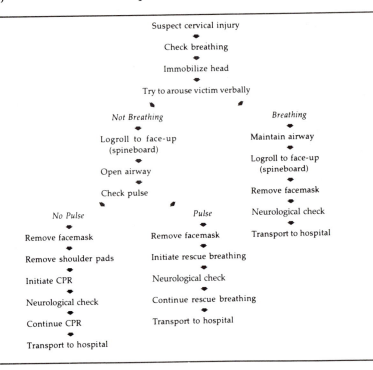

*Fig. 8.1* Field decision making – head and neck injuries of an unconscious athlete.

If the athlete is not breathing or stops breathing, the airway must be established. If he is face down, he must be brought to a face-up position. The safest and easiest way to accomplish this is by a logroll. In an ideal situation, your medical-support team is made up of five members: the leader, who controls the head and gives commands only; three members to roll; and a fourth to help lift and carry when it becomes necessary. If time permits and the spineboard is on the scene, the athlete should be rolled directly onto it. However, breathing and circulation are much more important at this point.

With all medical-support team members in position, the athlete is rolled toward the assistants: one at the shoulders, one at the hips and one at the knees. They must maintain the body in line with the head and spine during the roll. The leader maintains immobilization of the head by applying slight traction and by using the crossed-arm technique. This technique allows the arms to unwind during the roll (Figs 8.3–8.7).

Once the athlete has been moved to a face-up position, quickly re-

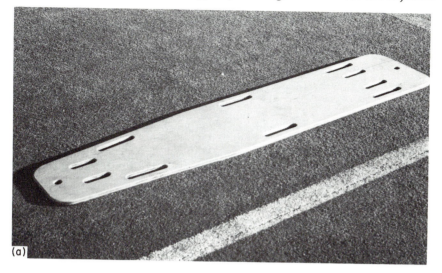

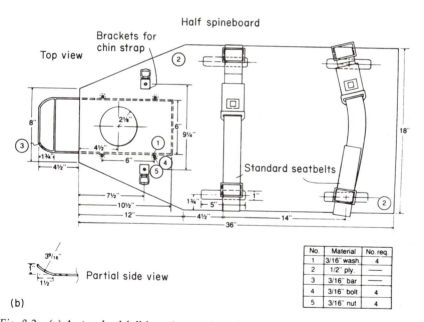

Fig. 8.2 (a) A standard full-length spineboard made of 1.80 cm (¾ in.) plywood; body straps are not shown. (b) The Purdue University (West Lafayette, Indiana) spineboard can be constructed in any school wood shop. The board is made from 1.80 cm (¾ in.) plywood; body straps are standard seat belts or luggage straps.

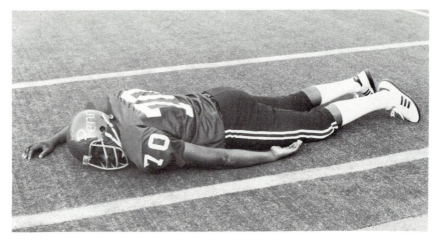

*Fig. 8.3* Athlete with suspected cervical spine injury may or may not be unconscious. However, all who are unconscious should be managed as though they had a significant neck injury.

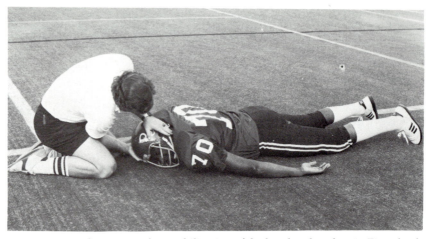

*Fig. 8.4* Immediate manual immobilization of the head and neck unit. First check for breathing.

evaluate breathing and pulse. If there is still no breathing, or if breathing has stopped, the airway must be established (Fig. 8.8).

'The jaw-thrust technique is the safest first approach to opening the airway of a victim who has a suspected neck injury, because in most cases it can be accomplished by the rescuer grasping the angles of the victim's lower jaw and lifting with both hands, one on each side, displacing the

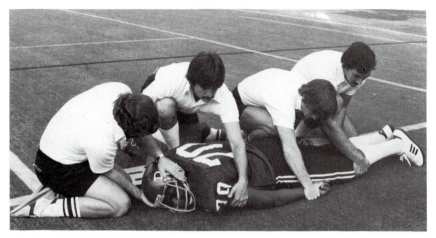

*Fig. 8.5* Logroll to a spineboard. This manoeuvre requires four individuals: the leader to immobilize the head and neck and to command the medical-support team. The remaining three individuals are positioned at the shoulders, hips, and lower legs.

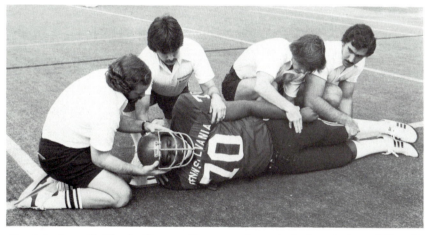

*Fig. 8.6* Logroll. The leader uses the crossed-arm technique to immobilize the head. This technique allows the leader's arms to 'unwind' as the three assistants roll the athlete onto the spineboard.

mandible forward while tilting the head backward. The rescuer's elbows should rest on the surface on which the victim is lying' (American Heart Association, 1977).

If the jaw thrust is not adequate, the head tilt–jaw lift should be substituted (Fig. 8.9). Care must be exercised not to overextend the neck.

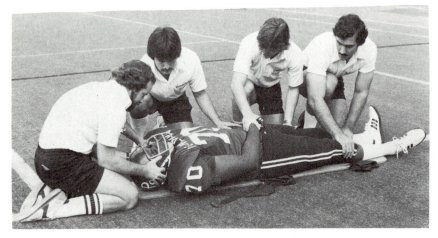

*Fig. 8.7* Logroll. The three assistants maintain body alignment during the roll.

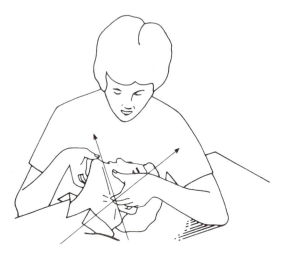

*Fig. 8.8* Jaw-thrust manoeuvre for opening the airway of a victim with a suspected cervical spine injury. (Reprinted with permission from the American Heart Association.)

The fingers of one hand are placed under the lower jaw on the bony part near the chin and lifted to bring the chin forward, supporting the jaw and helping to tilt the head back. The fingers must not press the soft tissue under the chin which might obstruct the airway. The other hand presses on the victim's forehead to tilt the head back.

If opening the airway does not restore breathing, the facemask must be

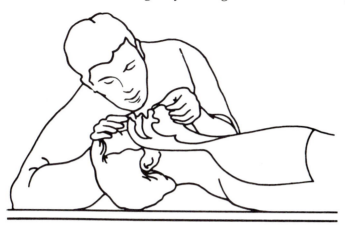

*Fig. 8.9* Head tilt–jaw lift manoeuvre for opening the airway. Used if jaw thrust is inadequate or if a helmet is being worn. (Reprinted with permission from the American Heart Association.)

removed from the helmet before rescue breathing can be initiated (Figs 8.10 and 8.11).

The transportation team should be familiar with handling a victim with a cervical spine injury. They should be receptive to taking orders from the

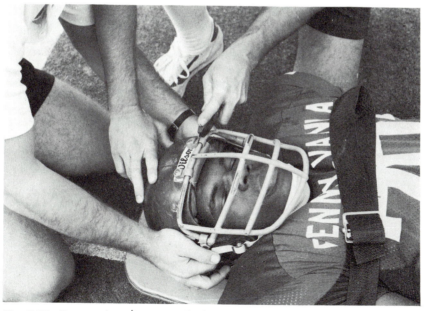

*Fig. 8.10* Remove 'cage'-type masks by cutting the plastic loops with a utility knife. Make the cut on the side of the loop away from the face.

Injuries to the cervical spine

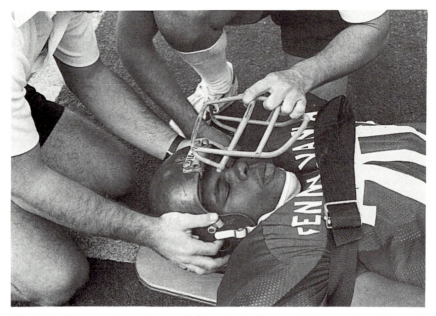

*Fig. 8.11* Remove the entire mask from the helmet so it does not interfere with further resuscitation.

'leader'. It is extremely important not to lose control of the care of the athlete. Therefore, be familiar with the transportation crew that is used. In an athletic situation, prior arrangements with an ambulance service should be made.

Lifting and carrying the athlete requires five individuals: four to lift and the leader to maintain immobilization of the head (Figs 8.12 and 8.13). The leader initiates all actions with clear, loud verbal commands.

The same guidelines apply to the choice of a medical facility as to the choice of an ambulance: be sure it is equipped and staffed to handle an emergency neck injury. There should be a neurosurgeon and an orthopaedic surgeon to meet the athlete upon arrival. Radiographic facilities should be standing by.

### 8.6   Cervical vertebra subluxation without fracture

Axial compression–flexion injuries incurred by striking an object with the top of the head can result in disruption of the posterior soft-tissue supporting elements with angulation and anterior translation of the superior cervical vertebrae. Fractures of the bony elements are not demonstrated on radiographs, and the patient has no neurological

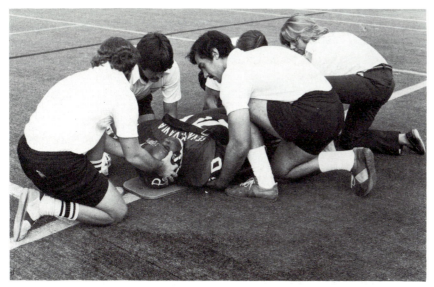

*Fig. 8.12* Four members of the medical-support team lift the athlete on the command of the leader.

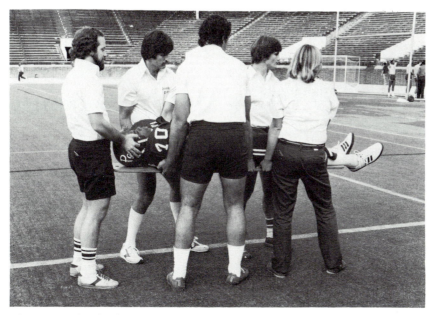

*Fig. 8.13* The leader maintains manual immobilization of the head. The spineboard is not recommended as a stretcher. An additional stretcher should be used for transporting over long distances.

# Injuries to the cervical spine

deficit. Flexion–extension radiographs demonstrate instability of the cervical spine at the involved level manifested by motion, anterior intervertebral disc space narrowing, anterior angulation and displacement of the vertebral body, and fanning of the spinous processes (Fig. 8.14). We believe that demonstrable instability on lateral flexion–extension radiographs in a young, vigorous individual requires vigorous treatment. When soft-tissue disruption occurs without an associated fracture, it is likely that instability will result despite conservative treatment. When anterior subluxation greater than 20% of the vertebral body is due to disruption of the posterior supporting structures, a posterior cervical fusion is recommended.

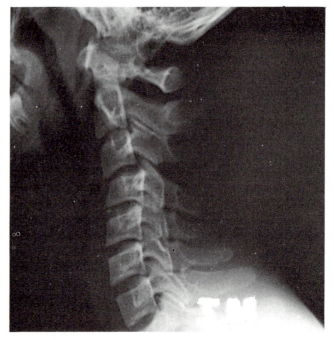

*Fig. 8.14* Radiograph demonstrates C3–C4 subluxation as manifested by anterior intervertebral disc space narrowing, anterior angulation, and displacement of the superior vertebral body, and fanning of the spinous processes.

## 8.7 Cervical fractures and dislocations

### 8.7.1 GENERAL PRINCIPLES

Fractures or dislocations of the cervical spine may be stable or unstable and may or may not be associated with neurological deficit. When

134

fracture or disruption of the soft-tissue supporting structure immediately violates, or threatens to violate, the integrity of the spinal cord, implementation of certain management and treatment principles is imperative.

The first goal is to protect the spinal cord and nerve roots from injury through mismanagement. It has been estimated that many neurological deficits occur after the initial injury. That is, if a patient with an unstable lesion is inappropriately manipulated when being transported to a medical facility. Or if later mismanaged, further encroachment on the spinal cord can occur.

Secondly, the traumatically malaligned cervical spine should be reduced as quickly and gently as possible to effectively decompress the spinal cord. When dislocation or anterior angulation and translation are demonstrated radiographically, immediate reduction is attempted with skull traction. We favour using Gardner-Wells tongs. These tongs can be easily and rapidly applied under local anaesthesia, without shaving the head, in the emergency room or in the patient's bed. Since these tongs are spring-loaded, it is unnecessary to drill the outer table of the skull for their application. The tongs are attached to a cervical-traction pulley, and weight is added at a rate of 5 lb per disc space or 25 to 40 lb for lower cervical injury. Reduction is attempted by adding 5 lb every 15 to 20 minutes and is monitored by lateral radiographs.

Experience indicates that unilateral and bilateral facet dislocations, particularly at the C3–C4 level, are not always reducible using skeletal traction. In such instances, closed skeletal or manipulative reduction under nasotracheal anaesthesia may be necessary. The expediency of early reduction of cervical dislocations must be emphasized.

It has been proposed that the presence of a bulbocavernous reflex indicates that spinal shock has worn off and that except for recovery of an occasional root at the injury, neither the motor nor sensory paralysis will resolve regardless of treatment. The bulbocavernous reflex is produced by pulling on the urethral catheter. This stimulates the trigone of the bladder, producing a reflex contraction of the anal sphincter around the examiner's gloved finger. Although the presence of a bulbocavernous reflex is generally a sign that there will be no further neurological recovery below the level of the injury, this is not always true. The presence of this reflex does not give the clinician licence to handle the situation in an elective fashion. The cervical spine malalignments and dislocations associated with quadriparesis should be reduced as quickly as possible, by whatever means necessary, if maximum recovery is to be expected.

In most instances in which a vertebral body burst fracture is associated with anterior compression of the cord, decompression is logically effected through an anterior approach with an interbody fusion. Likewise, traumatic intervertebral disc herniation with cord involvement is best managed through an anterior discectomy and interbody fusion. In cervical fractures and dislocations, posterior cervical laminectomy is indicated only rarely when excision of foreign bodies or bony fragments in the spinal canal is necessary. Realignment of the spine is the most effective method for decompression of the cervical cord.

Indications for surgical decompression of the spinal cord have been delineated. A documented increase in neurological signs is the clearest mandate for surgical decompression. Further observation, expectancy, and procrastination in this situation is contraindicated. Persistent partial cord or root signs, with objective evidence of mechanical compression, are also an indication for surgical intervention. However, in this instance, the procedure may be delayed seven to fourteen days. There is no evidence that a ten-day delay will impair the final return of neurological function, and mortality and morbidity is decreased by this period of re-equilibration.

Management of cervical spine fractures and dislocations requires the generous use of parenteral corticosteroids (dexamethasone) to decrease the inflammatory reactions of the injured cord and surrounding soft-tissue structures. Drugs that inhibit norepinephrine synthesis or deplete catecholamines have been advocated to prevent autodigestion of the cord, but there is no evidence as yet that this is of value in improving the prognosis for cord recovery. Procedures such as durotomy, myelotomy, and rhizotomy require extensive laminectomy, add further instability to the spine, and are contraindicated.

The third goal in managing fractures and dislocations of the cervical spine is to effect rapid and secure stability to prevent residual deformity and instability with associated pain and the possibility of further trauma to the neural elements. The method of immobilization depends on the post-reduction status of the injury. Thompson and associates have concisely delineated indications for non-surgical and surgical methods for achieving stability (Thompson, Morris and Jane, 1975). These concepts for managing cervical spine fractures and dislocations may be summarized as follows.

(1) Patients with stable compression fractures of the vertebral body, undisplaced fractures of the lamina or lateral masses, or soft-tissue injuries without detectable neurological deficit can be adequately treated with traction and subsequent protection with a cervical brace until healing occurs.
(2) Stable, reduced facet dislocation without neurological deficit can also be treated conservatively in a Minerva jacket brace until healing has been demonstrated by negative lateral flexion–extension radiographs.

(3) Unstable cervical spine fractures or fracture-dislocations without neurological deficit may require either surgical or non-surgical methods to insure stability.

(4) Absolute indications for surgical stabilization of an unstable injury without neurological deficit are late instability following closed treatment and flexion–rotation injuries with unreduced locked facets.

(5) Relative indications for surgical stabilization in unstable injuries without neurological deficit are anterior subluxation greater than 20%, certain atlantoaxial fractures or dislocations, and unreduced vertical compression injuries with neck flexion.

(6) Cervical spine fractures with complete cord lesions require reduction followed by closed or open stabilization as indicated.

(7) Cervical spine fractures with incomplete cord lesions require reduction followed by careful evaluation for surgical intervention.

The fourth and final goal of treatment is rapid and effective rehabilitation started early in the treatment process.

A more specific categorization of athletic injuries to the cervical spine can be made. Specifically, these injuries can be divided into those that occur in the upper, mid- and lower cervical spine.

### 8.7.2 UPPER CERVICAL SPINE FRACTURES AND DISLOCATIONS

Upper cervical spine lesions involve C1 to C3. Although rarely occurring in sports, there are several specific injuries that can occur to the upper cervical vertebrae that deserve mention. The transverse and alar ligaments are responsible for atlantoaxial stability. With rupture of these structures resulting from a flexion injury, and with translation of C1 anteriorly, the spinal cord can become impinged between the posterior aspect of the odontoid process and the posterior rim of C1. Such a lesion is potentially fatal. The patient gives a history of head trauma and complains of neck pain, particularly with nodding, and may or may not present with cord signs. Lateral radiographs of the C1–C2 articulation demonstrate an increase in the atlantodens interval. This interval is normally 3 mm in the adult. With transverse ligament rupture it may increase up to 10–12 mm, depending on the status of the alar and accessory ligaments. Note that an increase in this interval may only be seen with the neck flexed. Fielding states that atlantoaxial fusion may be the 'conservative' treatment for this lesion. He recommended C1–C2 fusion with wire fixation and iliac bone graft (Fielding, Fietti and Mardam-Bey, 1978).

Fractures of the atlas were described by Jefferson in 1920. There may be two types: posterior arch fractures and burst fractures. Posterior arch fractures are the more common of the two, and with a brace support go on to satisfactory fibrous or bony union.

The burst fractures result from an axial load transmitted to the occipital condyles, which then disrupt the integrity of both the anterior and posterior arches of the atlas. Radiographs demonstrate bilateral symmetric overhang of the lateral masses of the atlas, in relationship to the axis, with increase in the para-odontoid space on the open-mouth view. The patient is injured by striking the top of his head and characteristically demonstrates pain and limitation of the nodding motion. Treatment, as recommended by Fielding, includes head-halter traction until muscle spasm resolves, followed by brace support. If flexion–extension radiographs subsequently demonstrate significant instability, fusion may be indicated (Fielding, Fietti and Mardam-Bey 1978).

Fractures of the odontoid have been classified into three types by Anderson and D'Alonzo (1974). Type I is an avulsion of the tip of the odontoid at the site of the attachment of the alar ligament and is a rare and stable lesion. Type II is a fracture through the base, at or just below the level of the superior articular processes. Type III involves a fracture of the body of the axis. When not displaced, tomograms may be required to identify the lesion.

The mechanism of odontoid fractures has not been clearly delineated. However, these fractures appear to be due to head impact. All routine cervical spine radiographic studies should include the open-mouth view to identify lesions involving the odontoid as well as the atlas. If these are negative, and if a lesion in this area is suspected, tomograms or bending films may further delineate pathological changes in this area.

Managing Type II fractures is a problem. It has been reported that between 36% and 50% of these lesions treated initially with plaster casts or reinforced cervical braces fail to unite. Cloward has reported that 85% of his patients heal within three months when treated with the halo brace (Cloward, 1980).

It is necessary to stabilize surgically fibrous unions or non-united fractures of the odontoid if instability is demonstrated on flexion and extension views. Stabilization may be effected either through posterior C1–C2 wire fixation and fusion or anterior fusion of C1–C2 by a dowel graft through the articular facets, as described by Cloward (1980).

Fractures through the arch of the atlas are also known as traumatic spondylolisthesis of C2, or hangman's fracture. These are relatively rare lesions. The mechanism of injury is generally recognized to be hyperextension. However, there are instances in which a compression fracture of C3 is associated with traumatic spondylolisthesis of C2, indicating that the lesion was due to flexion. This injury is inherently unstable. However, it has been shown to heal with predictable regularity without surgical intervention. After reduction is affected with traction, a halo cast is applied and the fracture immobilized until healing occurs, which usually takes twelve to sixteen weeks. At that point, flexion and extension lateral radiographs are obtained. If instability is demonstrated, or the patient has persistent pain because of disruption of the C2–C3 inter-vertebral disc, fusion may be necessary. The anterior C2–C3 approach is recommended. To obtain stability by posterior fusion requires stabiliza-tion of C1 to C3, thus blocking C1–C2 rotation.

### 8.7.3 MIDCERVICAL SPINE FRACTURES AND DISLOCATIONS

Acute traumatic lesions of the cervical spine at the C3–C4 level are rare and are generally not associated with fractures (Torg *et al.*, 1977). These lesions are classified as follows:

(1) Acute rupture of the C3–C4 intervertebral disc.
(2) Anterior subluxation of C3 on C4;
(3) Unilateral dislocation of the joint between the articular processes.
(4) Bilateral dislocation of the articular process (facet).

Acute onset of quadriplegia with a motor-sensory level of the fourth cervical nerve root in an athlete who has sustained head impact with a negative cervical spine radiograph suggests acute rupture of the C3–C4 intervertebral disc. The syndrome of acute anterior spinal cord injury, as described by Schneider, may be observed. A cervical myelogram substan-tiates the diagnosis (Schneider, 1951; Schneider, Cherr and Pantek, 1954). Anterior discectomy and interbody fusion may be the most effective treatment of this lesion.

Anterior subluxation of C3 on C4 is a result of a shearing force through the intervertebral disc space which disrupts the interspinous ligament, as well as the posterior supporting structure. Radiographs demonstrate narrowing of the intervertebral disc space, anterior angulation and translation of C3 on C4, an increase in the distance between the spinous processes of the two vertebrae, and instability without fracture of the bony elements (Fig. 8.14). A posterior C3–C4 fusion may be necessary for adequate stabilization in such cases, in contrast with cervical spine instability caused by a fracture in which adequate reduction and sub-sequent bony healing result in stability. When the patient has posterior instability, posterior fusion is preferable to an anterior interbody fusion.

Unilateral facet dislocation at C3–C4 may result in immediate quadriparesis. This injury involves the intervertebral disc space, the interspinous ligament, the posterior ligamentous supporting structures, and the one facet with resulting rotatory dislocation of C3 on C4 without fracture (Fig. 8.15). At this level, strong skeletal traction does not yield a

139

# Injuries to the cervical spine

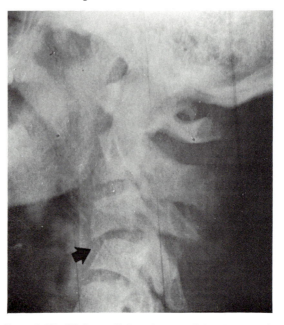

*Fig. 8.15* Unilateral C3–C4 facet dislocation resulting in complete motor and sensory deficit distal to the lesion. There is fanning of the spinous processes of C3 and C4 and more than 20% anterior displacement of the body of C3 on C4.

successful reduction, and closed manipulation under general anaesthesia is necessary to disengage the locked joint between the articular processes. Manipulation may be done with the patient supine on a Stryker frame, with the head and neck maintained in axial alignment, and a sandbag placed under the shoulders. Traction is applied through Gardner-Wells tongs with gentle lateral bend away from the dislocation joint, combined with extension and rotation toward the site of the lesion. Reduction is associated with a subtle click. In two reported cases, the initial neurological findings resembled those of acute anterior spinal cord injury. However, the recovery pattern was that of an acute central cervical spinal cord injury. Presumably, the injury involved initial compromise of the anterolateral cord function associated with central cervical cord oedema and haemorrhage. Following immediate reduction and subsequent anterior decompression and interbody fusion, six to nine months elapsed before there was significant motor improvement.

Bilateral facet dislocation at the C3–C4 level is a grave lesion (Fig. 8.16). Skeletal traction does not reduce the lesion, and the prognosis for this injury is poor.

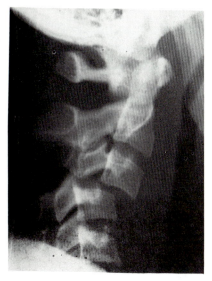

*Fig. 8.16* Bilateral facet dislocation at the C3–C4 level demonstrates anterior angulation as well as translation greater than 50% of the width of the vertebral body associated with spinous process fanning. The lesion resulted in quadriplegia.

### 8.7.4 LOWER CERVICAL SPINE FRACTURES AND DISLOCATIONS

Lower cervical spine fractures or dislocations are those involving C4 through C7. In those injuries that result from various athletic endeavours, the majority of fractures or dislocations of the cervical spine, with or without neurological involvement, involve this segment. Although unilateral and bilateral facet dislocations occur, they are relatively rare. The vast majority of severe athletically incurred cervical spine injuries are fractures of the vertebral body with varying degrees of compression or comminution.

*(a)   Unilateral facet dislocations*

Unilateral facet dislocations are the result of axial loading flexion–rotation type mechanisms. The lesion may be truly ligamentous without associated vertebral fracture. In such instances, the facet dislocation is stable and is not usually associated with neurological involvement. Radiographs demonstrate less than 50% anterior shift of the superior vertebra on the inferior vertebra. Attempts should be made to reduce the facet dislocation by skeletal traction. However, as with similar lesions described at the C3–C4 level, it may not be possible to effect a closed reduction. In this instance, open reduction under direct vision through a posterior approach with supplementary posterior element bone grafting should be performed.

Injuries to the cervical spine

## (b) Bilateral facet dislocations

Bilateral facet dislocations are unstable and usually associated with neurological involvement. These injuries are associated with a high incidence of quadriplegia. Lateral radiographs demonstrate greater than 50% anterior displacement of the superior vertebral body on the inferior vertebral body. Immediate treatment, as previously described, is closed reduction with skeletal traction. Such lesions are generally reducible by skeletal traction and are then treated by halo-cast stabilization and posterior fusion. It should be noted that instability is directly related to the ease with which the lesion is reduced since the easier it is to reduce, the easier it is to redislocate. If skeletal traction is unsuccessful, either manipulative reduction under sedation or general anaesthesia or open reduction under direct vision is recommended. When the dislocation is reduced closed and the reduction is maintained, immobilization should be effected by use of the halo-cast for eight to twelve weeks. Corrective bracing should continue for an additional four weeks.

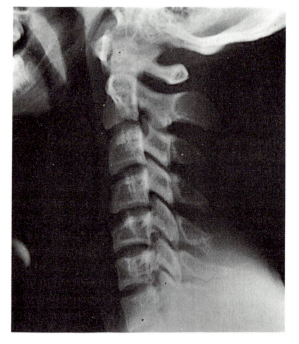

*Fig. 8.17* Type I vertebral body wedge compression fracture involving the anterior aspect of C5. There is no evidence of subluxation at the joints between the articular processes. Also, there is absence of fanning of the spinous processes. The small fragment at the superior aspect of the vertebral body is of no significance. This is a stable lesion that can be effectively managed with a cervical collar or brace.

142

*(d)  Vertebral body compression fractures*

Compression fractures of the vertebral body result from axial loading. Vertebral body fractures of the cervical spine can be classified into five types.

*Type I,* simple wedged compression fractures of the cervical vertebrae, are common injuries that respond to conservative management and rarely, if ever, are associated with neurological involvement (Fig. 8.17). It is important to differentiate these lesions from compression fractures that are associated with disruption of the posterior element soft-tissue supporting structures. The latter lesions are unstable and frequently associated with neurological involvement, including quadriplegia.

*Type II,* comminuted burst vertebral body fractures without displacement, are not usually associated with neurological involvement (Fig. 8.18(a) and (b)). However, settling of these fractures may result in late cervical instability. These patients should be considered for anterior exploration, decompression, and fusion.

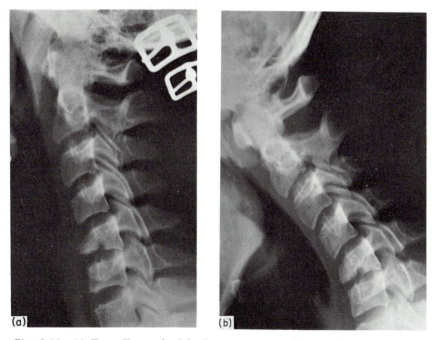

(a)  (b)

*Fig. 8.18*  (a) Type II vertebral body compression fracture demonstrates the characteristic comminuted burst fracture of the vertebral body without displacement into the vertebral canal. (b) Lateral flexion radiographs of the lesion demonstrate maintenance of adjacent disc space height, as well as a lack of subluxation or spinous process fanning. With no disruption of the posterior elements, this is a relatively stable lesion.

143

## Injuries to the cervical spine

*Type III*, comminuted burst vertebral body fractures, with displacement of bony fragments into the vertebral canal, are serious injuries that place the spinal cord in jeopardy and should be treated accordingly (Fig. 8.19).

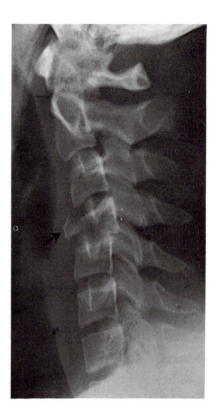

*Fig. 8.19*   Type III comminuted burst fracture of C4 with displacement of fragments into the vertebral canal.

*Type IV*, comminuted burst vertebral body fractures associated with disruption of the posterior elements are extremely unstable lesions with anterior subluxation or dislocation of the superior vertebral segments and associated quadriplegia (Fig. 8.20). The prognosis is poor. Combined anterior and posterior procedures may be necessary to effect stabilization.

*Type V*, comminuted burst vertebral body fractures are associated with fractures of the elements of the neural arch. Subsequently, there are both anterior and posterior instability. There is posterior displacement of the superior vertebral segment because of the disruption of the posterior bony elements (Fig. 8.21). As would be expected, quadriplegia is associated with this lesion. It should be noted that a posterior dislocation of the vertebral body cannot be realigned effectively without surgical intervention. Because of both anterior and posterior instability, combined anterior

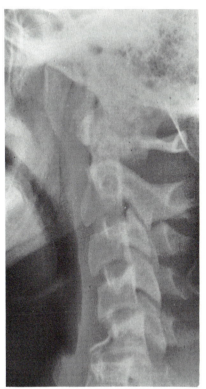

*Fig. 8.20* Type IV comminuted burst fracture of the vertebral body of C5 with associated fanning or widening of the spinous processes between C5 and C6 indicating disruption of the posterior soft tissue structures. The combined anterior and posterior instability has resulted in settling and posterior displacement of the superior vertebral segment. This lesion is the result of a compression–flexion injury.

and posterior operative procedures may be necessary to effectively stabilize the spine.

### (e) Transient quadriplegia

An infrequently occurring and not well-documented phenomenon is that of transient quadriplegia. This characteristically occurs to an athlete, most often a football player, who sustains either forced hyperextension or hyperflexion to his neck and cervical spine. A painless paralysis ensues which may manifest itself as weakness or complete absence of motor function in all four extremities. The episode is brief, lasting from five to ten minutes. The involvement of sensory function has not been established. Radiographs do not demonstrate findings indicating acute trauma to the cervical spine. However, examination of the lateral films reveals either a congenital fusion or a developmental decrease in the sagittal diameter of the spinal canal which is increased on lateral flexion and extension radiographs.

Injuries to the cervical spine

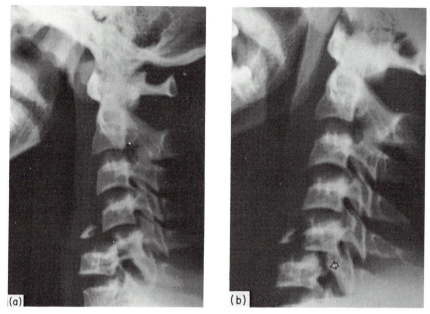

*Fig. 8.21* (a) Type V comminuted burst fracture of the vertebral body associated with fractures of the neural arch. There is settling and posterior displacement of the superior vertebral segment. (b) Distraction of the superior vertebral segment with skeletal traction permits visualization of fractures through the pedicles (arrow) of C6 in addition to the burst fracture of the body of C5.

## 8.8   Cervical spine instability

Late cervical spine instability following injury is a necessary considera-tion when an athlete is injured. If possible, it is well to avoid subsequent permanent or transient narrowing of the spinal canal with compression of the neural elements. For each particular injury it is not possible to predict accurately whether late instability will result in structural malalignment, with or without neurological deficit. However, the recent work of White and Panjabi in establishing guidelines regarding this problem is note-worthy (White and Panjabi, 1978). They performed a series of cadaver studies in which the various supporting structures were systematically cut and resulting instabilities in the spine were noted.

The supporting structures of the lower cervical spine can be divided into two groups: anterior and posterior. The anterior group includes soft-tissue supporting structures both anterior to and including the posterior longitudinal ligament. These are the anterior and posterior longitudinal ligaments, the intervertebral disc, and the annulus fibrosus. The pos-

146

terior group consists of the facet capsular ligaments, ligamentum flavum, and the interspinous and supraspinous ligaments. On the basis of this work, instability occurs when either all the anterior or all the posterior structures are disrupted. Therefore, we may define, on an anatomical basis, an anterior cervical spine instability and a posterior cervical spine instability.

Radiographically, cervical spine instability manifests itself by more than 3.5 mm of horizontal translation of one vertebra relative to an adjacent vertebra in lateral flexion–extension films. Instability also exists if radiographs demonstrate more than 11° of angular displacement of one vertebra relative to another on the lateral views.

## 8.9 Activity restrictions

Physicians involved in the management of athletes who have sustained significant cervical spine injuries are ultimately faced with the question of whether or not the patient can return to his or her activity. Since few, if any, attempts have been made to address this question formally, the following guidelines are offered which are based on clinical experience.

Youngsters who have been diagnosed and successfully treated for cervical sprains, intervertebral disc injuries without neurological involvement and stable wedge compression fractures may return to all activities when they are symptom-free, have a full range of cervical motion, full muscle strength and stability of the cervical spine as demonstrated by flexion and extension films.

Those with lesions of the cervical spine resulting in subluxation without fracture should be precluded from further participation in contact sports despite lack of motion on lateral flexion–extension films. Flexion and extension films are a static demonstration of stability and not an adequate measure of the stability of the spine when it is subjected to the forces involved in contact sports.

Individuals who have undergone a successful one-level anterior interbody decompression and fusion for herniated nucleus pulposus or anterior instability may return to all activities provided they have a full range of motion and strength. However, they should be fully aware of the possibility of intervertebral disc herniation at an adjacent level.

Individuals who undergo more than one-level anterior fusion or posterior fusion for cervical spine injury should be evaluated on an individual basis with regard to return to non-contact sports. However, these individuals should not be permitted to return to contact activity regardless of how 'solid' the fusion appears on the radiographs. Altered biomechanics of the cervical spine with more than a two-level fusion

# Injuries to the cervical spine

presents several problems. The decrease in motion will, in itself, deprive the spine of its capability of dissipating force through motion. Also, it would appear that there is a higher risk of injury because of the increased torque on the lever arm on the level above and below the fusion mass. The effect of cervical fusion as a precipitating cause of degenerative disease at other levels is also a question that is unanswered but should be considered.

## References

Albright, J. P., Moses, J. M., Feldick, H. G. *et al.* (1976) Nonfatal cervical spine injuries in interscholastic football. *J. Amer. Med. Assoc.*, **236**, 1243.

American Heart Association (1977) *A Manual for Instructors of Basic Cardiac Life Support*, Dallas.

Anderson, L. D. and D'Alonzo, R. T. (1974) Fractures of the odontoid process of the axis. *J. Bone Joint Surg.*, **56A**, 1663.

Clancy, W. G., Brand, R. L. and Bergfeld, J. A. (1977) Upper trunk brachial plexus injuries in contact sports. *Amer. J. Sports Med.*, **5**, 209.

Cloward, R. B. (1980) Acute cervical spine injuries. *Ciba Clin. Symp.*, **32**, 2.

Fielding, J. W., Fietti, V. G. and Mardam-Bey, T. H. (1978) Athletic injuries to the atlanto-axial articulation. *Amer. J. Sports Med.*, **6**, 226.

Jefferson, G. (1920) Fracture of the atlas vertebra. *Brit. J. Surg.*, **7**, 407.

Roaf, R. (1960) A study of the mechanics of spinal injuries. *J. Bone Joint Surg.*, **42B**, 810.

Roaf, R. (1972) International classification of spinal injuries. *Paraplegia*, **10**, 78.

Schneider, R. C. (1951) A syndrome in acute cervical injuries for which early operation is indicated. *J. Neurosurg.*, **8**, 360.

Schneider, R. C., Cherr, G. and Pantek, H. (1954) The syndrome of acute central cervical spinal cord injury. *J. Neurosurg.*, **11**, 546.

Thompson, R. C., Morris, J. N. and Jane, J. A. (1975) Current concepts in management of cervical spine fractures and dislocations. *Amer. J. Sports Med.*, **31**, 159.

Torg, J. S., Truex, R. L., Hodgson, M. J., Quedenfeld, T. C., Spealman, A. D. and Nichols, C. E. (1977) Spinal injury at the level of the third and fourth cervical vertebrae from football. *J. Bone Joint Surg.*, **59A**, 1015.

White, A. A. and Panjabi, M. M. (1978) *Clinical Biomechanics of the Spine*, J. B. Lippincott, Philadelphia.

# 9 Thoracic and cardiac injuries

TERENCE LEWIS

The central components of the cardiothoracic system, the lungs, heart and origins of the great vessels, are enclosed within and protected by a cage of bone and muscle. These contents, principally the heart, great vessels and lungs, can be damaged by penetration from without or by blunt trauma. Penetrating wounds are surprisingly difficult to achieve as the ribs provide a most effective barrier but the two points most at risk are from below up through the diaphragm, especially in relation to the xiphisternum, and at the root of the neck where the bony cage is incomplete. This latter route is the most common point of entry into the chest encountered in fencing injuries.

Blunt trauma to the chest can not only produce direct damage to the lung and anterior surface of the heart, but rapid deceleration of the bony skeleton allows the less firmly anchored structures within the chest to swing forward within the cavity, hinging on their more robust points of attachment. Thus the heart and aortic arch may swing forward leaving the descending aorta behind where it is more firmly attached deep to the parietal pleura and this may cause laceration and even transection at this point just distal to the subclavian artery.

Injuries or problems relating to the cardiothoracic system are rare in young healthy adults and children but when they do occur in relation to sporting activities the results may be catastrophic or fatal. This is particularly significant as the vogue for exercise, often violent, in the middle-aged becomes more widespread.

## 9.1 Pulmonary injuries

### 9.1.1 PNEUMOTHORAX

Air trapped between lung and chest wall, or more accurately between visceral and parietal pleura, must lead to an equal reduction in total lung volume, that is to say to a degree of pulmonary collapse. The clinical state

149

# Thoracic and cardiac injuries

that this produces is termed a pneumothorax which may be spontaneous or traumatic.

### (a) Spontaneous pneumothorax

This occurs usually in young adults, of either sex, and often during exercise (Fig. 9.1). Typically the person involved is tall and thin and there may have been previous episodes. The underlying pathological process is usually an area of emphysematous bullae with adhesions to the chest wall at the apex of the lung or, more rarely, the apical segment of the lower lobe, in the lingula, or the middle lobe.

Why these should occur is unknown but it has been suggested that these may be areas of local alveolar necrosis because of poor blood supply to the apex of a 'long lung' in a low pressure system. This however does not explain why bullae are occasionally seen in areas other than the apex. Presumably some abnormal shearing force, either overinflation or blunt trauma, causes a small bulla to burst and to leak air into the potential space between lung and chest wall. As the lung falls away, adhesions will further tear the parenchyma and in addition may cause bleeding, leading to a haemopneumothorax. This leakage of air does not usually last for

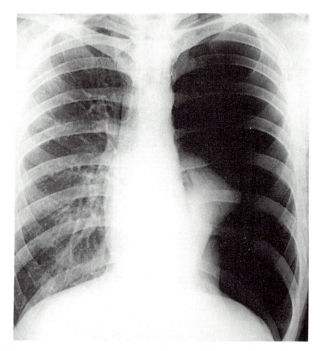

*Fig. 9.1* Spontaneous simple pneumothorax with complete collapse of the left lung, but no mediastinum shift.

150

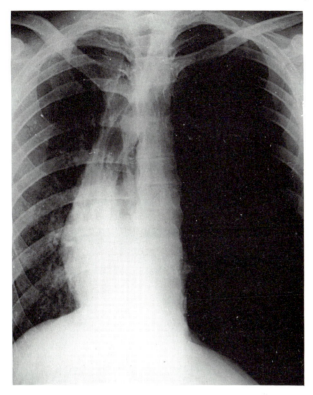

*Fig. 9.2* Tension pneumothorax with deviation of the mediastinum and compression of the contralateral lung.

long and probably most spontaneous pneumothoraces are small and not clinically important or even appreciated. The air leak may continue, however, and indeed the lung may completely collapse. Rarely a valve-like process occurs whereby with each inspiration more air is sucked into the pneumothorax cavity which enlarges under pressure pushing the surrounding mobile structures of the mediastinum, principally the heart, away compressing the other lung. This is termed a *tension pneumothorax* (Fig. 9.2) and is a life-threatening, although rare, phenomenon. Potentially equally dangerous, but luckily very uncommon, is the occurrence of pneumothoraces on both sides simultaneously.

*(b)   Traumatic pneumothorax*

This is less common but obviously seen with injuries that penetrate the chest wall. Outside air can enter through any gaping wound but usually damage to the lung itself leads to progressive leak of air by the same mechanism as a spontaneous pneumothorax, but often faster and with a less benign outlook. A pneumothorax must always be suspected in fencing accidents especially if the entry is the neck, as the tip readily enters the apex of the lung.

More commonly, traumatic pneumothoraces are caused by non-penetrating violence from blows to the chest while boxing, playing rugby, falling from a horse or any violent deceleration injury such as is sometimes seen in motor racing. Blunt trauma to the left lower chest especially when rib fractures are present are often associated with rupture of the spleen and, as shock secondary to blood loss from this intra-abdominal organ is sometimes delayed, these patients must be watched carefully. If there is the slightest doubt a laparotomy should be performed, preceded by a diagnostic abdominal paracentesis. Small pneumothoraces not associated with significant blood loss often resolve if left alone, especially in young people, but usually sufficient trauma to cause a pneumothorax also produces a haemothorax, especially if fractured ribs have been responsible for the damage to the lung. This situation requires drainage of both air and blood separately, although in emergency a single properly placed drain of sufficient size is usually enough.

Finally it must always be remembered when faced with the victim of a major and overwhelming injury, especially if caused by deceleration or collision, that pneumothorax is sometimes bilateral, is commonly associated with substantial blood loss into the chest and consequently the most life-threatening problem. First aid procedures such as adequate drainage or plugging a gaping chest wound can be life saving if appreciated and executed in time.

### 9.1.2 INSERTION OF A CHEST DRAIN

This has been well described in detail by Firmin and Welch (1980). The classical site of insertion of a drain is anteriorly through the second interspace in the mid-clavicular line (Fig. 9.3). This approach, however, requires passage of the drain through the pectoralis muscle in well muscled young men and is cosmetically unsightly in the long-term, especially for women.

Most urgent chest drains are inserted to relieve pneumothorax and for this the ideal situation is the fourth interspace in the mid-axillary line. This is behind the easily palpable free border of the pectoralis major and results in a kink-free course for the tube to pass to the apex of the lung. In this site the tube is easily managed, allows for safe transportation and is cosmetically more attractive after removal.

Chest drains should be inserted in the most aseptic manner that circumstances allow. Careful injection of 1% or 2% plain lignocaine in

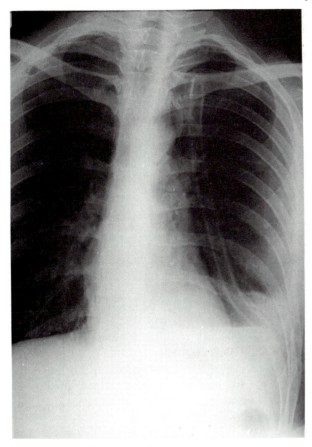

*Fig. 9.3*   Chest X-ray of patient seen in Fig. 9.2 with adequate sized drain inserted into classical anterior site with good position at the apex of the chest cavity and good re-expansion of the lung.

sufficient quantities – up to 20 ml throughout the whole thickness of the chest wall including the parietal pleura – results in pain-free insertion of the tube, which nowadays should be of the Argyle type. Following an adequate incision in the skin and subcutaneous fat, the chest cavity should first be entered by blunt dissection using a Spencer Wells or similar instrument. This avoids the inherent dangers of forcing a sharp lance-like trocar of the Argyle into the chest cavity with a sudden, uncontrolled lurch and occasionally transfixing the heart or great vessels.

With care, insertion of an intercostal drain should be quick, safe, and pain-free. Once inserted, the chest drain should ideally be connected to some form of underwater seal drain although, in an emergency, one of the commercially available flutter valves is usually quite satisfactory, provided that the valves are not stuck together by blood. Any drain inserted with less than perfect sterility, and possibly all chest drains, should be covered with antibiotics, ideally ampicillin and cloxacillin if the patient is not sensitive to penicillins.

Chest drains can and should be removed as soon as they are no longer performing their function, that is as soon as either air or blood ceases to drain. Prolonged chest drainage carries a very real risk of infection within the chest cavity which is a serious complication.

### 9.1.3 DECOMPRESSION PROBLEMS

Decompression problems, commonly known as the bends, are well appreciated by all divers, whether commercial or sporting, and are very well described and discussed elsewhere. It is sufficient here to say that inappropriate decompression must always be considered a possibility and if suspected the nearest fully equipped centre contacted via the police or coastguard. It behoves everyone involved in diving to be aware of the local facilities available to deal with decompression problems, even though these rarely involve the amateur sportsman or woman who does not generally dive to great depth. There is one context, however, which must always be borne in mind by even shallow water 'scuba divers': subclinical decompression problems are greatly magnified by reduction of the atmospheric pressure and therefore all diving, at any depth, must be avoided for at least twenty-four hours before travelling by aeroplane. Diving in the last hours before flying home from holiday is dangerous.

### 9.1.4 LUNG CYSTS

Lung cysts are not uncommon and are usually asymptomatic. They can cause problems by expanding at low atmospheric pressures and they must be excluded by routine chest X-ray of mountaineers and those intending to go to very high altitudes in poorly pressured aircraft or balloons.

## 9.2 Cardiac problems

Cardiac problems discussed in a book on sports injuries may at first glance seem somewhat inappropriate. After all it is *rare* for a javelin to puncture the chest and pierce the heart and if this does happen it is normally a matter for observation rather than treatment. However, sudden death, for cardiac reasons, during or shortly after exercise must be considered by anyone concerned administratively with many forms of sport, especially energetic or violent exercise involving the over 30s. Sudden death or acute myocardial infarction, whilst not often seen flyfishing or during archery, is distinctly common on the squash court and whilst jogging.

The majority of those who have a cardiac arrest and die during or shortly after exercise have established coronary artery disease of which they may or may not have been aware before the event. Myocardial infarction occurring during exertion with an oxygen debt already in existence is very difficult to treat and the rhythm disturbances – finally ventricular fibrillation – are often refractory. Probably the group at most risk in this way are overweight, competitive, but unfit, males in their 30s and 40s. Even if the myocardial infarction is survived, the extent of heart muscle damage is usually substantial which bodes badly for the future.

Pre-existing but undiagnosed aortic stenosis is regularly seen at autopsy in sportsmen dropping dead during exercise. In this country, routine screening at school picks up the majority of these people, most of whom have a congenitally bicuspid aortic valve. The story is different in less well developed countries, however, and a feature of the disease can be the absence of symptoms until the end. Resuscitation under these circumstances is often quite impossible due to the practical difficulties of massaging an adequate cardiac output through a tightly stenosed valve from a woody, non pliant, hypertrophied ventricle. Hypertrophic obstructive cardiomyopathy (HOCOM) can present in the same way for the same reasons.

Very occasionally sudden death occurs in young fit people with no underlying fixed obstruction to the coronary tree or with no cardiac valvular lesions and presumably these are rhythm disturbances occurring either spontaneously or in association with a cardiomyopathy or an underlying predisposition to dysrhythmia. Most ventricular ectopics are benign and get better with exercise, but some are aggravated by exertion and the stress of competition and these are potentially dangerous.

Sudden death will be encountered from time to time in all forms of sport, both amongst competitors and supporters, and there must be an appreciation of the possibility with provision of appropriate basic facilities to deal with it, such as an airway, oxygen and ideally an Ambubag. Staff and administrators must make it their business to understand first aid, artificial respiration and cardiac massage, and must appreciate that these two manoeuvres can keep a young adult alive for long periods while being transported to a place where there are more sophisticated facilities including drugs, electronic monitoring and defibrillating apparatus. This is particularly true in the case of drowning, which is often associated with self-induced hypothermia, thus allowing full recovery after a very long

155

period of cardiac arrest and resuscitation, especially in children, who appear to pass into a state of metabolic semi-hibernation.

There is an ever increasing army of patients who have either survived a myocardial infarction or who have successfully undergone coronary artery surgery and who have adopted a new life of weight reduction, no smoking and exercise. While this is an entirely proper course of action and is by no means locking the stable door after the horse has bolted, these patients will still be more likely to have cardiac events than others, and will present problems to the medical profession, mostly in terms of advice as to the most appropriate sports to follow. Full and regular screening including an exercise E.C.G. should be a regular part of these people's lives as indeed it probably should for all people approaching middle age and still exercising actively.

## 9.3 Chest wall problems

Chest wall problems are sometimes encountered by thoracic surgeons and may cause acute alarm.

### 9.3.1 THE STERNUM

Sternal abnormalities such as pectus excavatum or carcinatum are often first noticed and identified as being abnormal in the changing rooms. These variations in the normal chest wall, sometimes severe, can produce acute apprehension and embarrassment. They rarely, if ever, even in their most marked forms, cause any real physiological disturbance at all. The problems are usually psychological although none-the-less real. All that is normally required is positive reassurance. Certainly the various operations on the bony skeleton are far from being without risk and require prolonged immobilization and often seem cosmetically and functionally worse after the operative interference than before. For purely cosmetic reasons, tailor-made silastic implants are the least invasive choice for certain types of deformity but reassurance is the most sensible form of treatment.

### 9.3.2 ACUTE COSTOCHONDRITIS

Acute costochondritis as ascribed to Tietze is far from rare and presents as pain, sometimes acute, localized over a costochondral joint, usually the second, third or fourth anteriorly (Tietze, 1921). This can be incapacitating and alarming principally because it is often misinterpreted by the individual as being cardiac pain. Once it is understood that this is a costochondritis often secondary to trauma which is usually self-limiting, although local tenderness may continue on and off for years, it is more easily tolerated. Local injection of steroids may help. Occasionally there is a lump palpable and visible which may need biopsy to exclude a rare neoplasm of bone or cartilage.

### 9.3.3 RIB FRACTURES

Fractured ribs are commonly seen in sports involving collision with objects or other people. Very rarely do they create problems in the young and fit, other than pain, although rib fractures are occasionally associated with damage to underlying lung or spleen.

Uncomplicated rib fractures are best treated with analgesics. Strapping seldom helps and may hinder movement of the rest of the chest wall. Operative fixation converts a closed fracture into a compound fracture with no real benefit. Extensive multiple fractures may disarticulate a number of adjacent ribs anteriorly and fractures at the angles posteriorly results in a flail segment. This may well cause severe respiratory problems especially if associated with trauma to the underlying lung. These are best dealt with in an appropriate unit able to employ positive pressure ventilation which may be required for a number of weeks until the flail stabilizes and the underlying 'shocked' lung has recovered. Associated rupture of the diaphragm, usually the left side, requires operative correction via thoracotomy (Fig. 9.4).

### 9.3.4 JOGGER'S NIPPLE

Friction of the clothes may result in irritation of the delicate epithelium of the nipple in both men and women (Levit, 1977). This will cause inflammation and sometimes bleeding with associated discomfort. A Vaseline gauze cover under a dry dressing anchored with elastoplast will rapidly settle the problem.

### 9.3.5 SKIER'S NIPPLE

This condition, which is similar to jogger's nipple, is due to the braces sometimes worn with the old fashioned ski trousers. Modern ski clothes – the cat suit and the salopet – do not produce the problem.

### 9.3.6 BREAST INJURIES (BOUNCING BREAST SYNDROME)

If inadequately supported, the breast, especially if well developed, can bounce against the chest wall with such force as to produce haematoma

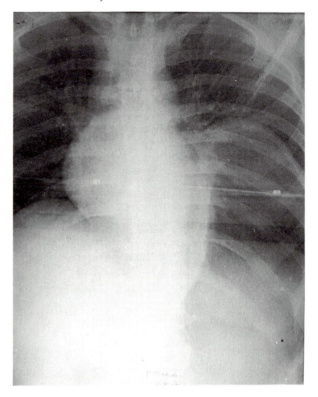

*Fig. 9.4* Rupture of the left hemi-diaphragm due to deceleration injury showing a grossly dilated stomach occupying the left chest and pushing the mediastinum into the contralateral chest cavity.

and surface bruising. It is also vulnerable to external trauma in games such as hockey and fast moving racquet sports. Further, unsupported breasts will stretch their suspensory ligaments. Advice regarding adequate brassiere support is important. 'Sports' brassieres should have wide shoulder straps and so support the breast that the side view will demonstrate a convexity from the top of the breast to the nipple. The cups should be seamless and there should be a wide chest band below breast level.

### 9.3.7   RUPTURE OF STERNAL HEAD OF PECTORALIS MAJOR

This can occur particularly in butterfly swimmers, weight lifters, in arm wrestling and in parachutists (Fig. 9.5). It usually tears at its insertion into the lip of the bicipital groove. If repair has to be carried out it is necessary to raw the insertion, drill the bone and suture the tendon back. It will have

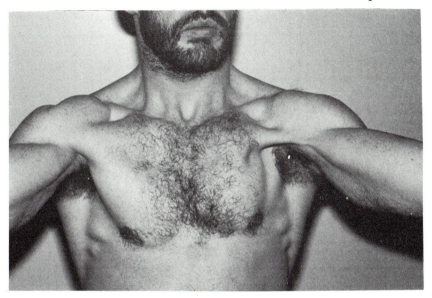

*Fig. 9.5*  Rupture of the sternal head of left pectoralis major.

to be protected for twelve weeks before any vigorous activity is permitted.

A unique case of bilateral pectoralis rupture has been described by the patient, a well known orthopaedic surgeon and sportsman (Buck, 1973). Park and Espiniella (1970) reviewed the literature and found that twenty-nine described cases amongst athletes needed surgical repair.

### 9.3.4  PECTORALIS MINOR SYNDROME

Compression of the axillary vein can occur due to compression by a hypertrophied pectoralis minor muscle producing venous claudication. This may cause weakness and discomfort in the arm together with venous engorgement and is particularly common in baseball pitchers. The diagnosis is confirmed by venography (Nakada, Knight and Mani, 1982).

### 9.3.5  WINGING OF THE SCAPULA

The mechanism of the abnormal protuberance of the inner edge of the scapula, which is called winging, is paralysis of the serratus anterior muscles, supplied by the long thoracic nerve. It may not be obvious in repose but if suspected a forward push of the arms by the patient will reveal it clearly.

The lesion is only rarely caused by injury, which is a direct blow to the nerve where it is rather exposed on the lateral chest wall. In these cases the damage is neuropraxia and recovery is complete. There is no treatment other than to maintain a full range of shoulder motion. Far more common is the atraumatic winging. This is of course often identified in the changing room as young sportsmen are not slow to point out something wrong with a colleague. This may follow a period of intense pain felt in the shoulder, lasting perhaps two weeks and at the end of which the winging is noticed. This is called neuralgic amyotrophy. Although recovery is usually complete a small proportion retain some degree of winging. Despite that, the functional recovery is full as far as the patients are concerned. They and the parents can be reassured and again the only treatment is to maintain motion while awaiting recovery. There is usually no need to restrict sporting activities.

## References

Buck, J. E. (1973) Bilateral rupture of the pectoralis major, B.A.S.M. Joint, p. 7070.

Firmin, R. K. and Welch, J. (1980) Hospital Update, 6, 481.

Levit, F. (1977) Joggers' nipple, J. Amer. Med. Assoc., 257, 1127.

Nakada, T., Knight, R. T. and Mani, R. L. (1982) Pectoralis minor syndrome. Ann. Neurol., 11, 433.

Park, J. Y. and Espiniella, J. L. (1970) Rupture of pectoralis major muscle, J. Bone Joint Surg., 52A, 577.

Tietze, A. (1921) Uber eine eigenartige haufung von fallen mit dystrophie der rippenknorpel. Berl. Klin. Wochnshr., 58, 829.

# 10 *Abdominal injuries*

ALASTAIR WILSON and ANTHONY GOODE

The diverse nature of sporting activity means that any abdominal injury encountered in surgical practice may occur as a result of sport. Specific sports are nonetheless associated with specific patterns of injury. The attending physician must recognize the risks involved in the relevant sport, and maintain a high index of suspicion whenever there is a possibility of abdominal injury (Walkden, 1981).

In general, sports injuries are blunt or non-penetrating. The scuba diver who has harpooned himself or the javelin thrower who has impaled himself on his javelin are obvious exceptions. These are rare. This chapter will consider blunt trauma.

The abdomen has a musculoskeletal function as well as providing a protective container for the viscera (Fig. 10.1). Diagrammatically it consists of a dome at either end of a hollow tube (Fig. 10.2). Both domes consist of a muscular diaphragm within a bony cage (Figs 10.3–10.5).

Aristotle noticed that even the slightest blow could rupture an intestine without any sign of injury to the skin. The severity of the injury may be out of all proportion to the cause and may be masked by the excitement and tension involved in sport. Also, if the muscles are relaxed, it takes little force to rupture gut or solid organs and the patient may have no recollection of the original injury.

When an abdominal injury occurs on the field of play ill-informed bystanders may give advice. This should be resisted and an assessment made as to whether there is serious abdominal injury when intravenous fluids may be a priority. Always beware of a confused history. There may be medicolegal complications, and the patient may be trying to protect or implicate others.

## 10.1 History

When the initial assessment has been made a history can be taken. The detailed nature of the injury and the point of traumatic contact may be the

# Abdominal injuries

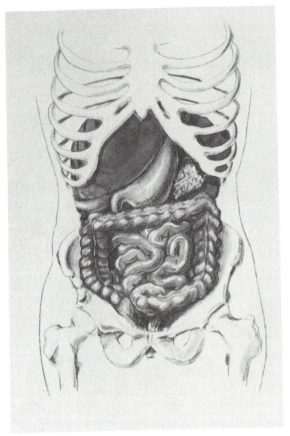

*Fig. 10.1* The abdomen provides a protective container for the viscera.

best indicator of damage to particular organs. The symptoms and reactions of the subject at the time of the injury and the development of symptoms until the time of examination often give clues as to the severity of the injury. Any concomitant disease or previous medical history, including any medications, may be important in subsequent management. The time the patient last ate or drank should be noted.

## 10.1.1 REFERRED PAIN

Sometimes pain is referred to sites distant from the primary intra-peritoneal injury. For example, left shoulder pain in patients with a ruptured spleen (Kehr's sign) occurs because of irritation of the peritoneum under the left diaphragm. Similarly, right sided shoulder pain occurs with rupture of the liver, though occasionally a rupture

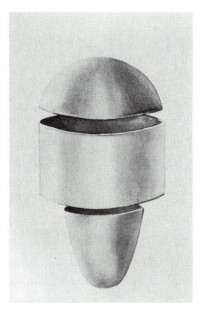

*Fig. 10.2* Diagrammatically, the abdomen consists of a muscular dome at either end of a hollow tube.

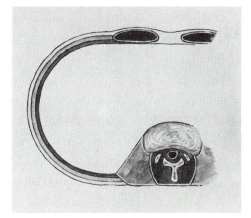

*Fig. 10.3* The tube consists of the spinal column, three investing muscle layers and the rectus muscles anterior.

involving the left lobe of the liver may cause pain in the left shoulder. If a splenic bleed is suspected Kehr's sign may be induced by tipping the patient into a steep head-down tilt for several minutes. Testicular pain may occur as a result of a retroperitoneal bowel perforation.

163

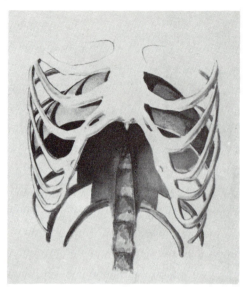

*Fig. 10.4*  The upper dome. Diaphragm within and ribs without.

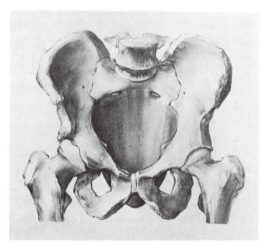

*Fig. 10.5*  The lower dome. Pelvis without and muscular pelvic diaphram within.

## 10.2  Examination

The initial assessment should have indicated the necessity for urgent resuscitative measures. Fluid replacement should never be delayed by

164

attending to minor detail and the airway, breathing, circulation and the level of consciousness must always be assessed first.

The clinical presentation is seldom simple, several organs may have been damaged together with muscles and bones. This 'complex' of injuries will give rise to 'complex' presenting features. It is helpful to reduce the findings into four simple possibilities.

(1) Has there been physical distortion and tearing of tissue?
(2) Has the injury given rise to haemorrhage (haematuria should be included here).
(3) Has the injury caused a leakage of visceral contents?
(4) Is there peritonitis?


## 10.3 Approach

There may be visible signs of abdominal trauma with marks and bruises on the skin indicating the point of contact of blunt trauma, but there may be a confusing array of grazes, bruises and cuts. Generally, bruising is found over bony prominences. Bruising over the softer anterior abdominal wall, perhaps with pattern imprinting of the clothes, suggests that there has been considerable compression of the anterior abdominal wall against the spine or pelvis. Intervening viscera are likely to have been damaged.

Localized swelling results from a haematoma or muscle rupture. If rupture is complete, it may be possible to demonstrate a gap where the muscle has sprung apart. When the rupture is partial, the muscle is very tender and there will be considerable spasm and rigidity. Immediate distension or generalized abdominal swelling indicates bleeding into the peritoneal cavity. Girth measurements should be recorded to monitor distension. If swelling is delayed in onset, it is more likely to indicate gaseous distension due to ileus.

Localized tenderness which is not related to guarding and rebound rigidity is usually attributable to superficial abdominal wall injury. Tenderness which begins to spread, or is associated with reflex muscle spasm, suggests that peritonitis is developing. Rebound tenderness is a sign of peritonitis, however, release tenderness can also occur over distended gut or in the presence of ruptured muscle tissue.


## 10.4 Nasogastric tubes

Nasogastric tubes have a diagnostic function as well as being a therapeutic aid. For example, aspiration not only empties the stomach (an

# Abdominal injuries

essential prerequisite for anaesthesia), but also allows examination of the aspirate for blood. The tube should not be aspirated before the abdominal X-rays because this removes the stomach air bubble. The site of this may be important in assessing the presence of a splenic haematoma.

## 10.5 Laboratory investigations

### 10.5.1 BLOOD

Blood should always be taken for haematological and biochemical examination in addition to cross-matching. Unexpectedly low haemoglobin and haematocrit levels indicate occult bleeding. White cell counts are unhelpful. Counts of $15\ 000 \times 10^9\ l^{-1}$ and above are common soon after injury. However, a leucocytosis occurring later may indicate peritonitis.

Estimations of urea and electrolytes are required to assess renal function and the intravenous fluid requirement. Serum amylase may be misleading. In pancreatic trauma elevation occurs in only about 70% of cases, even if the pancreas is transected. High values also occur with perforations of the gastrointestinal tract.

### 10.5.2 URINE

Urinalysis is essential. A note must be made of any blood, protein or sugar in the sample.

### 10.5.3 X-RAYS

X-rays are of value, but abdominal exploration may be the priority. The erect posteroanterior chest X-ray gives valuable information about the abdomen. A high diaphragm or displacement of the stomach bubble may indicate the location of a haematoma or mass. Fracture of the lower ribs occurs with rupture of the spleen or liver. The plain supine antero-posterior film of the abdomen may be considered in isolation or together with an erect or lateral decubitus view.

X-rays should be evaluated according to a regular plan. The bony contours should be traced with particular attention to the area of injury. Fractured transverse processes may reveal underlying organ damage. Avulsed spicules of bone should be noted. The size, position and outline of the liver, spleen, kidneys and bladder should always be checked and, in particular, distortion of their contours should be noted. Free gas indicates the rupture of a hollow viscus. This collects under the diaphragm in the erect abdomen, under the lateral abdominal wall in the

166

lateral decubitus view and as a 'dome' sign in the supine view. The gut may appear to have a double wall if there is gas on both sides of it. Retro-peritoneal gas can be detected as localized bubbles adjacent to the line of the duodenum, the rectum or caecum.

A dilated 'sentinel' loop of small bowel, with fluid levels, is seen as a result of localized peritonitis. Bowel is incorporated into the mass which forms about a perforation or organ rupture. Extra-gut fluid levels occur when there is both gas and free fluid within the peritoneal cavity. Intra-gut gas acts as a contrast medium and reveals the characteristic features of normal gut and its position. Occasionally gas may be seen in the biliary tree.

The psoas shadow may be absent when a retroperitoneal haematoma extends over its margins. There will be separation of tissue planes in association with local muscle trauma or in the inflammatory response to extraperitoneal leakage. Gas in the soft tissues must be recognized.

Excretion urography is useful, provided that there is no circulatory collapse and the renal blood flow is adequate. The importance of establishing the presence of a functioning kidney on the opposite side cannot be over-stressed and the examination may also demonstrate extra-vasation of dye or non-functioning renal tissue on the injured side.

Norell first used aortography in 1957 to diagnose a splenic rupture (Norell, 1957). Selective arteriography is much better than the 'high-flush' technique and has been used to establish ruptures of the spleen, kidney, liver, pancreas and duodenum. C.T. scanning and abdominal ultrasound are both used in picking up occult perforations and collections.

## 10.6 Peritoneal lavage

The signs of blunt trauma may develop more slowly and continuous assessment of vital signs is mandatory. Occasionally, and especially in the presence of head injuries, a dilemma arises because the clinician may be uncertain if there is intra-abdominal bleeding, but does not want to perform an unnecessary laparotomy.

Abdominal paracentesis is often unsatisfactory but peritoneal lavage will, in most cases, indicate abdominal injury (Root, Hauser and McKinley, 1965; Olsen and Hildreth, 1971). A dialysis catheter is inserted under local anaesthetic through a small subumbilical mid-line incision. The peritoneum is opened under direct vision and the catheter is inserted without a hazardous blind stab. If blood is withdrawn, then a laparotomy is indicated. If no blood is aspirated, 1 litre of normal saline is run through the catheter. The fluid is now allowed to drain out by gravity and the fluid collected.

## Abdominal injuries

Counts of above 100 000 red cells/mm$^3$ or 500 white cells/mm$^3$, an amylase concentration in excess of 100 Somogyi units per 100 ml or the presence of bile or intestinal contents in the lavage fluid indicates that a formal laparotomy should be performed. More usually the find is grossly contaminated with blood. An accuracy of 90–97% can be obtained. Over half the patients with indeterminate counts have abdominal injuries and one-third of pelvis fractures have a positive result.

Peritoneal lavage should be considered in the presence of serious head injuries or if the patient requires an anaesthetic for another reason, but not if the patient's condition is stable.

## 10.7 Shock

Shock is an acute surgical emergency and demands urgent intravenous colloid or blood replacement and then laparotomy. The patient becomes pale and sweaty, the skin being cold and clammy. The pulse rises to well over a hundred. Blood pressure falls below 100/50 mmHg and the patient may feel anxious and uneasy. Respiratory rate increases until consciousness is lost. Urinary output is a sensitive monitor of renal perfusion and should be recorded on an hourly basis following bladder catheterization.

A fit young subject is initially able to compensate for considerable blood loss with few signs of shock. Cardiac function is excellent and peripheral vasoconstriction is well able to compensate for the diminishing circulating blood volume. This delays the onset of shock. The older patient is less able to compensate and signs of shock develop earlier.

## 10.8 Winding

Immediately after a blow to the abdomen, there is a characteristic response. Winding is often caused by a punch in the 'solar plexus'. It is probably caused by a sudden compression of the stomach and intestines. This acute stretching of smooth muscle gives rise to considerable vagal afferent activity. The subject experiences a characteristic cramping pain. There is a subjective need to gasp for air yet a complete objective inability to do so. There can also be reflex spontaneous defaecation or micturition and occasionally fits of coughing.

## 10.9 Injury to the abdominal wall

It may be difficult to distinguish between injury involving the abdominal wall alone and more serious intra-abdominal pathology. Tenderness and spasm occur routinely after a muscle tear and are easily confused with the tenderness and guarding of peritonitis. A mass associated with a muscle haematoma can be indistinguishable from an intra-abdominal mass.

### 10.9.1  BRUISES AND CONTUSIONS

Bruises are commonest where the pelvis and ribs are immediately under the skin. Any blow over a bony prominence, such as the iliac crest, is arrested immediately. The skin will be bruised or torn, but unless the blow is sufficient to fracture the underlying bony structure, the injury is unlikely to be severe. If there has been a contusion at the point of attachment of muscle to bone there may be disproportionate disability. Any movement involving muscles attached to such a point will cause pain and may delay healing.

Blunt trauma to the muscular areas of the abdomen which do not overlie bone produces an unpredictable result, because of their elasticity and resilience. Even the hardest of blows may be absorbed. When sufficient force is applied to a tightly contracted muscle, there may be bleeding and bruising within the muscle fibres, some disruption of muscle fibres themselves or total disruption of the muscle group.

Contusions can involve skin, subcutaneous fat, muscle and periosteum. Tetanus toxoid should be administered if the skin is broken unless the patient has had a booster dose within the previous three years. Grazes which are contaminated with mud must be scrupulously cleaned since this may be associated with clostridial infection.

Mild muscle contusions are treated by applying ice-packs and compression. Later, heat may be applied and long acting local anaesthetic with hyaluronidase injected to give relief from pain and to prevent later adhesion formation. The area should be protected against further injury with padding.

### 10.9.2  MUSCLE TEARS

The rectus muscle is the commonest to be injured and may be associated with a number of well defined symptoms and signs. It is usually contracted against a force (as in a tennis player serving the ball) and this alone may be enough to tear muscle fibres. The added force of the racquet hitting the ball may complete the tear. If, at the same time, the abdomen

169

is hit by a ball, or other extraneous force, tearing may be worsened.

Tears may be partial or complete. Partial tears are associated with localized swelling at the site of the injury. Ability to use the muscle may be retained, but will give considerable pain. If there is an abdominal mass which is palpable when the patient tenses his rectus muscle and which ceases to be mobile when the rectus is tensed (Bouchacourt's sign), this indicates that the mass is within the abdominal wall. Complete tears may be associated with retraction of muscle and this may also appear as a mass.

Bleeding may occur from small arteries within the rectus muscle, but occasionally bleeding occurs from the inferior epigastric vessels and this can lead to hypovolaemia and shock. The posterior rectus sheath is absent below the arcuate line, which explains why blood tracking behind the sheath irritates the peritoneum in the lower one-third and this mimics peritonitis. Bruising is unlikely to be seen unless the anterior rectus sheath has been breached.

If there is any doubt whatever about the nature of such a haematoma, or if it is thought that the underlying pathology is being masked, it is safer to explore. Provided the haematoma is small, a conservative approach may be adopted with bed-rest and local heat. If the haematoma is larger, or if it is suspected that epigastric arteries are involved, the rectus sheath should be opened as for a paramedian incision. The haematoma is evacuated and the bleeding points ligated.

## 10.10 Injury to the abdominal contents

### 10.10.1 THE SPLEEN

The spleen is the most commonly injured intra-abdominal organ (Dickerman and Dunn, 1981). In health it lies under the left costal margin, protected by the dome of the diaphragm and the lower ribs. Direct blunt trauma may be sufficient to rupture it without fracturing the ribs. If, however, the overlying ribs are broken, rupture of the spleen is more likely. Spontaneous ruptures of the spleen may occur. Violent pressure changes in the abdominal cavity, such as occur with vomiting or straining, can be enough to cause rupture. The spleen is more vulnerable when enlarged, for example due to infective mononucleosis (Alberty, 1981). Thalassaemia, some haemoglobinopathies, viral infections and thrombocytopenic purpura, are all causes of splenic enlargement. Splenomegaly is an absolute contraindication to participation in contact sports.

Splenic rupture may lead to catastrophic haemorrhage and death within minutes (especially in the presence of splenomegaly). A period of initial shock is usually followed by recovery and low blood pressure, together with the confining omentum, prevents further bleeding. When the resulting splenic mass bursts shock is profound. There is tenderness, possibly with bruising and skin marking over the point of impact and in the left hypochondrium. Abdominal rigidity may be marked and localized to the left hypochondrium. Kehr's sign will be positive. This can also be induced by elevating the foot of the bed. Shifting dullness in the right flank, constant dullness in the left flank, is due to a left sided mass composed of coagulated blood and omentum, and free blood in the right flank (Ballence's sign). The abdomen may be observed to distend as a paralytic ileus develops. Presentation of a splenic rupture may be delayed for up to several days but sometimes even longer.

A chest X-ray may show an indentation of the left side of the stomach together with fractures of the lower ribs. Elevation of the left cupola of the diaphragm may be present. An abdominal X-ray may show no splenic outline and the psoas shadow may be obliterated. Occasionally free fluid can be detected between gas filled loops of intestine. Ultrasound and C.T. scanning are of value in the diagnosis.

Resuscitation initially consists of intravenous replacement with blood, or, if not immediately available, with Hemacel or Dextran. Splenectomy is the safest procedure to control haemorrhage after splenic rupture; although splenic repair operations have been advocated (Sherman, 1981). After splenectomy, the patient is susceptible to septicaemia, typically due to infection with penumococcus or salmonella organisms. Sudden death from disseminated intravascular coagulation may complicate the infection (Francke and Neu, 1981; Ferguson, 1982). The family practitioner must be aware of the patient's susceptibility to rapidly fulminating infection. Long-term penicillin therapy should be considered. In unexplained fever antibiotic therapy should be started immediately after blood cultures have been taken.

## 10.10.2 THE PANCREAS

The pancreas is seldom injured in sport, and diagnosis may be difficult. It lies immediately anterior to the thoracic spine behind the peritoneum. Any pressure which pushes the anterior abdominal wall towards the spine may transect the pancreas (Dickerman and Dunn, 1981). There may be an associated splenic rupture. Pancreatic injury may be difficult to diagnose because the organ is retroperitoneal and rupture gives rise to few physical signs. Indeed, the injury may not be noted at all until a pseudocyst of the pancreas later develops.

Amylase levels are elevated in most cases, though the rise may not occur immediately. Persistent elevation suggests pseudocyst formation. If pancreatic trauma is suspected, its localization and extent can be determined by ultrasound, C.T. scanning, and endoscopic retrograde cholangiopancreatography (E.R.C.P.). Urgent laparotomy may be required to control haemorrhage of the pancreas and may entail the excision of dead tissue or the suture of smaller lacerations. Pseudocysts and pancreatic abscesses may be found and should be drained into the stomach.

### 10.10.3  THE DUODENUM AND BOWEL

In duodenal trauma there is frequently delay in diagnosis as the injury is often thought to be trivial (Moncur, 1973). There is epigastric pain which may radiate to the right iliac fossa. Nausea and vomiting may occur. On examination the epigastrium is tender and the patient may be shocked. Blood examination will reveal raised bilirubin and amylase levels. The abdominal X-ray may show air in the retroperitoneal space. It has been postulated that the duodenum can perforate after only minimal blunt force because a blind loop of bowel can be excluded and compressed to the right side of the spine (Cooke and Meyer, 1964). Unless duodenal rupture is specifically looked for at laparotomy, the condition will be missed and the mortality rate can rise to as much as 70%.

Injuries to the intestines may involve tears at the points where the retroperitoneum confines the bowel. The rectum is occasionally injured as a result of high pressure injection of water during water-skiing, or in direct blunt trauma in the perineal region (Morton, 1970; Tweedale, 1973). Damage is usually below the peritoneal reflection and can be treated by primary repair in expert hands.

### 10.10.4  THE LIVER

The liver, though well protected by the upper dome of the diaphragm and ribs, is still commonly injured (Dickerman and Dunn, 1981). Rupture may present with the same features on the right side as the spleen produces on the left. If hepatic rupture is suspected, early laparotomy is indicated.

### 10.10.5  THE ANUS

The anus is a frequent site of trouble in sportsmen. Excessive sweating in the perineal region, together with poor hygiene, can lead to pruritis ani or to infections of the skin. In cyclists this is known as saddle sore. Fungal infections of the anus are also common in sportsmen and local irritation may be exacerbated by the soft stool of the beer drinker. Scrupulous hygiene must be encouraged and infections treated appropriately.

## 10.11  Abdominal trauma in different sports

### 10.11.1  TEAM GAMES (RUGBY FOOTBALL AND SOCCER)

Abdominal injuries depend on the quality of bodily contact. A rugby player is more likely to rupture a spleen than a soccer player because there is much more violent physical connection in the appropriate anatomical area. Abdominal trauma in rugby accounts for about 3% of all injuries. J. P. Sparks at Rugby School has published his statistics of injuries accrued during half a million hours of rugby football, over a period of thirty years (Sparks, 1981). In a total of 9885 injuries there were only two ruptured spleens, four ruptured kidneys and nine contused scrota. This represents 0.2% of all injuries.

O'Connell's statistics (see the section on further reading) shown in Table 10.1 show an incidence of 2.5% of abdominal injuries in a sample of 600 injuries. Unfortunately the sample of abdominal injuries (15 patients) allows only general observations about precipitating factors. Injuries occur more frequently towards the end of a game as players get tired. Foul play is often the cause of trauma. Certain players are more prone to injury than others and the full-back position is most at risk.

Table 10.1  Incidence of abdominal injuries in rugby players (O'Connell)

| Injury | Number in sample | % |
|---|---|---|
| Ruptured spleen | 4 | 0.66 |
| Ruptured liver | 1 | 0.16 |
| Ruptured kidney | 1 | 0.16 |
| Rectus muscle tear | 2 | 0.33 |
| Strangulated hernia | 1 | 0.16 |
| Testicular bruise | 2 | 0.33 |
| Scrotal tears | 2 | 0.33 |
| Foreskin tears | 1 | 0.16 |
| Ruptured urethra | 1 | 0.16 |
| Overall | 15 | 2.50 |

It is remarkable how often soccer players are winded and yet it is rare that serious intra-abdominal damage is sustained. Again, certain players may be most at risk. The goalkeeper, as he stretches for the difficult ball, will be unprotected and vulnerable.

The team physician must be confident about his diagnosis and treat-

173

# Abdominal injuries

ment of the player injured on the field. It is dangerous to allow a player to finish a match if the integrity of his viscera is in doubt.

## 10.11.2 COMBAT SPORTS

McLatchie has reported illustrative cases which are typical of serious abdominal injury in combat sports (McLatchie, 1980, 1981). A woman with a subcapsular liver haematoma required surgery six weeks after injury to evacuate the haematoma. Two patients presented with profound shock having sustained splenic ruptures after round-house kicks. Splenectomy was performed on both. McLatchie reported a case of acute traumatic pancreatitis with an amylase of over 12 000 i.u. and with recovery after conservative management.

## 10.11.3 EQUESTRIAN INJURIES

McLatchie has carried out a prospective study of equestrian injuries in one geographical area presenting at one casualty department (McLatchie, 1979). There were 115 injuries of which 5% were visceral and included two ruptured spleens and one ruptured liver.

No matter how rigorous the rules and how intense the supervision there will inevitably be intra-abdominal injuries. Records should be kept in each case to ensure that adequate safety precautions have been maintained and to act as a reference back for future assessment.

The possibility of other disease processes presenting in the guise of a 'sports' injury should be remembered. Children will often date the pain associated with a torsion of the testis to a fall astride a bike. The abdominal pain which is related to a blow in the abdomen may have quite a different cause.

## References

Adams, I. D. (1977) Rugby football injuries. *Brit J. Sports Med.*, **11**, 1, 4.

Alberty, R. (1981) Surgical implications of infective mononucleosis. *Amer. J. Surg.*, **151**, 559.

Cooke, W. M. Jr and Meyer, K. K. (1964) Retroperitoneal duodenal rupture. *Amer. J. Surg.*, **108**, 834.

Dickerman, R. M. and Dunn, E. L. (1981) Splenic, pancreatic and hepatic injuries. *Surg. Clin. N. Amer.*, **61**, 1.

Ferguson, A. (1982) Hazards of hyposplenism. *Brit. Med. J.*, **285**, 375.

Francke, E. L. and Neu, H. C. (1981) Post splenectomy infections. *Surg. Clin. N. Amer.*, **61**, 1, 135.

# References

McLatchie, G. R. (1979) Equestrian injuries. A one year prospective survey. *Brit. J. Sports Med.*, **13**, 29.

McLatchie, G. R. (1980) Injuries in karate. A case for medical control. *J. Trauma*, **20**, 11, 956.

McLatchie, G. R. (1981) Karate and karate injuries. *Brit. J. Sports Med.*, **15**, 1, 84.

Moncur, J. (1973) Fatal football injury – ruptured duodenal diverticulum. *Brit. J. Sports Med.*, **7**, 162.

Morton, R. C. (1970) Gynaecological complications of water skiing. *Med. J. Aust.*, **2**, 1256.

Norell, H. G. (1957) Traumatic rupture of the spleen diagnosed by selective arteriography. *Acta Radiol.*, **48**, 449.

Olsen, W. R. and Hildreth, D. H. (1971) Abdominal paracentesis and peritoneal lavage in blunt abdominal trauma. *J. Trauma*, **11**, 824.

Root, H. D., Hauser, G. W. and McKinley, C. R. (1965) Diagnostic peritoneal lavage. *Surgery*, **57**, 633.

Sherman, R. (1981) Rationale for methods of splenic preservation following trauma. *Surg. Clin. N. Amer.*, **61**, 1, 127.

Sparks, J. D. (1981) Half a million hours of rugby football. *Brit. J. Sports Med.*, **15**, 1, 30.

Tweedale, P. G. (1973) Vaginal laceration in water-skiers. *Can. Med. Assoc. J.*, **108**, 20.

Walkden, L. (1981) Immediate management of injuries, *Brit. J. Sports Med.*, **15**, No. 68.

## Further reading

Symposium on liver, spleen and pancreas. *Surg. Clin. N. Amer.*, **61**, No. 1, February, 1981.

Symposium on trauma. *Surg. Clin. N. Amer.*, **62**, No. 1, February, 1982.

O'Connell, T. C. J. *Injuries in Rugby Football and Other Team Sports*. Published by the Irish Rugby Football Union.

# 11 Sportswomen – gynaecological and other aspects

MIKE EMENS

The obstetrician is in a unique position of being able to observe the very nature of a woman's specific function, that of bearing and rearing the young, and, despite all claims to the contrary this is fundamentally her biological role, whereas for the male it is the protection and support and provision of the family unit. In work-sharing societies, of which homosapiens offers the highest example, these clear-cut divisions of labour may be to some degree obscured. This is a matter of quiet convenience rather than in-built necessity.

Sport, historically, derives from the preparation of male members of society for the essentially and traditionally masculine roles of hunting and fighting. It comes as no surprise, therefore that the majority of sports, based as they are on primitive training rituals for the chase and war, seek to glorify characteristics which we recognize in nature as particularly masculine. This is not necessarily to deny women fleetness of foot nor strength of arm. In classical mythology, Atlanta and Hippolyte respectively offer examples of appropriate female athleticism but nevertheless they were regarded as the exception rather than the rule.

It is only recently that with the growth of organization in society a degree of role reversal has become possible today. There has been a huge increase in the numbers of women participating in a wide range of sports and along with this there has been some acceptance of this fact by the largely masculine ruling bodies. In 1970 only one woman entered the New York City marathon – and she did not finish the race. In 1980 2578 women entered that marathon and 1621 ran the distance! This is an impressive upsurge of participation in an activity once considered too strenuous for the allegedly weaker sex.

There is still, however, much resistance from society in general, often due to an unwillingness of spectators to be confronted by women involved in what is traditionally an unfeminine situation. Rightly or wrongly, society in general does not like to see its womenfolk sweaty and bedraggled, caked in mud, black of eye or bloody in nose. What is

177

# Sportswomen – gynaecological and other aspects

acceptable in some societies is not universally acceptable. Though social concepts change and evolve, Western society has traditionally extended to its women a peculiar code of courtesy and consideration based essentially upon the acceptance that women cannot compete with men on equal terms across the board. It is this recognition that women would be at a positive disadavantage in open competition with men in many fields of life – not the least of which is sport – that has led to the parallel development of women's sport as a separate entity. What price then women's liberation and where do women find their place in sport?

## 11.1 Sex characteristics

The normal female has 46 chromosomes, 44 autosomal and XX. The male sex chromosomes are XY. There are a variety of chromosomal abnormalities, among them Klinefelter's syndrome XXY, Turner's syndrome XO and XXX, the so-called 'super female'. Individuals may also have a mosaic pattern, the cells containing chromosomes which have developed from two or more stem lines. All females competing in the Olympic Games and in international competitions must undergo a sex test. Problems arise if an individual has an unexpected chromosome abnormality, for example the rare testicular feminizing syndrome when the individual has XY sex chromosomes and has testes but looks and acts as a female.

## 11.2 Anatomical differences from males

Women tend to be smaller and lighter than males and have a lower centre of gravity. The female pelvis differs from that of the male in many particulars and the distinctive sex characteristics are already present in the fetal pelvis by the third or fourth month of intrauterine life. The female pelvis is wider in all its diameters, particularly the inferior aspect. The pelvic cavity is rounder, roomier, shorter and less funnel-shaped than that of the male; the sacrum is shorter, wider and less curved; the subpubic angles are greater than 90° in the female. The acetabulum is smaller in the female but the distance between the acetabulum and the pubic symphysis is greater, thus increasing the width of the pelvis.

Because of the wider pelvis in the female there is a greater tendency to genu valgum, or knock-knees. The normal pull of the quadriceps tends to pull the patella laterally, a tendency magnified by the wider pelvis and chondromalacia patellae is relatively common. Thomas (1974) suggests that the relationship between the width of hips and running speed is low and should not be an inhibiting factor. The shoulders are narrower and

178

the bones of the upper limbs are shorter in the female. The carrying angle measured when the forearm is fully extended, the hand is supinated and the forearm is directed laterally, is 167° in the female and 173° in the male. The angle disappears on flexion of the elbow but is a disadvantage to females in throwing events.

The average female has twice as much measurable fat as the average male (de Vries, 1981), 20 to 25% for females compared to 10 to 14% for males. There is also a wide variation amongst trained female athletes. Novak et al. (1977) found swimmers to have relatively more fat, 18% more, than runners and gymnasts. It is well documented that the trained female has relatively less fat than normal sedentary controls. The relationship of percentage body fat and the maintenance of the normal menstrual cycle will be discussed later. The greater average relative fat of females compared to males has been proposed as one of the factors responsible for the sex differences and distance running performances (Wilmore, Brown and Davis, 1977). In swimming, sex differences and body composition tend to be advantageous, the reduction in body drag leading to less energy expenditure per unit of distance swum (Prendergast et al., 1974).

Although there are numerous references to structural and functional changes in the heart of male athletes there is little information on the female athlete. It is known that females have smaller hearts than males and this is reflected in their smaller left ventricular mass, left ventricular dimensions and stroke volume. However from studies involving a variety of athletic participants (Zeldis, Morganroth and Rubler, 1978; Rerych et al., 1980) it would seem that women adapt to training in a similar manner to males. More recent work (Rubal, Rosentsweig and Hamerly, 1981) has shown significant differences between moderately enduranced, conditioned games players and their controls, with changes in favour of the athletes in left ventricular and diastolic dimension, diastolic volume, total left ventricular volume, left ventricular muscle volume and muscle mass.

## 11.3  Iron metabolism

There are marked differences in the number of red blood cells, haemoglobin concentration and blood volume in males and females. Blood volume and Hb differences are approximately 25% in untrained populations and 12% in trained athletes in favour of the male. Menstruating females experience greater losses of body iron than the average male. Serum iron levels are lower in trained women athletes than in their sedentary counterparts. Serum iron levels decrease only if iron lost exceeds storage. Iron losses appear to be associated with training. However some subjects may have sufficient storage iron to absorb

179

training effects (Writh *et al.*, 1978). For the haemoglobin level to fall there has to be an advanced stage of serum iron deficiency. This has been demonstrated with athletes who have exhibited a normal haemoglobin level during intensive training with a corresponding low serum iron (Strauzenberg and Kabner, 1980). These investigators advocate iron supplementation of the female athletes.

## 11.4  Menstruation

One clear disadvantage that women have in comparison with their male athletic counterparts is the monthly phenomenon of menstruation. The effects of menstruation on the individual subject may vary enormously. If there are any abnormalities in the pathway involving the hypothalamus (Fig. 11.1), pituitary, ovary and uterus problems may arise. These may result in irregular, infrequent, or even in the absence of periods.

Many factors may be responsible for dysfunction. Age is an important factor. In the young pubertal woman anovulatory and irregular cycles are normal. In 5% of girls the menstrual loss is heavy and prolonged. If

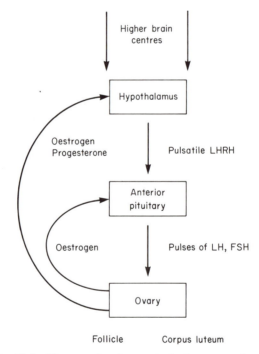

*Fig. 11.1*  Neuroendocrine control of menstrual cycle.

menstrual bleeding remains excessive for more than a few months it should be investigated and treated by appropriate hormone therapy.

In the adult female dysfunctional uterine bleeding is the commonest abnormality. This means abnormal uterine bleeding due to oestrogen/progesterone aberrations for reasons not known. This term may only be applied after exclusion of systemic disease, infection, foreign body (e.g., intrauterine contraceptive device, I.U.D.) or tumour.

### 11.4.1   PATTERNS OF DYSFUNCTIONAL BLEEDING

There are a number of typical clinical presentations of abnormal menstrual bleeding: (a) A normal regular cycle with excessive loss (menorrhagia). This is more common in women over thirty who have had children. (b) Normal menstruation occurring too often (epimenorrhoea). This is usually caused by a shortening of the luteal phase, due to early degeneration of the corpus luteum and may occur in the younger woman. (c) Menstrual bleeding lasting too long with spotting or bleeding at inappropriate times (metropathia).

### (a)   Amenorrhoea

Amenorrhoea means absence of menstrual bleeding. It is called primary amenorrhoea if the patient has never menstruated and it is helpful to distinguish this from secondary amenorrhoea which follows a period of more or less normal menstruation. However, most causes of amenorrhoea can apply to either type. If a woman has not menstruated by the time she is eighteen her condition should be investigated. There are many causes of amenorrhoea but pregnancy is by far the commonest cause and must always be considered first in any female aged twelve to fifty.

### (b)   Psychological factors: stress

Any type of stress can act on the hypothalamus to inhibit GnRH releasing hormone secretion although some menstrual irregularity, oligomenorrhoea (very scanty periods) is more usual than complete amenorrhoea. Women athletes involved in distance running, particularly where they are training more than 48 km (30 miles) a week, are more prone to menstrual irregularities. Training is a stress factor.

Severe fasting, leading to emaciation, is a problem associated with a rejection by the female of the responsibilities of adulthood as well as a rejection of the associated problems of female sexuality. Anorexics need expert psychiatric advice.

Finally, there are a variety of endocrine disorders which may be responsible for amenorrhoea. These involve diseases and tumours of pituitary, thyroid, adrenal and ovarian organs and are beyond the scope

181

of this chapter. Genetic and chromosomal abnormalities are also causal factors.

The stopping of oral contraception, usually with a view to pregnancy, is sometimes followed by amenorrhoea for a year or more. Usually no treatment is required in these patients, but they occasionally require investigation if they wish to become pregnant.

Any subject with amenorrhoea should be investigated until a cause is found and the patient advised or treated accordingly.

### 11.4.2 TREATMENT OF DYSFUNCTIONAL UTERINE BLEEDING

The root cause of dysfunctional bleeding is often psychological and no treatment aimed at the uterus will cure the patient. Also there is a tendency, especially in the younger woman, towards a spontaneous return to a normal cycle. The patient should be investigated to exclude systemic disease, including a blood examination and if possible estimation of pituitary hormones. Endometrium should be obtained for examination to eliminate organic disease by curettage under general anaesthesia (D and C) or by an outpatient method requiring neither anaesthesia or cervical dilatation, for example, Vabra curettage. This is where a sample of endometrium is obtained by suction through the cervix by a fine curette the size of a drinking straw.

Once the diagnosis is certain it is usual to attempt medical treatment which will improve the condition and allow time for spontaneous cure. Anaemia, if present, should be corrected by iron supplements. In the younger women oestrogen/progesterone combinations such as oral contraceptives are probably the best treatment for dysfunctional bleeding. Prostaglandin inhibitors such as aspirin, naproxen or Ponstan, are also helpful when given during the menstrual period for reducing blood loss and discomfort.

### 11.4.3 DYSMENORRHOEA

Dysmenorrhoea implies pain during menstruation and most women experience some degree of pain at least on the first day of their period when the loss is heaviest. Some authors report more dysmenorrhoea among athletes, others less. Explanations on either side are conjectural. The causes of dysmenorrhoea are complex but they are probably related to prostaglandin release within the myometrium. Many women will also describe varying sorts of discomfort before the period starts but this symptom should be regarded as a manifestation of the premenstrual tension syndrome. The pain may be secondary to organic disease such as endometriosis or infection but primary dysmenorrhoea which is being discussed here occurs in the presence of a normal genital tract.

Pain is usually described as having two components. A continuous lower abdominal pain attributed to vascular congestion which radiates through to the back and sometimes down the thighs and an intermittent cramping pain. Primary dysmenorrhoea is commoner in the young, nulliparous girl, usually between sixteen and twenty-six, and it may produce considerable disability at the time of her periods, at work or school, and total inability to train. There is no characteristic personality or physique in the woman who suffers from dysmenorrhoea. Childbirth does not abolish dysmenorrhoea but may reduce its severity.

Pain is a subjective experience and its perception is highly variable. Generally, however, athletic and otherwise active women are less disabled by pain than are sedentary women. The selfdiscipline and pain tolerance developed during athletic training could explain this finding as could the athlete's innate resistance to pain or her diminished perception of it – perhaps because activity is distracting. Whatever the reason, exercise offers short- and long-term benefits to women who experience dysmenorrhoea. Primary drug treatment includes most prostaglandin inhibitors as already described for menorrhagia. The contraceptive pill is also extremely effective in dysmenorrhoea as this is very unlikely to occur in the absence of ovulation, probably because of the pseudo-atrophy of the endometrium.

## 11.4.4 THE PREMENSTRUAL SYNDROME

The premenstrual syndrome is a term describing a group of symptoms which occur in some women, usually during the pre-menstrual phase of the cycle. A vast number of symptoms have been described with varying degrees of severity. The average age of patients seen suffering with the syndrome is thirty-five years, but it can also be incapacitating in the younger woman. The symptoms can either be physical or psychological, the most common being headache, depression, irritability, breast swelling and tenderness, loss of concentration, abdominal bloating, lethargy, swelling of fingers and ankles, and anxiety.

A large number of hypotheses have been put forward as to the causation of the syndrome but unfortunately it continues to be an enigma. Most of the recent research on the topic would suggest a slight abnormality in hormones which control the menstrual cycle.

As stated earlier the symptoms can vary in severity from being unpleasant to incapacitating. This is therefore bound to have an effect on the woman's personality and efficiency. This in turn can lead to a disruption in the family and also of relationships with friends.

# Sportswomen – gynaecological and other aspects

The effect that the syndrome has on women has been studied in detail. Dalton (1960a) showed that in a survey of 124 women, 84 of whom menstruated regularly, 44 were involved in an accident during menstruation or the four days before menstruation. This accident proneness occurred not only at home, but on the road and in factories while women were performing routine actions. She suggested that the increased lethargy during the premenstrual phase and menstruation was responsible for both a lowered judgement and slow reaction time.

Dalton (1960b) has also shown that schoolgirls have a deterioration in work and an increase in forgetfulness and non-punctuality during menstruation. Dalton (1968), studying the examination results, also showed that the results were lower in both O- and A-level examinations when these were taken in the premenstrual phase or during menstruation.

Psychiatric admissions and the number of suicide attempts are also known to be increased during the premenstruum (Glass et al., 1971).

In view of the lethargy, loss of concentration and clumsiness associated with the syndrome, it would not appear, therefore, to be the optimum time for performing tasks which require a certain amount of dexterity or concentration, this being particularly relevant to the skilled athlete.

There has been some work published on the relationship between physical exercise and the premenstrual syndrome, and also in relation to dysmenorrhoea. Timonen and Procopé (1971) studied 748 female university students with the aid of questionnaires. It was shown that a sport had a favourable effect, especially for the various symptoms of tension, e.g., irritability, anxiety, headache and depression, etc. The finger and ankle swelling, and breast tenderness showed no benefit whatsoever. In comparison, gymnasts did not obtain as much relief from their symptoms.

Dysmenorrhoea was far less frequent among the athletes than among the gymnasts, the difference however being not as large as for the premenstrual syndrome. This study showed interestingly that the incidence of premenstrual pain is not affected by the practice of sports. Ingman (1953) has also reported a favourable effect of sports in fourteen cases of dysmenorrhoea in a series of 107 athletes. More recent work by Shangold (1981) confirmed the above work and also reported that muscular co-ordination was poorer just before and during menstruation.

There is, however, much difference of opinion regarding the effect on athletic performance by the premenstrual syndrome and menses. Dividing the menstrual cycle into four weekly phases is convenient but does not reflect accurately the hormonal changes. Dalton (1977) used the seven phases illustrated in Fig. 11.2. Matthews (1980) has summarized some of Dalton's work and also added some information regarding training

184

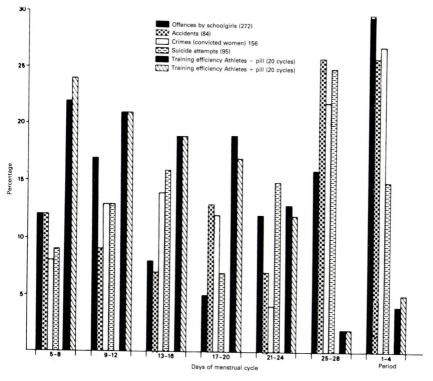

*Fig. 11.2* Cyclical influence of menstruation.

efficiency which was based on a single cycle recorded by 40 international track and field athletes who were asked to score their daily training on a menstrual chart with a score of 2 for good, 1 for average and 0 for bad. Twenty were using oral contraceptives and these were matched with twenty who were not. The scores for each day were added up and expressed as a percentage of the total. The pre menstruum and menstruation scored the lowest marks and the preovulatory phases the highest. There were no significant differences between the two groups (Fig. 11.2).

Figure 11.3 approaches the subject in a slightly different way. A total of 61 international athletes were asked to mark the days on which they would 'most like to compete' and the days on which they would 'least like to compete'. Statistical analysis is not possible because some girls marked only one or two days and others as many as twenty. Nevertheless it has some merit as an illustrative exercise. Of the 1708 days covered 602 were good, 341 bad and 765 not mentioned at all. The favourite was day 5 and the one to be avoided was day 1 closely followed by days 28 and 27. Of the

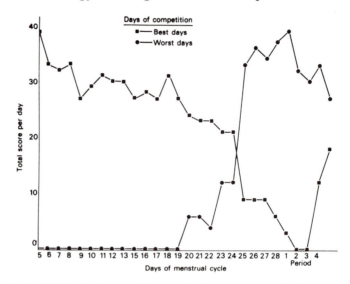

*Fig. 11.3*  Athletes' choice of days in their menstrual cycle for competition.

total, 39 girls were taking oral contraceptives and 22 were not. As there was little difference in the pattern they were grouped together.

*(a) Treatment*

Treatment of the premenstrual syndrome is empirical and three drugs are at present commonly used. Progestogens are usually given in the second half of the cycle. Drugs such as dydrogesterone (Duphaston) 10 mg, twice daily, or norethisterone (Primolut N) 5 mg, daily, can be given in tablet form. The response to progesterones is extremely variable but on balance appears to be beneficial. Pyridoxine (vitamin B6) can be given at a dose of 100 mg on a daily basis and appears in some women to exert a beneficial effect but has the clear advantage of having very few, if any, side effects. The logic behind its use is that endogenous depression is accompanied by reduced brain 5-hydroxytryptamine as a result of disordered tryptophan metabolism and pyridoxine is supposed to correct this.

Oral contraceptives have certainly revolutionized the treatment of premenstrual syndrome, particularly in the younger girl, and currently about 80% of international athletes use the pill. Over half of these are using the pill for menstrual regulation and not for contraceptive purposes. Matthews' work has shown that although the premenstrual discomfort and the loss itself are reduced, it is the predictability of the period that counts.

## 11.4.5 SHOULD THE MENSTRUAL CYCLE BE ADJUSTED?

Many consider hormonal manipulation of the menstrual cycle is imprudent, and that the side effects of the drugs themselves are as deleterious as those caused by the menstrual cycle (Wearing *et al.*, 1972). Other authors consider the giving of oestrogen and progesterone combinations may be associated with impaired control when these hormones are withdrawn (Shangold, 1981). Like Matthews (1980) I feel that whatever the truth may be the athletes now appear to have decided the issue themselves. As yet no sinister results have been published or even forecast. Anecdotal evidence points to the fact that a majority of pill-taking athletes are much happier both with the effects of the pill and the predictability of menstruation. It is simply one factor less to worry about. A further percentage of athletes who consider their performance is affected by menstruation of any type, whether a withdrawal bleed or natural, suppress menstruation by taking continuous oral contraception for three or four months during the peak season. Occasional withdrawal bleeding which may occur during this regimen is usually scanty, free from symptoms and does not affect performance. Athletes with dysmenorrhoea in particular benefit from a few months absence of menstruation and may well be free from dysmenorrhoea when menses are resumed.

Following continuous suppression by hormones normal menstruation usually restarts within a couple of months. However, if menstruation is delayed longer than six months a five day course of clomiphene will stimulate the hypothalamus and restart the cycle so that menstruation may be expected after a three week interval. Those who stop hormone therapy and are anxious to conceive should be advised to start recording their early morning temperatures to discover whether they have ovular or anovular cycles; if the latter then clomiphene is again indicated even though the menstruation may be regular. Non-athletic patients on continuous therapy may report the gradual development of loss of libido. This does not seem to be the experience with athletes. As regards the legality of taking progestogens – although they are testosterone analogues there is no objection to their use, either alone or in the contraceptive pill in competitive sport. They may well possibly be added to the list of drugs banned to competing sportswomen in the future.

## 11.4.6 THE EFFECTS OF TRAINING ON THE MENSTRUAL CYCLE

The effect that sport and training have on the menstrual cycle is equally controversial. Some investigators have reported a higher incidence of menstrual irregularity among athletes than among non-athletes but most of these studies overlooked pretraining menstrual patterns. Obviously, irregular menses cannot be blamed on exercise if there was irregularity before the training commenced. Shangold (1981) reports the survey of the 1841 women who entered the 1979 New York marathon and indicated that exercise did not appear to be the cause of oligomenorrhoea or amenorrhoea in most of the 394 respondents. In this sample most of those who had a regular menses before training reported continued regularity while training, and most who had been oligomenorrhoeic or amenorrhoeic before remained so during training. Bausenwein (1960) and others observed that girls who started intensive training before the menarche later showed a higher percentage of menstrual disorders than those who started after puberty. Erdelyi (1962) agrees with Shangold and noted that menstrual disorders in general remained unchanged in 85% of athletes, improved in 5.6% and deteriorated in 9.3%. She also noted that dysmenorrhoea was the most common complaint and this improved in most athletes other than those involved in swimming and other water sports.

Frisch *et al.* (1981), in a study of 400 track, field and cross country college athletes, found an association between the weekly training mileage and the incidence of amenorrhoea. Amenorrhoea occurred in 43% of the 'high mileage' girls and in only 6% of the 'low mileage'. None of these subjects were taking oral contraceptives. It was agreed that stress was probably the causal factor. Increasingly intensive training could lead to both better performance and more stress which in turn could cause the amenorrhoea. These authors have a long term programme for the study of the relation and possible cause of exercise and menstrual abnormalities. Their recent report clearly shows the age of the menarche and the subsequent menstrual cyclicity is influenced by the age at which the individual begins intensive athletic training. There seems to be a delay of 0.4 months per year of training. Dale, Gerlach and Wilhite (1979) compared runners (more than 48 km (30 miles) a week) with joggers (8 to 48 km (5 to 30 miles) a week) and with non-runner controls. More menstrual irregularity occurred in the runners, 34%, and in the joggers 23% who nevertheless had a significantly higher incidence of irregularity than did the non-runners, 4%. This report again suggests that the degree in frequency of menstrual dysfunction is directly proportional to the level of physical exertion as judged by the miles run per week. The Dale group also found that the runners are significantly lower in body weight for height and with less body fat than the non-runners. Investigators suggest that these factors correlated with the runners' oligomenorrhoea or amenorrhoea.

Several different problems may lead to menstrual irregularity in many athletes, but two main clinical pictures emerge. In one the subject has a hormonal pattern similar to that of women in the early follicular phase of the cycle with low oestrogen levels. In the other the pattern resembles that of women in the late follicular phase but with oestrogens higher but still in the normal range. Women with very low weight, low body fat, low nutritional status or combinations of these are subject to hypo-oestrogenic amenorrhoea resulting from inadequate gonadotrophin stimulation. Amenorrhoeic athletes of very low weight, low body fat or both often have depressed oestrogen levels. The cause could be exercise alone or could involve emotional stress of training and competing, weight loss, low weight, insufficient body fat or a combination of all three. The task of separating and analysing these variables is complex and it is difficult to pinpoint specific causes. This problem may thus resemble a condition observed in patients with anorexia nervosa. Anorexic patients revert to pre- and mid-pubertal gonadotrophin secretion patterns. The abnormal patterns that characterize this condition often resolve when the psychiatric problem is corrected and the patient gains weight.

Chronic stress can also produce a syndrome of anovulatory amenorrhoea marked by normal oestrogen levels resembling those of the late follicular phase. This condition may be similar to the polycystic ovary syndrome (PCO) which is also distinguished by anovulation. In this syndrome the ovaries, adrenals or both secrete excessive androgens. This surplus induces a self-perpetuating cycle of chronic anovulation with continuous production of androgens and oestrogens. The surfeit of hormones activates a positive feedback mechanism that signals the pituitary to respond with non-stop production of LH.

The analogous stress-induced anovulatory amenorrhoea in athletes is not completely understood but it seems that the LH surge is inhibited by some neurological endocrine influence. However, as with stress-related hypo-oestrogenic amenorrhoea, the cause could be exercise alone, the emotional stress of training and competing, weight loss, low weight, low body fat or combinations of these.

Shangold (1981) issues a warning in her article that although anovulation and hypo-oestrogenism may be very common in athletes the cause of these conditions should not be overlooked and that athletes and non-athletes should be evaluated with equal fairness and it should never be assumed that because a woman is an athlete her amenorrhoea is exercise-related. Colt, Wardlaw and Frantz (1981) have recently explained one possibility of the shortening of the length of the luteal phase: a decrease in plasma progesterone, to be associated with the increased secretion of beta endorphin. Beta endorphin is associated with hypoprolactinaemia and decreased LH. Although Colt and his colleagues dispute the fact that the small increase in beta endorphin levels in the peripheral circulation could result in euphoria, this seems to be to be a non-sequitur. It would certainly seem to be an obvious explanation of the 'high' that is felt after completing a particularly arduous training schedule.

## 11.5 Anabolic steroids

The taking of drugs by athletes has had a long and colourful history going back into Roman times. The use of anabolic steroids is a relatively recent problem which has come to plague our sport. The first use of these drugs to induce weight gain in athletes rather than in undernourished or anorexic patients is attributed to the body builders of California. Unconfirmed reports of their use by certain heavyweight event athletes from the USA were circulating in 1960 and by the Olympics of 1964 many large competitors had become not only larger but very much more aggressive. Records in the men's field events were broken with great frequency. From 1966 more and more British athletes began to experiment with steroids. One of the typical explanations given by an athlete confessing that he had taken drugs is that he was 'just experimenting', always against his better judgement!

Up until 1968 the world women athletes, and in particular the British women athletes, were relatively innocent. In the last decade there has been a great upsurge of female sporting success in East Germany and a slower rise in West Germany. Discussions with defectors from East Germany, both athletes, scientists and doctors of sports medicine have shown that the use of anabolic steroids and other drugs is part of the state's scientifically and medically controlled sports training programme.

Detection of anabolic steroids taken by female athletes from East European countries has taken place up to and including the last European athletics championships. Many women have been disqualified for this reason, and yet more found to be positive for anabolic steroids and not disqualified. It is to be expected that women would gain a relatively larger performance advantage from taking anabolic steroids than men. However, there are, as far as I know, no objective data on this. Ryan (1976) reviewed the world literature dealing with experimental evidence for the effect of anabolic steroids on muscle size and strength in human subjects and found twenty-three reports of studies on men but none in women.

Whether anabolic steroids are effective or not is beyond the scope of this chapter. There is now considerable literature concerning both the use and effectiveness of anabolic steroids and the long-term side effects. Hervey (1982) concludes in his chapter that in the long run taking anabolic steroids in the doses used by athletes seems certain to be harmful and one of the most consistently demonstrable effects of long-term use is evidence of damage to the liver. The abnormal appearance of athletes on steroids is obvious, producing the Cushingoid appearance of facial puffiness and increase in trunk girth. The androgenic effects in women are just as serious and much more visible. Women naturally have about 0.1 mg of testosterone in their bodies, about $\frac{1}{2}$ to 1% the amount in men. Even a low dose anabolic steroid can cause outward signs of masculinization in women – whiskers, baldness, deepening of the voice and clitoral enlargement – and these effects may be irreversible. In addition steroids frequently cause acne in women users as well as menstrual irregularities and amenorrhoea.

Testing athletes for drugs and disqualifying them if the tests were positive began officially at the Mexico City Olympics in 1968. Steroid testing, a complex two-part procedure, began officially at the 1976 games in Innsbruck and Montreal. Several women athletes have been steroid positive and disqualified. Very few of the women who have been disqualified have disappeared from international competition. Many have been reinstated. There are many ways to cheat on anabolic steroid tests, either by discontinuing steroid intake weeks before testing or by taking testosterone by injection. Detection of the administration of the natural male hormone presents a novel problem in detection but Brooks (1982) has developed a method of measuring the ratio and concentration of testosterone to that of luteinizing hormone. This urine ratio may form an effective screening test. Out of season 'random' drug testing has now been established (January 1986) by the British Amateur Athletic Board with the intention to 'random test' athletes likely to be selected for international competitions. This will be a very effective deterrent against all forms of drug abuse by athletes.

## 11.6  Pregnancy

There is no evidence that a normally established pregnancy in a fit woman is threatened by exercise at any particular level. It is my policy to actively encourage my pregnant patients to participate in some form of exercise. In some women with poor obstetric histories or with impaired health, however, the obstetrician may prescribe rest or reduction in the amount of exercise taken.

There is little doubt that physical fitness during pregnancy contributes to ease of parturition. Certainly what evidence has been accumulated suggests that childbirth is generally easier if individuals are of an athletic disposition (Zahavieva, 1972). Of all the forms of sporting activity available, swimming is probably the most satisfactory and is much to be encouraged for mothers-to-be. Following delivery a certain amount of physical activity will assist the process of involution of the uterus but such activity should be relatively light. Heavy training and high-powered competitive activity should be contraindicated for several months. This is particularly the case if the mother is breast-feeding since the lactating breast is relatively larger and more cumbersome than its normal counterpart and is therefore, to some extent, liable to injury, quite apart from producing mechanical problems.

Following the joys and tribulations of childbirth there is no physical reason why sporting activities should not be taken up again and indeed there are many famous women champions who gained their titles after childbirth.

### 11.7   Injury to female genital organs

Unlike the male, where genital injuries are fairly common, injuries to the perineum and vulva are few. Vulval haematomas and lacerations can occur resulting from direct trauma. These are commonly experienced in gymnastic vaulters and in other sports involving jumping. Treatment is usually by ice packs and measures to prevent excessive haemorrhage. Occasionally a vulval haematoma is large enough to require surgical treatment and the patient should be referred to a gynaecological specialist unit.

Water-skiing is one of the few sports where the female is particularly prone to gynaecological injury. Forceful retrograde vaginal douching occurs mainly in inexperienced skiers due to their difficulty in standing up after starting their run (Malton, 1970). This is specially noticeable in multiparas. Vaginal lacerations of sufficient severity to cause serious haemorrhage requiring surgical control have been described. The consequence of retrograde douching is salpingitis, peritonitis and the development of pelvic abscesses. The wearing of suitable protective clothing is the simple way to prevent all these injuries. The wearing of tight-fitting, wet-suit pants should be mandatory for all female participants in this sport.

### 11.8   Summary

Where then do women find their place in sport? Despite a male antithesis to women participating in all aspects of sport there has been in the last two decades an enormous increase in female participation with increasing opportunities and superlative performances. Accumulating evidence points to women's immense potential in the stamina events and the strong possibility of their equality with, if not superiority, to the men in endurance events. This is particularly so in long distance sea swimming where the two-way Channel swim record and the England to France record are both held by women. Elizabeth Ferris (1980) points out 'that no matter how brilliantly women perform it appears that society is unable to accept the extraordinary athletic potential women possess, so deeply embedded is the view that females are inherently limited in this area'. She goes on to state 'that many female athletes are held back and do not achieve what is possible for them to achieve because they don't believe they can'. I think that women's attitudes are changing as are the attitudes of their male counterparts. I look forward to increasing participation and success of women in all aspects of sport.

# References

Bausenwein, I. (1960) *Sportarztl Prax.*, **3**, 12.

Brooks, R. V. (1982) in *Science and Sporting Performance. Management or Manipulation?* (eds B. Davies and G. Thomas), Clarendon Press, Oxford, pp. 111–19.

Colt, E. W. D., Wardlaw, S. L. and Frantz, A. G. (1981) The effects of running on plasma B endorphin. *Life Sci.*, **28**, 1637.

Dale, E., Gerlach, D. H. and Wilhite, A. L. (1979) Menstrual dysfunction in distance runners. *Obst. Gynaecol.*, **54**, 47.

Dalton, K. (1960a) Menstruation and accidents. *Brit. Med. J.*, **2**, 1425.

Dalton, K. (1960b) Schoolgirls' behaviour and menstruation. *Brit. Med. J.*, **2**, 1647.

Dalton, K. (1968) Menstruation and examinations. *Lancet*, **2**, 13.

Dalton, K. (1977) *The Pre-menstrual Syndrome and Progesterone Therapy.* Heinemann, London, pp. 26–29.

de Vries, H. (1981)*Physiology of Exercise for Physical Education and Athletics*, 3rd edn, Saunders College Publishing.

Erdelyi, G. J. (1962) Gynacological survey of female athletes, *J. Sports Med. Phys. Fit.*, **2**, 174.

Ferris, E. (1980) Are women liberated in sport? *Medisport*, **2(9)**, 259.

Frisch, R. E., Gotz-Welbergen, A. V., Albright, T., Witschi, J. *et al.* (1981) Delayed menarche and amenorrhoea of college athletes in relation to age of onset of training. *J. Amer. Med. Assoc.*, **246**, 1559.

Glass, G. S., Heninger, G. R., Lansky, M. and Talan, K. (1971) Psychiatric emergency related to the menstrual cycle. *Amer. J. Psychiat.*, **128**, 705.

Hervey, G. R. (1982) in *Science and Sporting Performance. Management or Manipulation?* (eds B. Davies), Clarendon, Oxford, p. 120.

Ingman, O. (1953) Menstruation in Finnish top class sportswomen. In *Proceedings of the International Symposium of the Medicine and Physiology of Sports and Athletics at Helsinki 1952* (ed. M. J. Katronen), Finnish Association of Sports Medicine, Helsinki.

Malton, B. C. (1970) Gynaecological complications in water skiing. *Med. J. Aust.*, **2**, 12–56.

Matthews, A. (1980) Sport and the menstrual cycle. *Medisport*, **2(9)**, 275.

# Sportswomen – gynaecological and other aspects

Novak, L. P., Woodward, W. A., Bestit, C. and Mellerowicz, H. (1977) Working capacity, body composition and anthropometry of Olympic female athletes. *J. Sports Med.*, **17**, 275.

Prendergast, D., Wilson, D., di Pramper, O. P. and Rennie, D. (1974) Energy cost of swimming. *Med. Sci. Sports*, **6**, 86.

Rerych, S. K., Scholz, D. M., Sabiston, D. C. and Jones, R. H. (1980) Effects of exercise training on left ventricular function in normal subjects: A longitudinal study by radionuclide angiography. *Amer. J. Cardiol.*, **45**, 244.

Rubal, B. J., Rosentsweig, J. and Hamerly, B. (1981) Echocardiographic examination of women collegiate soft-ball champions. *Med. Sci. Sports Exer.*, **13**, 176.

Ryan, A. J. (1976) in *Anabolic-androgenic Steroids* (ed. C. D. Kochakia) Springer-Verlag, Berlin, pp. 515–34.

Shangold, M. (1981) Do women's sports lead to menstrual problems? *Contemp. Obst. Gynaecol.*, **17(3)**, 52.

Strauzenberg, S. E. and Kabner, R. (1980) Iron deficiency in female athletes. In *Abstracts from the International Congress: Women and Sport*, Rome, p. 160.

Thomas, C. (1974) Special problems of female athletes. In *Sport and Medicine* (eds A. Ryan and F. Olman), Academic Press, New York, pp. 347–73.

Timonen, S. and Procopé, B. J. (1971) Pre-menstrual syndrome and physical exercise. *Acta Obst. Gynecol. Scand.*, **50**, 331.

Wearing, M. P., Yuhosz, M. D. and Campbell, R. *et al.* (1972) The effect of the menstrual cycle on tests of physical fitness. *J. Sports Med. Phys. Fit.*, **12**, 38.

Wilmore, J., Brown, G. H. and Davis, J. A. (1977) Body physique and composition of the female distance runner. *NY Acad. Sci.*, **301**, 775.

Writh, J. C., Lohman, T. G., Avallone, J. P. *et al.* (1978) Effects of physical training on the serum iron levels of college age women. *Med. Sci. Sport Exer.*, **10**, 223.

Zahavieva, E. (1972) Olympic participation by women: effects on pregnancy and childbirth. *J. Amer. Med. Assoc.*, **221**, 992.

Zeldis, S. M., Morganroth, J. and Rubler, S. (1978) Cardiac hypertrophy in response to dynamic conditioning in female athletes. *J. Appl. Physiol.*, **44**, 849.

# 12    *Urological problems*

JOHN P. BLANDY

Major injury to the urogenital system is not common in sport, but many problems arise that refer to the system in dealing with young men and women who take active exercise. This chapter therefore does not limit itself to the injuries of the urinary and genital system, but attempts to embrace a rather wider field.

## 12.1    Proteinuria

Nearly every young man or woman embarking in serious sport will undergo a routine medical examination, during which the urine will be tested, usually with a 'stix' type of test, for protein and blood. A common problem is therefore to know what to do when the stix test shows a positive reaction.

The stix tests are performed with paper impregnated with an indicator dye, tetrabromophenol blue. This is yellow in acid, blue in alkaline urine. The paper strip is buffered so that the pH is very acid (pH 3), at which the colour normally stays yellow. But protein forms a complex with the indicator that makes it blue even in the acid environment, and the more protein the more the colour changes from yellow through green to deep blue.

If the urine is stale, or very infected, so that bacterial action has converted urea to ammonia and the pH has risen, the buffer in the paper is insufficient to keep it acid and the indicator will turn blue. Some contaminants that find their way into a urine sample also make it go blue, notably traces of disinfectants such as chlorhexidine.

Similarly, if acid has been added to the urine, e.g. in the container used to measure the calcium content in suspected hypercalciuric cases, the pH is kept in the yellow range.

If the stix test is positive, a semi-quantitative estimate of the protein in the urine can be easily performed by adding 5 drops of 25% salicylsul-

195

# Urological problems

Symptomless proteinuria

The stix tests for protein

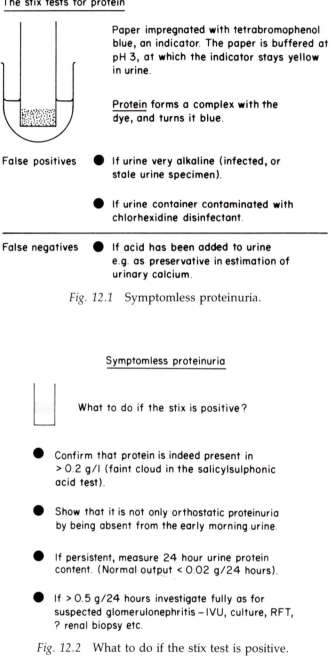

Paper impregnated with tetrabromophenol blue, an indicator. The paper is buffered at pH 3, at which the indicator stays yellow in urine.

Protein forms a complex with the dye, and turns it blue.

False positives
● If urine very alkaline (infected, or stale urine specimen).

● If urine container contaminated with chlorhexidine disinfectant.

False negatives
● If acid has been added to urine e.g. as preservative in estimation of urinary calcium.

*Fig. 12.1* Symptomless proteinuria.


Symptomless proteinuria

What to do if the stix is positive?

● Confirm that protein is indeed present in > 0.2 g/l (faint cloud in the salicylsulphonic acid test).

● Show that it is not only orthostatic proteinuria by being absent from the early morning urine.

● If persistent, measure 24 hour urine protein content. (Normal output < 0.02 g/24 hours).

● If > 0.5 g/24 hours investigate fully as for suspected glomerulonephritis – IVU, culture, RFT, ? renal biopsy etc.

*Fig. 12.2* What to do if the stix test is positive.

phonic acid to 1 ml of urine. A faint cloud signifies that there is about 0.2 g $l^{-1}$ of protein present: a heavy flocculent precipitate signifies about 5 g $l^{-1}$. Either response must be taken seriously, for the normal protein content of urine is less that 0.05 g $l^{-1}$.

The next step is to collect a 24 hour specimen of urine, and have the laboratory measure the protein. If it is more than 0.5 g per 24 hours, then the patient should be referred to a nephrologist as a probable example of the nephrotic syndrome. The laboratory will probably proceed to make specific measurements of the type and quantity of different proteins present in the urine, for upon their relative amounts one may be able to predict whether the glomerulonephritis will or will not respond to steroids.

### Symptomless proteinuria

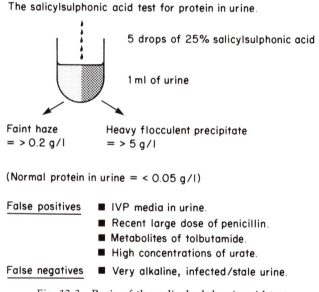

The salicylsulphonic acid test for protein in urine.

5 drops of 25% salicylsulphonic acid

1 ml of urine

Faint haze = > 0.2 g/l

Heavy flocculent precipitate = > 5 g/l

(Normal protein in urine = < 0.05 g/l)

False positives
■ IVP media in urine.
■ Recent large dose of penicillin.
■ Metabolites of tolbutamide.
■ High concentrations of urate.

False negatives
■ Very alkaline, infected/stale urine.

Fig. 12.3    Basis of the salicylsulphonic acid test.

At the same time, a simple test is made to see whether the proteinuria is dependent upon posture: the so-called orthostatic proteinuria (Parfrey, 1982a,b). It is easy to ask the patient to let you have the first specimen passed in the morning after a night's rest. If this is consistently free from protein, one can be confident that there is nothing seriously wrong. Orthostatic or effort proteinuria is very common, especially in adolescents. Its cause is not clear; it is thought to be related to alterations in renal blood flow brought about as a compensation for the alteration in posture. It is typically intermittent, not present every day. One should have a tiny feeling of caution about dismissing orthostatic proteinuria if it is present every time it is sought. In about half the patients who have persistent orthostatic proteinuria, minor glomerular lesions may develop during the subsequent five years (Robinson, 1970).

## 12.2 Haematuria

The stix test commonly used for routine testing of the urine also signifies the presence of 'blood'. The test relies on the presence of haemoglobin, which acts as a catalyst for cumene peroxidase present in the paper strip, along with colourless orthotoluidine. The peroxidase, catalysed by haemoglobin, converts orthotoluidine into the blue compound indigo. Because the test depends on the catalytic activity of haemoglobin, it is slightly more sensitive to free haemoglobin than to red cells. Myoglobin also acts in the same way as do other peroxidases present in bacteria, and other oxidizing agents that contaminate the urine, e.g. povidone iodine and hypochlorite.

The normal adult male loses about 40 000 red blood cells (RBCs) per hour in the urine; this results in about 8 RBCs per high power field. The 'high power field' is by no means a constant volume and if one needs to quantify the rate of red cells loss accurately it is necessary to centrifuge down a standard volume of urine and resuspend it in a known volume of diluent and count the cells in a haemocytometer. In fact the stix text is

### Haematuria

● Normal rate of passage of red cells in urine
20 000 RBC per hour – children
40 000 RBC per hour – adults

● 95% of males have < 20 000 RBC/ml urine
= < 8 RBC per high power field in centrifuged urine
= < 40 RBC in centrifuged and resuspended urine

● Stix test is + ve with > 50 000 RBC/ml

i.e. Any positive stix test is well above normal and must be investigated.

*Fig. 12.4* Haematuria is never innocent.

positive when there are about 50 000 RBC ml$^{-1}$ urine i.e. double the normal upper limit (20 000 RBC ml$^{-1}$). Hence any positive stix test must be investigated.

The first check is to carry out urine microscopy, to see that red cells are in fact present in more than 8 per high power field. If there are no red cells, then one must assume that the stix has responded to free haemoglobin or myoglobin.

## 12.2.1 ATHLETES' HAEMOGLOBINURIA

'March' haemoglobinuria is caused by the destruction of red cells passing through the capillary bed in the soles of the feet. It can be prevented by using well-padded shoes, or by running on soft grass rather than hard pavement. It may persist (Woodhouse, 1982). It is entirely innocent.

In athletes after severe trauma myoglobin may appear in the urine as well, giving rise to a positive stix test. It is rare that the amount of crushed muscle will be enough to produce the 'crush syndrome' of wartime bomb casualties, and if the test is repeated after a short period of rest then anxieties may be laid at rest.

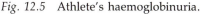

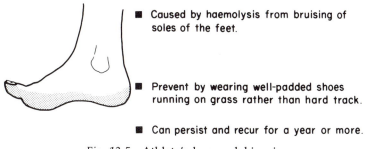

**Haemoglobinuria in athletes**

■ Caused by haemolysis from bruising of soles of the feet.

■ Prevent by wearing well-padded shoes running on grass rather than hard track.

■ Can persist and recur for a year or more.

*Fig. 12.5* Athlete's haemoglobinuria.

## 12.2.2 WHAT TO DO WHEN THE STIX TEST IS POSITIVE

The first check is to microscope the urine as above. If an excess of red cells is present, then the result must be taken very seriously indeed. Every patient must be as fully investigated by a urologist as if he or she had noticed frank blood in the toilet on passing urine: i.e. they need urine cytology (send ordinary urine diluted with an equal volume of 10% formalin to the cytology laboratory). They should have an excretion urogram, and they must have a cystoscopy performed.

The urine should be cultured, and if more than 50 000 organisms per ml are grown, then the patient must be considered to have a urinary infection. The appropriate antimicrobial therapy will be given, and in a male even the first episode of infection will be followed by a comprehensive urological investigation including an excretion urogram and a cystoscopy.

### Haematuria

> ### What to do when stix test is positive
>
> ● Confirm by microscopy that RBC are present (more than 10 per high power field, or, centrifuge and resuspend and check again < 40/HPF).
>
> ● Investigate fully by
>     urine Papanicolaou
>     IVU
>     cystoscopy.
>
> ● 20% will have major lesion, of which half will have cancer of bladder, prostate or kidney.
>
> ● Negative investigations. Watch out! 2% will develop a serious lesion within 3 years.

*Fig. 12.6*  What to do when the stix test is positive.

If microscopy of the urine has, in addition to the red cells, shown the presence of pus cells, but the culture of the urine is sterile, then it is necessary to exclude cancer of the bladder and tuberculosis. The former is excluded only by cystoscopy, the latter by sending at least three early morning urine specimens for staining with Ziehl-Neelsen's stain for acid and alcohol fast bacilli, and culturing for six weeks on Loewenstein-Jensen media.

By this systematic examination of every patient with haematuria major lesions such as cancer of the kidney, prostate and bladder will not be missed. Stones will be discovered – and it is important to be aware that stones are common in fit young people of either sex, particularly when they are involved in dehydrating and exhausting exercise.

In men and women from Africa or the West Indies and Brazil, where schistosomiasis is endemic, haematuria may mean that ova of the parasitic worm are present in the submucosa of the bladder. Mid-day urine should be examined as soon as possible for the presence of the characteristic ova. In cases of doubt, cystoscopy should be performed, and a tiny mucosal biopsy of the bladder removed with cup forceps, crushed between a slide and a cover-slip and examined for the ova which are often very numerous.

The sickle-cell trait or disease is also an important cause of haematuria in black people, being precipitated by jet travel in incompletely pressurized compartments, as well as by anoxia and trauma.

While every athlete must have these major and important causes of haematuria thoroughly excluded, there remain a few cases where haematuria follows exercise so regularly that one can almost be sure that it is the cause of the bleeding. In marathon runners haematuria is quite common: in one study eight out of fifty doctors participating in a long-distance run showed haematuria for up to forty-eight hours afterwards (Siegel et al., 1979). Here there have been several possible causes suggested. It may be that there is relative ischaemia of the kidney, or that the renal vein is compressed, but most convincingly Blacklock (1977) has described a characteristic contusion on the trigone in runners. I have seen it (and have biopsied the lesion) twice in joggers (both doctors). Blacklock suggests that the bladder vault is allowed to rub against the trigone during exercise. Whatever the mechanical explanation there is a typical reddened area on the trigone with thickening of the mucosa and new and old submucosal haemorrhages. This cannot be the only explanation for this haematuria after exercise is seen in rowing and swimming, but the

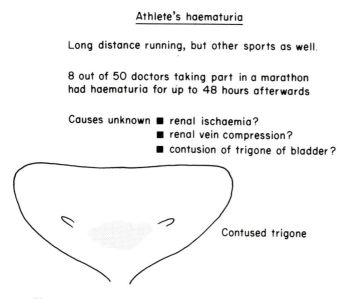

Fig. 12.7  Athlete's haematuria (Siegel et al., 1979).

writer has not had the opportunity to cystoscope any such patient immediately after the offending exercise.

## 12.3   The solitary kidney and the athlete

A not uncommon question confronts the specialist in sports medicine who is asked to advise a young person in whom a diagnosis of a solitary kidney is made, or who (increasingly nowadays) has donated a kidney to a sibling. Should they indulge in sport, and what precautions should they take?

There is good evidence (Santiago *et al.*, 1972; Davison, Uldall and Walls, 1976; Hamburger and Crosnier, 1968) that the patient with a single kidney has a normal life expectancy, and many urologists think it is quite unnecessary to forbid any activity. My own subjective feeling is that such patients would be better not to indulge in skiing, whether on land or water, since each season seems to yield its sorry harvest of renal trauma. Similarly in Britain the rugby football field seems to occasion its share of traumatic haematuria. In all other respects, however, and in all other activities there is no reason why they should not lead a normal life.

## 12.4   Renal colic in sportsmen

Minor exercise may provoke bleeding if there is a calculus in the kidney, and a small stone may be dislodged after exercise. So on both accounts stones do give rise to many clinical problems to the specialist in sports medicine. When there is haematuria it is always necessary to rule out other more sinister causes for the bleeding as outlined above. But when a young athlete presents with ureteric colic, what should be done?

It is important that the doctor and the patient should get the matter in perspective: in temperate climates at least 10% of people get ureteric colic sooner or later, and in the tropics the proportion is higher. It is even higher in certain occupations where much fluid is lost by sweating, and athletes are at higher risk in this respect if they do not pay extra attention to replacing lost fluid by adequate water intake. Dietary fads and fancies, common among athletes, may cause them to take unnecessary amounts of milk (in the belief that it is good for them) or vitamin D on the assumption that vitamins have some magical property. As a result they may put out an excessive amount of calcium in the urine because they take in an excessive amount in the diet.

Every patient with a stone should be screened for hyperparathyroidism (at least two careful measurements of the plasma calcium should be

202

performed by a trustworthy laboratory). The majority will be normal. What should be done?

During the attack of colic, a plain radiograph should be taken to show where the stone is situated. If there is any doubt as to the diagnosis, i.e. if there is a suspicion that the pain may be from an acute appendix or a ruptured ectopic pregnancy, then an excretion urogram should be obtained as an emergency. But it is important that the often bizarre and frightening appearances of these emergency urograms should be correctly interpreted by an experienced urologist. At the height of an attack of ureteric colic, the kidney may seem not to be functioning, and to be grossly obstructed, with extravasation of contrast around the kidney and ureter. This is an appearance which is entirely compatible with spontaneous passage of the stone without any detectable damage to the kidney.

If the stone is a small one (as they usually are), i.e. 5 mm in diameter, then there is a 98% chance that it will pass on its own, after a few episodes of colic. Any surgical intervention carries some risk, and it is important to protect the patient from unnecessary and meddlesome instrumentation when the stone is likely to pass naturally.

The patient needs relief of pain. Morphine or pethidine are equally good, so long as they are given in an adequate dose. Diclofenae 100 mg i.v. or by suppository gives equal relief. Fluids should not be forced (a) because they will make the patient vomit and (b) because they merely increase the distension in the urinary tract upstream of the obstructing stone. Forcing fluids does not help to get the ureter to pass the stone.

After four weeks (so long as the patient is without pain) the radiograph should be repeated. Only if the stone is failing to travel down the ureter, or if the kidney is showing dilatation, is any surgical intervention necessary. It is particularly important that these anxious young men and women are not allowed to bully their physicians into agreeing to some procedure, such as the removal of the stone with the Dormia basket, merely to allow them to travel to an athletics contest. Kidneys have been sacrificed many times merely because the patient was importunate.

## 12.5 The athlete's groin

All young men are more or less obsessed with their genitals and the sports medicine clinic must be prepared to deal with a number of problems that concern these highly strung youngsters.

# Urological problems

## 12.5.1 HAEMOSPERMIA

Curiously absent from many undergraduate textbooks, haemospermia is a very common and completely innocent symptom. Because it is the universal experience of all those who have investigated it with care, that there is never any cause for alarm, investigations are virtually contra-indicated. A rectal examination should be made to rule out cancer of the prostate: the testicles should be examined carefully to rule out cancer. The urine should be tested for pus, and cultured to exclude an infection. In practically every case all these simple tests will be negative. It is important not to make bogus diagnoses such as 'prostatitis' which can seldom be supported by facts, and for which there is no real treatment. The patient should be heartily reassured and sent upon his way.

## 12.5.2 THE ATHLETE WITH A 'GROIN STRAIN'

Probably there are true 'strains' i.e. minor tears and minor haemorrhages into the origin of the adductor muscles along the pubic rami, but it is not uncommon that the patient notices pain 'somewhere in the groin', and cannot easily distinguish its exact site. In such a patient one may often discover a small indirect inguinal hernia, if the standard manoeuvre is used of inserting a finger-tip into the internal inguinal ring. These very small, and probably very early, herniae are notoriously easy to overlook, especially when the surgeon has a clinic in the morning. The prolapse of the peritoneum which constitutes the hernia may be much more easy to feel in the evening at the end of an exhausting day, when, incidentally, the patient is more likely to notice that the pain is worse. Such a hernia is easily repaired and the patient relieved of his 'strain'.

The symptom of ill-defined pain in the groin also deserves a meticulous examination of the testis and epididymis. Any swelling in the testis – any slight difference in consistence from the normal – must be referred at once to a urologist experienced in testicular tumours (see below). Swellings in the epididymis are nearly always tiny innocent cysts, but acute inflammatory changes are commonly seen in the epididymis, probably related to extravasation of sperm, and perhaps brought on by straining, e.g. the Valsalva manoeuvre may force urine down the lumen of the vas and so breach the walls of the tubules of the epididymis.

Epididymitis is usually obvious. If seen, and if it is possible clearly to distinguish epididymis from testis, one must search the urine for micro-organisms, including tubercle bacilli.

A varicocele is almost universally present in healthy young men to some degree, and there is no clear evidence that they do any harm. It is customarily believed today that varicoceles are a cause of subfertility.

204

Such controlled trials as have been reported (Nilsson, Edvinsson and Nilsson, 1979; Turner, 1983) do not support this widely held belief. Occasionally a varicocele is associated with severe aching pain in the 'groin' which will be relieved by dividing the testicular veins. But such cases are very uncommon, and one must always consider that dividing the testicular veins puts the testicular artery at hazard and is not a procedure without complications.

The patient with vague pain referred to the testicle may be suffering from a lesion in the lower thoracic vertebrae giving rise to pain referred along the root of T10.

### 12.5.3 THE UNDESCENDED TESTICLE

There is a far higher incidence of testicular cancer in association with maldescent of the testis, and when a testis is found that lies high in the inguinal canal, or at the external ring, in an otherwise healthy young man, the wisest advice is usually for the patient to have it removed. If he insists on keeping the organ, it may be moved down to the scrotum by the operation of orchidopexy, but this will not restore fertility (which will be absent from that testis) nor alter the chance of malignancy. Orchidopexy should be performed between the ages of two and four years, an age range out of the scope of this chapter.

### 12.5.4 LUMPS IN THE TESTICLE

Any hard lump in the testicle should be sent at once to the urologist: it is bound to be a malignant tumour. (There are no benign hard lumps in the testis.) If the hard lump is definitely in the epididymis rather than the testis, it may be sperm granuloma or tuberculosis. Tumours are very rare, but the patient needs careful investigation.

Cystic lumps in front of the testis are hydroceles: if they are behind the testis they are epididymal cysts. Small hydroceles can be left without treatment so long as it is possible to feel the underlying testis clearly. If not, they should be operated on, and the opportunity taken to rule out malignancy in the testicle and to cure the hydrocele once and for all. There is no place for aspirating hydroceles in healthy young men.

Cysts of the epididymis are diverticula of the vasa efferentia testis. Removing them usually results in blockage of the pathway for sperms from testis to epididymis, i.e. virtually performs a vasectomy on that side. Hence in young males who have not had their quota of children every effort should be made to desist from any operation on an innocent cyst of the epididymis.

# Urological problems

### 12.5.5 INFLAMMATIONS OF THE TESTICLE

Mumps orchitis does not attack males until after puberty. There is usually an epidemic of mumps in the vicinity, so the diagnosis is seldom in doubt. If seen early, there is some evidence that decompressing the testis may preserve its function, and its certainly relieves pain. Others have used steroids at this stage, but of course without any controls. When in doubt, the mumps orchitis should be explored if only to rule out the other far more serious condition that affects men in the 'sportsmen' age group – torsion of the testicle.

*Torsion of the testicle* occurs nearly always after a series of minor episodes of incomplete twisting of the testicle on its congenitally lax mesentery. Occasionally one may be lucky enough to hear the story of attacks of sudden pain and swelling in the testicle which go away as suddenly as they came. This is the classical story of torsion, and deserves operation. More often one only sees the patient when he comes up with a painful, hot, red, apparently inflamed scrotum. It is so oedematous that it is impossible to distinguish testis from epididymis. It is tempting to jump to the diagnosis of epididymitis, but epididymitis is usually obviously limited to the epididymis, and nearly always is preceded by urinary infection. In all other cases the testicle should be explored as an emergency. If one operates, one may be in time to untwist the testicle on its stalk, and preserve its function. It is wise to recall that the contralateral testicle is likely to be affected by the same type of arrangement of loose tunica vaginalis, and should be inspected and fixed at the same operation. Bilateral torsion leading to castration by neglect is all too common.

### 12.5.6 INJURY TO THE TESTIS

Fortunately serious injuries to the testicle are rare, but the natural history of testicular injury is insufficiently well appreciated even today. Closed trauma to the testicle splits the tunica albuginea of the testis, allowing blood to escape. The blood fills the cavity of the tunica vaginalis until bleeding stops as a result of tamponade. The blood does not clot, as a rule, but collects into small loculi, and attracts fluid. The tunica vaginalis swells, and the testicle is more and more compressed, until eventually it is atrophied to the form of a thin shell occupying one wall of the tunica.

It has been clearly shown (Atwell and Ellis, 1961; Cass, 1983) that *not* to explore such a testicle deprives it of its only chance to survive. Early intervention allows the surgeon to remove the clot, repair the rent in the tunica albuginea, and preserve testicular function. Time should never be lost in aspirating the swelling and hoping that time and nature will make the lump go away: they will – but so will the testicle.

## 12.5.7 THE RISK OF TESTICULAR CANCER

Whenever a young man is seen in the sports medicine clinic complaining of discomfort in the region of the testis, the first and over-riding concern of the doctor should be to make sure that the patient does not have a cancer of the testis. This is not rare; it is becoming more common; but it is still only referred to hospital too late. In Britain and in North America more than half the cases of testicular cancer have already developed metastases at the time of their first visit to hospital (Blandy, 1977; Oliver, 1985). When there is any suspicion at all, please give the patient the benefit of the doubt and get a second opinion from a urological surgeon with experience of this condition. Today we may expect to cure 100% of patients who come up without metastases, and we can cure a good proportion even of those with widespread tumour – but the patient has to suffer severe discomforts from lymph node dissection and chemotherapy if he is to be cured, and none of these treatments are required if the tumour is still localized to the testicle.

## 12.6   Injuries of the kidney

Suspect an injury to the kidney whenever a patient has been injured in the lower ribs and loin. Haematuria will be noted in the urine passed soon after the injury.

The natural history of closed injury to the kidney is very innocent. The tight strong fascia of Gerota surrounds the kidney like a cellophane bag. The split in the renal parenchyma loses blood, but tamponade soon controls it, and the bleeding usually ceases without any further ado. Occasionally the main renal artery is torn, and the tamponade of the fascia of Gerota is not enough to stop the bleeding. In such a kidney there may be such a loss of blood that to save life the kidney must be removed and the artery secured. The problem is that when the patient first comes to hospital, nobody knows (in the first few hours) what is going to happen.

So the first task is to make sure that the patient has the luxury of having two kidneys, and an IVP must be done as an emergency. It may not show a good kidney on the injured side, but the purpose of the X-ray is to make sure that the patient has two. Having done this, the patient is put to bed. His pulse and blood pressure are recorded every half-hour. Each specimen of urine that he passes is saved for inspection by the doctor (the colour should gradually fade and become more brown as fresh bleeding stops). The abdomen is regularly examined to make sure that no huge mass of blood is collecting around the kidney.

Urological problems

If there is evidence of internal bleeding, or if the loin becomes full, or if the IVP shows no kidney on the contralateral side, a renal angiogram is performed. At the angiogram, the radiologist should be prepared to stop the bleeding by injecting chopped-up muscle or gelfoam into the renal artery, to embolise it. This will save the patient an operation, and if only a renal artery branch is seen to be bleeding at the time of angiography, then it may well save him the greater part of his kidney.

If the patient is evidently bleeding very much, there may be no time for an angiogram. But there is always time for a pyelogram! Operations for renal injury usually end up removing the kidney. Partial nephrectomy and repair of lacerated kidneys by suture have been reported from time to time, but usually in cases where no operation was needed at all.

Such circumstances are the exception. Most patients get better with simple bed rest. An IVP should be done at three and at twelve months to make sure there are no late sequelae (such as hydronephrosis and pseudocyst), and the blood pressure should be measured regularly during the first year to detect the (very rare) Page kidney – where compression of the kidney by subcapsular haematoma (Conrad et al., 1976) leads to renin release and hypertension.

### 12.7 Injuries of the ureter

Closed injuries of the ureter are almost unknown. In sudden deceleration (e.g. motorcycle accidents) there may be a tear of the ureter just where it issues from the renal pelvis (Drago et al., 1981). In such a patient there is anuria: when the patient recovers from shock, an IVU shows extravasation of contrast from the kidney. Clinical deterioration obliges the surgeon to explore the loin.

### 12.8 Closed injury of the bladder

A drunk with a full bladder may perforate the distended dome of the organ spontaneously, or upon receipt of quite slight injury. The overdistended bladder splits, allowing urine to squirt into the peritoneal cavity. At first there is little reaction, since the urine is usually dilute (and therefore not a chemical irritant) and uninfected (and so not a cause of bacterial peritonitis). Neglected, or missed, the presence of a few litres of urine in the peritoneal cavity does in time give rise to pain, distension, absence of bowel sounds, and a curiously doughy feeling when the abdomen is palpated. There is a risk in that such a patient may be

208

discharged from hospital without any such late signs being noticed by his medical team.

If suspected, the diagnosis may be made by (a) a 4-quadrant needle aspiration of the peritoneal cavity, and having a urea measurement made of the fluid that is aspirated (no other body fluid contains more urea than the blood except for urine); (b) a cystogram is performed, but needs a large volume of fluid, or else the small leak will not be noticed; (c) cystoscopy will show the tear in the bladder if one seeks it carefully.

The treatment is simple: the bladder is catheterized and allowed to heal up on its own. Only if there are increasing signs of peritoneal irritation should laparotomy be performed, and the bladder sewn up and patched with omentum. Such injuries are not likely to be seen in clean-living young sportsmen, but injured spectators who have perhaps celebrated too well may be referred to the specialists in sports medicine!

## 12.9 Pelvic fractures and urological complications

### 12.9.1 PERINEAL TRAUMA

In the old days of sailing ships this was an injury of seamen who fell from tall rigging astride a spar or rail. Today it is almost always confined to sportsmen. They fall astride a bar, forcing the bulbar urethra hard up against the thin underedge of the symphysis pubis. The urethra is squashed, torn, and contused. If the lumen is pierced urine may escape: blood certainly escapes in large quantity, distending the space bounded by the fascia of Scarpa in the perineum.

The real danger of this injury is that if the urine that leaks is hypertonic or infected then the surrounding tissues of the perineum may undergo necrosis and slough. (This used to happen in days gone by.)

In times past also, surgeons were advised to explore these injuries and try to sew up the ruptured urethra. Today it is recognized that, left to itself, the urethra will usually heal, and often without any stricture. All that is needed is a suprapubic cystostomy to lead urine away from the perineum, and some simple drainage of any urine and blood that may have collected in the perineal space. Often, when seen early, there is no need even for a perineal incision.

After ten or twelve days the urethra is looked at with the urethroscope, and has usually healed. The patient must be followed carefully for the next year to ensure that a stricture does not develop at the site of injury. It is rare for a stricture to form, and today, if it does, it can usually be managed by internal optical urethrotomy. At the worst, a patch urethroplasty can be performed in one stage (Blandy, 1980).

### 12.9.2 PELVIC FRACTURE WITH SUSPECTED RUPTURE OF THE URETHRA

When a patient sustains an injury to the pelvis, and a plain X-ray shows a fracture of the pelvic girdle, one must suspect that the urethra has been injured. Blood may appear at the external urinary meatus – sometimes in large amounts – but it may have to be looked for carefully when the patient is admitted to hospital. The patient with a ruptured urethra cannot pass water. Any patient after a pelvic injury who has blood at the external meatus and cannot void is therefore a suspect.

There has been much debate and discussion as to the correct way to deal with these injuries. The clue to the problem is to understand the nature of the injury to the urethra.

There are two types of pelvic fracture that concern us. In the first, the 'spring-back' fracture, a segment of pelvic ring, like the keystone of an arch, is broken off, forced backwards, and then springs back into place (or nearly so) (Fig. 12.8). In the other type of fracture, there is a complete dislocation of one half-pelvis, and the entire innominate bone is forced upwards, dislocated at the symphysis and the sacroiliac joint (Fig. 12.9).

In the spring-back fractures the urethra is held firm by the close binding

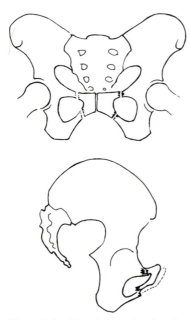

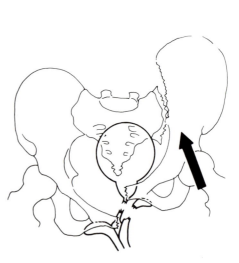

*Fig. 12.8* Simple undisplaced spring-back type of pelvic fracture.

*Fig. 12.9* Pelvic fracture with dislocation of entire half-pelvis. The prostate and urethra are tethered to one half of the pelvis, the bulbar urethra to the other.

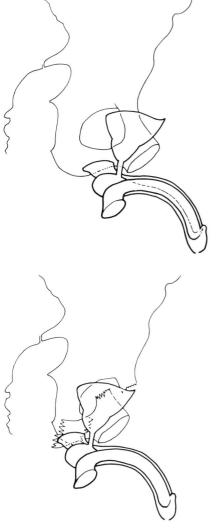

*Fig. 12.10* The attachments of the prostate and urethra: the prostate is fixed to the symphysis by the pubo-prostatic ligaments, the urethra fixed to the middle third of the ischiopubic ramus by the corpus cavernosum on each side.

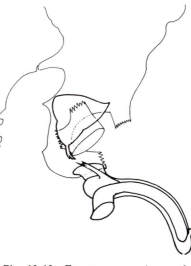

*Fig. 12.11* Fractures behind the mid-third of the ischiopubic ramus – the entire prostate and urethra are carried backwards, and the membranous urethra need not be stretched or torn.

*Fig. 12.12* Fractures anterior to the attachment of the corpus cavernosum – the bulbar urethra is fixed, the prostate carried back with the sym-physis and the membranous urethra stretched or torn.

of the bulbar urethra to the inner aspect of the ischial rami (Fig. 12.10). If the fracture lines run posterior to the middle third of the ischial rami, then the keystone segment of pelvic girdle may carry back the bulb as well as the bladder and prostate, and there is nothing to tear the prostate off the bulbar urethra (Fig. 12.11). On the other hand, if the fracture line runs anterior to this attachment of the corpora cavernosa, the bulb will be held down, and the prostate torn back; the urethra is then torn across at its weakest point (Fig. 12.12).

In the fracture with dislocation of the half-pelvis the bulb is held against one part of the pelvis by the attachment of the corpus cavernosum on that side, while the bladder and prostate are wrenched upwards by their attachment to the upriding innominate bone.

A glance at the X-rays and a glance at the condition of the patient should guide the surgeon as to the correct management in the early hours after the injury. Often there is no choice: the patient is severely injured, there are multiple lesions and there may be internal bleeding from torn liver, spleen and great vessels. Nothing more traumatic than a simple suprapubic cystostomy with a trochar and cannula is needed to divert the urine.

If there is a dislocation of the hemi-pelvis, the urethra is certain to be torn across and in the early days, again, only a suprapubic tube should be inserted. Later on the urologist, collaborating with the orthopaedic surgeon, will make every effort to reunite the distracted ends of the urethra, and the orthopaedic surgeon will reduce the dislocated pelvis using external fixation, if the fracture allows it.

In the patient who is otherwise reasonably fit, and who has no gross trauma that forbids early intervention, the fracture may be of the spring-back type. In such a case nothing is lost by a trained urological surgeon attempting to pass a narrow soft catheter no larger than 12 F. Such a catheter is never armed with a steel stilette, and no force at all is ever used. If it goes into the bladder and clear urine comes away, our own series (Blandy and King, 1983) shows that no harm comes of this manoeuvre. When the patient is comfortable and mobile, the catheter is removed, and one can predict that there will be no stricture.

If the catheter does not slide into the bladder so easily, one may choose between a temporary suprapubic cystostomy, or, if all the circumstances are right, attempt to look into the urethra with a urethroscope, to see the extent of the damage. If there is a complete separation between prostatic urethra and bulbar urethra, and if the patient is fit, the gap should be mended there and then. Early repair of the ruptured urethra has been shown (Blandy and King, 1983; Al-Ali and Husain, 1983) to give a good chance of healing without any stricture at all. But there may be good reasons why this early operative intervention ought to be postponed for a day or two, and in such a case, a temporary suprapubic tube should be inserted.

The worst thing that can be done to the patient is to leave the suprapubic tube *in situ*, and then do nothing, hoping that nature and time will bring the distracted ends of the urethra together again. It does not. In such patients (and the writer has had many referred to him from elsewhere) there is a long gap between one end of the urethra and the other. To bridge the gap requires a very difficult urethroplasty which is attended by complications, and runs the risk of causing incontinence. Far better to prevent this by early reduction of the fracture and reinstatement of continuity to the urethra (Patterson *et al.*, 1983).

## 12.10   Conclusions

In this chapter emphasis has been laid upon the common problems that raise doubt as to the health of the urogenital system, but in practice these are the problems: haematuria, proteinuria and, a 'strain in the groin' that disturb young sportsmen. The management of traumatic haematuria and the ruptured urethra associated with fracture of the pelvis is exceedingly complex in practice. Whenever possible, such patients should be transported to urological centres where familiarity and repetition have made complicated problems seem simple, and where teamwork and practice – just as in sport – give the best results.

## References

Al-Ali, I. H. and Husain, I. (1983) Disrupting injuries of the membranous urethra – the case for early surgery and catheter splinting. *Brit. J. Urol.*, **55**, 716.

Atwell, J. D. and Ellis, H. (1961) Rupture of the testis. *Brit. J. Surg.*, **49**, 695.

Blacklock, N. J. (1977) Bladder trauma in the long-distance runner: '10 000 metres haematuria'. *Brit. J. Urol.*, **49**, 129.

Blandy, J. P. (1977) Testicular tumours. In *Recent Advances in Surgery – 9* (ed. S. Taylor), Churchill Livingstone, Edinburgh, pp. 249–68.

Blandy, J. P. (1980) Surgery for urethral stricture. In *Modern Technics in Surgery* (ed. R. M. Erlich), Futura Publishing, New York, p. 22.

Blandy, J. P. and King, J. B. (1983) Management of the fractured pelvis with urethral injury in the male. *World Urol. Update Ser.*, **1(37)**, 1.

Cass, A. S. (1983) Testicular trauma. *J. Urol.*, **129**, 299.

Conrad, M. R., Freedman, M. Weiner, C. *et al.* (1976) Sonography of the Page kidney. *J. Urol.*, **116**, 293.

Davison, J. M., Uldall, P. R. and Walls, J. (1976) Renal function studies after nephrectomy in renal donors. *Brit. Med. J.*, **1**, 1050.

Drago, J. R., Wisnia, L. G., Palmer, J. M. and Link, D. P. (1981) Bilateral ureteropelvic junction avulsion after blunt abdominal trauma. *Urology*, **17**, 169–71.

Hamburger, J., and Crosnier, J. (1968) In *Human Transplantation* (eds T. T. Rapaport and J. Dausset) Grune and Stratton, New York, p. 37.

# Urological problems

Nilsson, S., Edvinsson, A. and Nilsson, B. (1979) Improvement of semen and pregnancy rate after ligation and division of the internal spermatic vein: fact or fiction? *Brit. J. Urol.*, **51**, 591.

Oliver, R. T. D. (1985) Factors contributing to delay in diagnosis of testicular tumours. *Brit. Med. J.*, **290**, 356.

Parfrey, P. S. (1982a) Symptomless abnormalities: proteinuria. *Brit. J. Hosp. Med.*, **27**, 254.

Parfrey, P. S. (1982b) The nephrotic syndrome. *Brit. J. Hosp. Med.*, **27**, 155.

Patterson, D. E., Barrett, D. M., Myers, R. P. *et al.* (1983) Primary realignment of posterior urethral injuries. *J. Urol.*, **129**, 13.

Robinson, R. R. (1970) In *Proteins in Normal and Pathological Urine* (eds Y. Manualk, J. P. Revillard and H. Betuel), Karger, Basle, p. 224.

Santiago, E. A., Simmons, R. L., Kjellstrand, C. M. *et al.* (1972) Life insurance perspectives for the living kidney donor. *Transplantation*, **14**, 131.

Siegel, A. J., Hennekens, C. H., Solomons, H. S. and Van Boeckel, B. (1979) Exercise related hematuria. Findings in a group of marathon runners. *J. Amer. Med. Assoc.*, **241**, 391.

Turner, T. T. (1983) Varicocele: still an enigma. *J. Urol.*, **129**, 695.

Woodhouse, C. R. J. (1982) Symptomless abnormalities: microscopic haematuria. *Brit. J. Hosp. Med.*, **27**, 163.

# 13 Shoulder injuries

BASIL HELAL, JOHN KING and WILLIAM GRANGE

## 13.1 Introduction

Many sports involve vigorous shoulder movement. In some, the action of the arm is the chief activity of the sport, such as throwing or bowling. In these sports shoulder injuries are incapacitating. In other sports the arm moves passively. Such sports are running and soccer. At first sight shoulder injuries are less devastating in these people. However this is not so, for the pain and stiffness reduces mobility to such an extent that the sportsman's skill is greatly impeded.

The shoulder is uniquely dependent on muscular activity. It is grossly unstable in the presence of weakness or paralysis in the girdle muscles. Injury to the muscles is thus disproportionately significant, for both weakness and instability result. Muscle injuries which would cause a little pain and stiffness in another joint cause severe incapacity in the shoulder, often curtailing the sportsman's training or performance.

The outcome depends on the injury itself and on the treatment. The signal importance of the shoulder musculature means that treatment should be directed primarily at restoration of muscle function. Muscles waste and become adherent to their neighbours very quickly after injury, thus treatment must also be designed to anticipate and prevent this.

The bony anchorage of the muscles is often involved in shoulder injuries. Here two conflicting principles face the attending doctor. Bones heal by immobilization but muscles waste with immobilization. The skill and art of treating shoulder injuries rests with the establishment of a rational compromise between these two conflicting therapeutic demands.

Shoulder injuries may be classified into acute and chronic. Acute injuries follow a sudden unexpected load and usually immediately prevent further sporting activities. The pathology is a disruption of previously healthy tissue. The prognosis depends on the lesion and on the treatment: recovery may be complete; there may be permanent incapacity or the sportsman may be left with partial incapacity of a variable degree. Chronic injuries interfere with the sport but may not be the result of a single injury. Local degeneration may occur as a result of acquired or even congenital abnormality associated with repeated vigorous movement. Thus congenital coracoclavicular bars may cause acromioclavicular degeneration and secondary impingement of the rotator cuff. Similarly humeral head anteversion, a congenital abnormality, may cause recurrent subluxation of the shoulder during forceful external rotation or abduction.

In dealing with shoulder injuries, both chronic and acute, the attending doctor must bear the patient's sporting requirements in mind. Thus steroid injections, which are such useful permanent local analgesics in the elderly, must be used with great caution in the sportsman, for the local concentration may become cytotoxic, inviting rupture of the damaged tissue when heavy loads are applied. In the same way an operation to restore shoulder stability is useless to the patient if it so reduces shoulder mobility that he can no longer indulge in the sport which precipitated the symptoms.

Anatomical and pathological diagnosis is extremely important in shoulder injuries. A mistake may lead to serious errors of treatment and a disastrous outcome. Recurrent subluxation of the glenohumeral joint and acromioclavicular instability may cause similar symptoms. The treatment of one is completely different from that of the other. Care must therefore be taken in reaching a diagnosis. Diagnosis rests on a sound knowledge of structure and function.

Normally the scapula and the humerus move simultaneously during arm movement. The angular excursion of the thoracoscapular joint is about half that of the glenohumeral, so that the arm moves twice as fast as the scapula during abduction. In weakness of the rotator cuff scapular excursion exceeds glenohumeral and the shoulder hunches first before the arm ascends. In painful lesions of the rotator cuff the glenohumeral part of the shoulder's excursion is avoided if possible: at the extremes of movement, when scapular excursion has been exhausted, the glenohumeral joint adds its reluctant contribution with a painful jerk.

## 13.2 Predisposition to injury

Unexpected weakness in a muscle used for strenuous movement may result in partial rupture if loaded in the usual manner. It is not unusual for a sportsman to injure his shoulder after a period of voluntary or enforced inactivity. A vacation or unassociated injury may provide the opportunity for highly trained muscles to waste and weaken. The athlete may be unaware of this and may, for instance, hurl the discus, tearing the anterior belly of his deltoid during the passive extension of the wind-up. Explosive activities are all prone to this sort of injury, and throwers should be warned to build up to full effort gradually after a period of inactivity. Preferably, of course, wasting should not be allowed to occur. Careful coaching and supervision should prevent wasting even during rehabilitation from another injury. The attending doctor should be aware of this danger during recovery from injuries, and should bear it in mind when examining and treating recently injured athletes.

Environmental and temperamental factors may prevent a thrower from warming-up fully. On a cold day, or in a lazy athlete, or both, the muscles may fail to lengthen passively during vigorous explosive events. Partial tearing occurs with immediate severe local pain and tenderness. Nearby muscles then increase in tone, further increasing the chances of tearing.

Congenital ligament laxity predisposes to recurrent shoulder subluxation, particularly in swimmers. This is unfortunate, for most good swimmers have generalized ligament laxity: it is assumed that this condition is a requirement for excellence in this sport. Furthermore, the congenitally lax rely on muscle activity for joint stability more than others, and so muscle injury in these people causes more incapacity. Minor rotator cuff contusions, which would cause minimal symptoms in the normal sportsman, may cause severe instability in the congenitally lax with shoulder hunching on attempted abduction.

The normal stiffening of joints which occurs with age affects the shoulder as much as it affects other joints. The shoulder, however, because of its unique mobility, is particularly prone to injuries associated with this stiffening. The older golfer or tennis player may easily stretch the stiff soft tissues beyond their limits, causing painful partial tearing. In addition the fraying and thinning of the rotator cuff, which appears to be an age-related phenomenon, makes it more and more likely that the cuff will rupture under load in the older athlete. Steroid injections, frequently given to relieve local pain, may well accelerate the local weakening in the cuff, further increasing the chances of rupture.

The rotator cuff may impinge against minor congenital abnormalities in the subacromial space. This causes chronic attrition and predisposes to rupture. Common congenital abnormalities are the anterior acromial spur and the incomplete coracoclavicular bar. Similar impingement may take place beneath the displaced or expanded acromioclavicular joint following acromioclavicular injury (Fig. 13.1). Rupture of the cuff may take place suddenly and unexpectedly in patients with chronic impingement, although more usually pain and weakness gradually worsen as the cuff frays and the final rupture is then a relatively trivial event.

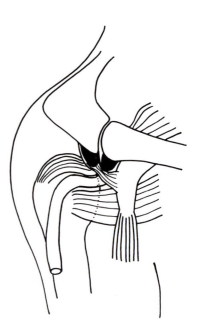

*Fig. 13.1* Attrition of the rotator cuff due to impingement on congenital or acquired abnormalities of the sub-acromial arch such as an acromial spur, an acromioclavicular osteo-phyte or displaced clavicle.

## 13.3 Diagnosis

Treatment should only follow an accurate diagnosis. This involves a careful history and a meticulous examination. Special investigations are also frequently required.

The mechanism of the injury should be identified. Violent passive movement is likely to cause soft-tissue tearing and stretching whereas direct blows are likely to cause bony injury. The premorbid state of the joint must be determined. Were there previous symptoms or signs? Was there a previous injury?

## 13.4 Examination

Examination is the most revealing. Acromioclavicular disorders cause local swelling and tenderness of the joint. Severe disruptions cause abnormal mobility between the clavicle and the acromion. Glenohumeral dislocation causes a characteristic combination of stiffness and deformity. However, the attending doctor may well miss subtle physical signs unless he examines the patient systematically, for many injuries are not as obvious as these.

The patient should be undressed to the waist and first examined whilst standing. Failure to expose the other shoulder may disguise an otherwise glaring abnormality. The shoulder should be inspected from the front and back with the torso vertical and both shoulders put through their full passive range of movement simultaneously: with the patient's arms straight, both should be gently lifted sideways until they meet over the patient's head. Then with the elbows flexed, the arms are rotated internally and externally at the shoulder. These movements are then performed actively by the patient. Gross difference between active and passive movement implies muscle weakness or rupture. In deltoid muscle weakness the shoulder hunches on attempted active abduction; the arm cannot be held in the abducted position after it is placed there passively; the muscle is palpably softer than its fellow during attempted abduction. In rotator cuff rupture abduction is similarly weak. However, the arm can be held in the abducted position once it is placed there passively and the deltoid muscle can be felt working as strongly as its fellow on the other side.

The bony contours of both shoulders must now be palpated simultaneously. The clavicle, the acromion and the spine of the scapula form a continuous arch. Local deformity or tenderness points to a bony injury. The head of the humerus can be felt only vaguely deep to the deltoid, but comparison with the other side and palpation during passive movement can give the examining doctor a great deal of information. This is easiest with the patient seated and the examiner behind the patient. Both tuberosities can then be felt to move beneath the examining fingers.

The neck and arms must always be examined. Many a neck injury is missed because it causes shoulder pain. Many a shoulder injury is complicated by denervation or devascularization in the arm.

Finally the soft tissues around both shoulders are carefully palpated. Tenderness will localize soft-tissue lesions most accurately this way. It is important to postpone this phase of the examination until last for it may cause so much pain that further examination becomes impossible.

## 13.5  Special investigations

Infiltration of the tender area with a small volume of short-acting anaesthetic frequently helps in localizing the source of the pain in cases of doubt. For instance, after a violent wrench the patient may have pain and tenderness over the acromioclavicular joint and the greater tuberosity. Active and passive abduction may be possible, but painful. Infiltration of the soft tissues near the greater tuberosity does not affect the pain if it is arising from the acromioclavicular joint, but allows full painless abduction if it is arising from the rotator cuff insertion into the tuberosity.

## Shoulder injuries

Radiography is the sheet-anchor of all the special investigations of the shoulder. If there is the slightest doubt about the diagnosis a radiograph will add a great deal of irrefutable information and even in cases of obvious injury radiographs reveal the extent of the bony lesion much more explicitly than any physical examination.

The standard radiographs are the anteroposterior and the lateral. Both views are extremely fallible. The anteroposterior may not reveal gleno-humeral dislocation or acromioclavicular dislocation because of difficulties in projection. The lateral view may be impossible to interpret because of superimposition of other structures. In cases of difficulty or doubt special views should be taken. An oblique 'anteroposterior' view with the film held against the scapula and in the plane of the scapula shows the glenohumeral joint in profile. The X-ray beam is perpendicular to the plate (Fig. 13.2).

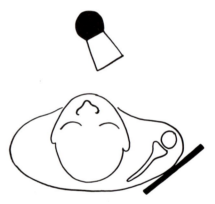

*Fig. 13.2* Oblique anteroposterior radiograph to show the glenohumeral joint.

The glenohumeral joint may be visualized in the axial view too. The beam passes vertically through the joint and the axilla. However, extremely painful shoulder lesions or severe fixed adduction deformity make this view impossible.

The acromioclavicular joint is often poorly shown on standard views. This is due to a combination of projection difficulties and overpenetration. When physical signs suggest an injury to this small joint the penetration should be reduced and the beam should be angled about 20° upward to pass through the joint from front to back with the plate angled perpendicularly to it. In this way minor, albeit significant, abnormalities of the joint are revealed which would otherwise be missed.

The value of arthrography in shoulder injuries is disputed. There are those who maintain that physical examination and plain radiography are always sufficient. There are others who argue equally strongly that this investigation is the only way to assess accurately the state of the rotator cuff. The truth probably lies somewhere between these extreme views.

It would seem wise to advise arthrography where the state of the rotator cuff is in doubt and where surgical exploration of the cuff is contemplated. A small volume of water-soluble radiocontrast is introduced into the joint under radiographic screening control. The normal joint will accept only about 5 ml. This volume fills the capillary space between the humeral head and the glenoid fossa as well as the small axillary pouch. In cases of chronic stiffness of the joint, such as frozen shoulder, not even this volume will flow into the joint. In cases of cuff rupture the contrast medium passes through the defect into the subacromial space which it outlines. The space will accommodate a large volume. It extends over the humeral head as far as the surgical neck and to a variable extent over the subscapularis muscle deep to coracoid process. The filling of the subacromial space must not be considered an immediate indication for operative intervention. Many patients have small asymptomatic defects in the cuff. The decision to operate is a clinical one; the arthrogram simply confirms a clinical impression and marks the size and position of the defect.

## 13.6 Acromioclavicular disruptions

A heavy fall on to the point of the shoulder may damage the acromioclavicular joint. The degree of damage varies from a minor sprain to complete disruption of the articulation between the clavicle and the scapula (Weaver and Dunn, 1972).

### 13.6.1 MINOR LESIONS

In these injuries the integrity of the coracoclavicular conoid and trapezoid ligaments is preserved. The joint is swollen and tender due to haemarthrosis, but the scapula and the clavicle remain firmly attached to one another. The outlook is good in the long-term, although local symptoms may prevent sporting activity for several weeks. The differentiation between minor and major injuries is important for some of the major injuries require surgical treatment and delay diminishes its effectiveness.

*(a) Diagnosis*

In minor injuries the acromion is stable on the clavicle. Local pain may make examination difficult. It is worth infiltrating the joint with local anaesthetic in these cases. This abolishes most of the local pain. The clavicle is grasped with one hand and the acromion with the other. Firstly the two bones are pushed and pulled in an effort to demonstrate

221

abnormal mobility between them. In cases of severe instability there is no doubt. In mild cases it may be necessary to test the uninjured side to establish whether instability exists.

### (b) Treatment

If no instability exists the joint may be mobilized rapidly within the limits of pain in the confident expectation that local signs and symptoms will resolve rapidly and that there will be no permanent sequelae.

In minor disruptions, where there is extreme urgency to return to the sportsfield, the joint may be numbed with long-acting local anaesthetic such as Marcain. Of course this is not ideal, for local signs will persist longer if rest is prevented while the acute phase resolves. However, it allows the athlete to take part in important competitions without seriously affecting the prospects of eventual full recovery. In less urgent cases the arm should be immobilized in a sling for a few days until local tenderness and pain begin to settle. During this time non-steroid anti-inflammatory drugs keep the pain under control and prevent reflex wasting and stiffness in other joints. Local ice-packs also help in controlling the inflammatory reaction. They are most effective in the first few hours following the injury.

Once the acute post-traumatic inflammatory reaction has begun to subside gentle mobilization should begin. This is best done under the supervision of a physiotherapist, for the enthusiastic athlete may initiate secondary tearing and bleeding in the soft healing capsule by over-vigorous active and passive movement. Analgesic drugs mask pain and may allow the patient to damage the joint at this stage: they should be used with great caution. Local steroid injections stop pain by their cytotoxic effect and invite late rupture of weakened tissue.

Short-wave diathermy gently warms the injured tissue and promotes healing. It is useful in cases of some urgency or when local wasting and stiffness appear to threaten rapid resumption of sport. The technique is not a replacement for active and passive mobilization, and its absolute effect is difficult to quantify. Nonetheless in the hands of an experienced practitioner there seems little doubt that it hastens return to the sportsfield.

Ultrasound treatment affects maturation of mesenchyme. In low doses it is a useful local analgesic. However, it should be used with great care for large doses cause local dissolution of bone. Short-wave diathermy is much safer.

Occasionally the joint is damaged in spite of the absence of rupture of the coracoclavicular ligaments. The damage usually consists of injury to the articular cartilage and the meniscus, although sometimes the bone on one or both sides of the joint is distorted. In these cases full recovery does not take place and the athlete has permanent late pain and stiffness. These symptoms are usually trivial but sports which involve full shoulder excursion, such as throwing sports and swimming, may be curtailed. It may be possible to keep symptoms under control with courses of short-wave diathermy and regular mobilizing exercises. However, in some cases the severity of symptoms warrants surgical intervention when conservative treatment fails.

Excision arthroplasty of the acromioclavicular joint is most effective as long as there is no doubt about the integrity of the coracoclavicular ligaments. The outer centimetre of the clavicle is excised through a skin cleavage-line incision over the joint. The surgeon should take care to remove the whole of the outer end of the clavicle: the joint is oblique and it is easy to leave a spike of bone posteriorly which continues to impinge against the acromion causing persistence of symptoms. He should also take care to close the defect in the aponeurotic tissue between the trapezius and deltoid muscles left by the removal of the outer centimetre of the clavicle. The gap otherwise formed allows the clavicle to click about painfully (Fig. 13.3). The arm should be rested in a sling for two to three weeks after the operation to ensure snug healing of the aponeurosis. During this period the hand and elbow should be exercised regularly to prevent stiffness weakness and ulnar neuropathy. Once the wound has healed, active and passive rehabilitation should be started. Complete recovery usually takes three to six weeks.

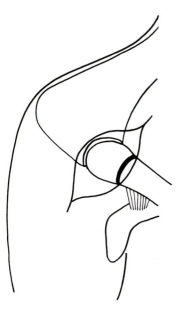

*Fig. 13.3* Excision arthroplasty of the acromioclavicular joint.

### 13.6.2 MAJOR LESIONS

In major injuries the stability of the joint is reduced by damage to the trapezius and deltoid muscles and to the conoid and trapezoid coraco-clavicular ligaments: there is abnormal mobility between the acromion and the clavicle. The degree of instability varies. It is important to distinguish between slight and severe instability, for the outcome of each is different. Slight instability will probably spontaneously heal but severe instability is almost certain to lead to late painful shoulder movement.

Cases of slight instability usually have less pain than severe ones. There is displacement of the outer end of the clavicle, but some contact between clavicle and acromion is maintained on the radiograph. Gentle manipulation usually distinguishes slight from severe, but it may be necessary to infiltrate the damaged tissues with local anaesthetic before there is confidence in the differentiation.

### (a)   Slight instability

Those with slight instability should be treated non-operatively with immobilization and analgesics until local pain, swelling and tenderness begin to subside. This generally takes two to three weeks. The most expeditious way of achieving this is to put the affected arm in a triangular sling. Local padding and strapping has been advised in an effort to reduce the displacement at the acromioclavicular joint. This is unwise, for pressure sufficient to maintain reduction almost always causes skin ulceration. In addition, there is no evidence that the outcome is related to the accuracy of the reduction in these cases.

Following resolution of the acute phase gentle active and passive exercises are encouraged within the limits of symptoms until a full range is achieved. It is important to warn the athlete to retrain his shoulder before exerting full strength in his sport: he may otherwise stretch or tear the fibrotic muscle. Usually recovery is full, but the patient may have an obvious residual deformity over the outer end of the clavicle. It is important to warn the sportsman about this before he becomes aware of it, for he may otherwise become erroneously convinced that something serious is amiss.

Sometimes late symptoms appear. These are due to secondary acromioclavicular degeneration and severe forms may be dealt with by excision arthroplasty, removal of the outer centimetre of the clavicle.

### (b)   Severe instability

Where severe scapuloclavicular instability exists there is little chance of spontaneous resolution. Untreated, most patients develop late severe pain and stiffness due to the replacement of the torn conoid and trapezoid ligaments by scar tissue which is much weaker. The best chance of full restoration of excursion and strength is early surgical repair.

Through an incision in a cleavage line between the acromioclavicular joint and the coracoid process the joint is reduced and a synthetic non-absorbable tape is passed over the clavicle and under the coracoid process. The tape is tightened so as to reduce the joint and is then sewn to itself in this position. A threaded pin is passed across the joint from the acromion to the clavicle. It is left protruding from the skin. The arm is rested in a sling for five weeks before the pin is removed and active mobilization is commenced (Fig. 13.4). Extensive new bone may form at the site of the torn conoid and trapezoid ligaments with or without repair.

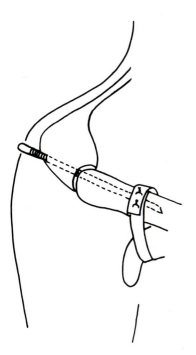

Fig. 13.4 Method of repair of severe-ly unstable acromioclavicular disruption.

## 13.7 Acute glenohumeral dislocation

Many a sportsman stumbles from the field with a very stiff, painful, deformed shoulder due to glenohumeral dislocation. The injury occurs in forced rotation, usually external, combined with abduction. The injury is common on the football field, either association, rugby or American. Other sports may produce the occasional case. Canoeists not infrequently dislocate their shoulders. Judo and wrestling have their crop too.

225

# Shoulder injuries

Young men are much more frequently affected than others. The humeral head is torn from the glenoid fossa and comes to lie either in front or behind the scapula. Anterior dislocation is about twenty times as common as posterior.

## 13.7.1 DIAGNOSIS

The diagnosis is strongly suggested if the patient's shoulder is extremely stiff in either external or internal rotation. The dislocation is probably anterior if fixed in external rotation and posterior if fixed in internal rotation. However, fixed rotational deformity is not the invariable rule: the humeral head may rotate back to the neutral position after the dislocation. Of more diagnostic importance is the characteristic square appearance of the shoulder produced by prominence of the acromion. The humeral head itself may be vaguely palpable near the coracoid process in cases of anterior dislocation and over the dorsal surface of the scapula in posterior dislocation. There may be denervation or devascularization in the arm: these complications are rare, but their effects are devastating. Speed in the treatment of both is important: the attending doctor should always look for these complications when he first sees the patient.

Radiological examination is essential to make the diagnosis. Manipulative reduction on the sports field without radiological confirmation of the diagnosis may worsen the injury for it may not be a simple dislocation. Two projections are required: the most useful are the anteroposterior and the axial. The axial may not be possible due to fixed adduction; in this case a lateral usually reveals the direction of the dislocation, anterior or posterior.

After confirmation of the anatomical diagnosis the doctor must decide on the nature of the dislocation, for the management is guided by the premorbid state of the shoulder.

## 13.7.2 CLASSIFICATION

The dislocation may be acute or recurrent. The recurrent variety may be traumatic or atraumatic and the atraumatic variety may be voluntary or involuntary. Finally there may be a variety of involuntary recurrent atraumatic dislocation complicating the voluntary form (Fig. 13.5).

A careful history usually suffices to establish the premorbid state. The young sportsman with no previous shoulder trouble almost certainly has an acute dislocation. Previous dislocations may have been traumatically induced, albeit by minimal force, indicating recurrent traumatic dislocation. Previous dislocation in the absence of injury suggests recurrence of

226

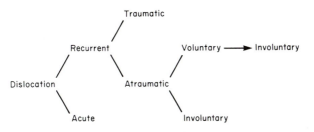

*Fig. 13.5* Classification of glenohumeral dislocation.

atraumatic dislocation. This may be completely beyond the patient's control, involuntary dislocation, or it may be done as a party trick or a neurotic tic, voluntary atraumatic recurrent dislocation. This condition may become involuntary if repeated often enough.

In cases of doubt in the classification, radiological examination may help. About 80% of cases of recurrent traumatic dislocation have a characteristic notch in the humeral head seen best in the anteroposterior projection with the arm internally rotated. This defect is not seen in atraumatic cases (Fig. 13.6).

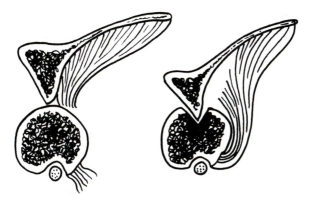

*Fig. 13.6* The difference between acute anterior dislocation in youth and senility. In youth the subscapularis muscle is stretched and stripped of the front of the scapula, leading to instability. In old age the muscle tears: on reduction it heals, abolishing the instability. The characteristic humeral head notch is shown in the young person's dislocation too.

When the dislocation is posterior careful enquiry into the patient's general health should be made. A large proportion of posterior dislocations are the result of a fit: the bitten tongue or the wet bed may be the only evidence. Electric shocks have the same effect.

## 13.7.3 TREATMENT

The atraumatic dislocations need no urgent treatment. Voluntary dislocation should be prevented for it may become involuntary, leading to
degenerative joint disease. Firm advice may be all that is required. Some
patients, however, need to be referred for psychiatric advice. Involuntary
dislocations are due to acquired or inherited structural abnormalities
which may require surgical correction.

Acute dislocations and recurrent traumatic dislocations both require
manipulative reduction. In general acute dislocations are the more difficult to reduce. Many patients who have recurrent dislocation learn how to
reduce the joint themselves.

The Hippocratic method is much older than Hippocrates: it is
illustrated in the Egyptian pyramids. The essential prerequisite is relaxation. This may be achieved on occasion by voluntary relaxation of the
patient. More often a general anaesthetic is required. As soon as sufficient
relaxation is achieved it is possible to distract the joint by gentle traction.
The arm is then adducted while the traction continues. Finally the arm is
internally rotated (for anterior dislocations, posterior dislocations need to
be externally rotated at this stage) and the joint reduces. Reduction may
be achieved before the manoeuvre is completed. It is important to have
radiographic proof of reduction before reversal of the anaesthetic; many
embarrassing mistakes are made for want of this simple step. ·

There is still debate in orthopaedic circles about the duration of
immobilization required after the reduction. There is evidence that the
tendency to recur is established at the moment of dislocation: the
younger the patient the more likely the humeral head is to strip the
subscapularis off the scapula, leading to instability of the joint and
recurrence of the dislocation. Very few old people develop recurrence
after acute dislocation for the humeral head tears through the
subscapularis rather than strips it off its origin; the tear heals after
reduction and recurrence does not take place (Fig. 13.6). Some surgeons
apply ruthless logic and mobilize the young patient's shoulder within the
limits of pain after the injury. Others insist that damage done at the time
of the injury, whatever its severity, stands a better chance of healing
satisfactorily by immobilization for three weeks after reduction. This is
the majority view: there is no firm evidence that early mobilization is
beneficial (Reeves, 1966).

After reduction of the dislocation the patient is instructed to keep the
arm in a sling for three weeks and then to mobilize the shoulder within
the limits of pain. Most acquire full active and passive excursion without
pain very quickly. Like any patient who wears a sling for more than a few
days, the patient should be asked to move the elbow and the hand a few

times a day without moving the shoulder to prevent stiffness elsewhere in the arm.

## 13.8   Recurrent traumatic glenohumeral dislocation

A large number of athletes suffer recurrent glenohumeral dislocation which interferes with their sport. The only treatment is surgical and this should be resorted to early rather than late, for there is nothing to be gained by waiting once the tendency to recur has been established; spontaneous healing does not take place.

### 13.8.1   DIAGNOSIS

Before making a final decision the surgeon should ensure that the diagnosis is correct. It is quite common for a neurotic sportsman to convince himself and attending doctors that he has recurrent dislocation of the glenohumeral joint when he does not. I have seen two patients who were booked for operations for recurrent glenohumeral dislocations; both were then found to have post-traumatic instability of the acromioclavicular joint and symptoms were abolished by surgical treatment of that condition. The anxious sportsman may seek the only operation he knows for serious disorders of the shoulder, and may attempt to help the surgeon by embroidering his history to fit the well-known symptoms.

The best concrete evidence is a radiograph showing an earlier dislocation. The next best is a radiograph showing the characteristic notch. It is important to have a comparable view of the other (normal) shoulder taken to exclude the frequent anatomical notch between the tuberosities seen on the same view. The history of repeated dislocations 'put back' by the patient or his intimates should not be relied upon. Only a brave surgeon would decide to operate on these flimsy grounds.

The finding of increased anteroposterior mobility (as compared with the other side) is very good evidence that glenohumeral dislocation is the cause of the patient's symptoms. Of equal weight is the positive apprehension test: vigorous provocative movement causes fear of dislocation.

The surgeon must also decide on the direction (anterior or posterior) of the dislocation. Usually the history and the position of the radiological notch will help him. Sometimes, however, he will have to postpone the decision until anaesthesia has been induced and an examination under anaesthesia can be performed.

Epileptics (usually with recurrent posterior dislocation) and neurotics with recurrent voluntary dislocation must be identified and treated before the surgical details can be finalized.

# Shoulder injuries

## 13.8.2 TREATMENT

Most sportsmen demand an operation which will abolish their symptoms and will allow them back onto the sportsfield. In this respect the sportsman is different from the rest of the population, for most patients do not demand to be able to do vigorous sports after their operations. The commonest and one of the most reliable operations for recurrent gleno-humeral dislocation is the Putti–Platt operation. The subscapularis muscle is shortened and this permanently restricts external rotation. This may cause no disability in a bank manager, an electrician or a surgeon, but will prevent permanently any thrower from fully winding-up before a throw. Of course the sprinter or the footballer would be able to continue. Operations which are equally reliable, but which do not limit external rotation are the Bristow and Bankart operations. In the Bristow procedure the tip of the coracoid and its attached muscles are pushed through a split in the subscapularis muscle and fixed to the front of the neck of the scapula with a screw (Fig. 13.7) (Lombardo *et al.*, 1976). The Bankart repair obliterates the space beneath the subscapularis into which the head of the humerus passes in anterior dislocation. This is done through a standard deltopectoral groove incision and in most cases the tip of the coracoid can be left undisturbed. The medial part of the clavicular origin

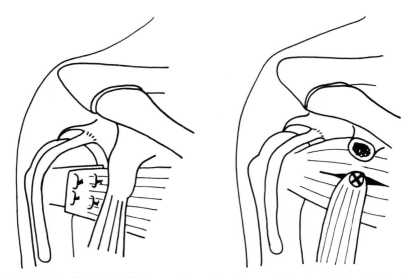

*Fig. 13.7* In the Putti-Platt operation the subscapularis is shortened. In the Bristow operation the tip of the coracoid and its attached muscles are fixed to the front of the neck of the scapula through a split in the subscapularis.
scapula through a split in the subscapularis.

of the deltoid may need elevation in the muscular athlete. The repair is performed with sutures through drill holes in the glenoid margin and the displaced labrum with minimal disruption of the anterior muscles and no loss of external rotation (Bankart, 1938).

After the Putti–Platt operation the patient is bandaged in a tight cocoon with the arm tightly adducted and internally rotated for three weeks. Rehabilitation is prolonged after this procedure and may take from four to eight weeks. After the Bristow procedure immobilization is much less rigid. A simple sling prevents excessive movement for two weeks before rehabilitation begins. Two or three weeks usually suffices to restore full strength and range. The postoperative treatment of a Bankart repair is similar, allowing no external rotation or abduction for four weeks and then passive and active supervised movements begun.

There is little doubt that the Bristow or Bankart operation is superior to the Putti–Platt for the sportsman. It is said that it is difficult to re-operate on a shoulder once a Bristow operation has been performed. This is a council of despiar, for all second operations are more difficult than first ones. It should not be used as an excuse to avoid the technically more demanding operation for the sake of the simpler, but less satisfactory one.


## 13.9 Recurrent glenohumeral subluxation

This condition, a frustrated form of recurrent traumatic glenohumeral dislocation, has only recently been placed in perspective amongst other shoulder injuries of the sportsman. The patient complains of episodic momentary severe instability and pain in the shoulder during vigorous movement. It has been called the 'dead arm syndrome'. The diagnosis is often arrived at late, sometimes even after the sportsman has given up his sport in despair. It affects all sports involving vigorous arm movement: throwers, bowlers, rugby players and tennis players. Crawl and butterfly swimmers may subluxate their shoulders posteriorly because of a build up of powerful internal rotator muscles (Boyd, 1972).


### 13.9.1 DIAGNOSIS

The diagnosis is notoriously difficult to make. Many patients are dismissed as neurotic. The increased anteroposterior laxity and the apprehension sign of recurrent dislocation are present. However the radiological notch is absent and since the joints never require manipulative reduction the casualty officer never confirms the diagnosis. The only effective diagnostic measure is examination under anaesthetic. Provocative external rotation causes the humeral head to slide anteriorly in an

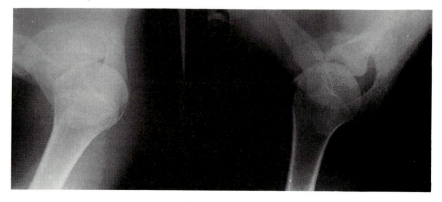

*Fig. 13.8* Radiographs of a swimmer showing posterior subluxation of the left shoulder.

unmistakable way. Very rarely recurrent posterior subluxation can be demonstrated (Fig. 13.8). Recurrent dislocation and acromioclavicular instability are the differential diagnoses.

### 13.9.2 TREATMENT

The Bankart or Bristow operation is as effective in this condition as it is in recurrent anterior dislocation. In the early stages of posterior subluxation in swimmers rehabilitation is possible by building up the external rotator muscles to counteract the powerful internal rotators.

### 13.10 Glenohumeral fracture-dislocation

Many glenohumeral dislocations are complicated by fracture of the humeral head. The commonest fracture is through the greater tuberosity, although other fractures such as those through the lesser tuberosity, the surgical neck, and the anatomical neck may occur. The fractures are often seen in combination producing two- three- and four-part fractures. This method of classification (Neer's) is very useful for it helps on decision making: the outcome depends on the degree of displacement, on the age of the patient, on the number of fragments and, of course, on the treatment (Neer, 1970).

### 13.10.1 DIAGNOSIS

This injury is less common in the sportsman than glenohumeral dislocation. Similar forces are involved and the two may be impossible to

232

distinguish clinically. However the patient usually has more pain and swelling after a fracture-dislocation. Abnormal mobility at the fracture site may be demonstrable.

Radiographs are diagnostic. However one projection may fail to reveal the fracture: never accept a single view of the shoulder before declaring the joint normal.

## 13.10.2 TREATMENT

Slightly displaced fractures heal satisfactorily as long as the joint is reduced and movement is prevented for a few weeks with a sling.

The very common displaced fracture of the greater tuberosity usually reduces almost perfectly when the dislocation is reduced. Sometimes the fragment does not reduce. If left in the unreduced position it causes a severe form of the impingement syndrome with late pain and stiffness in the shoulder. For this reason displaced fractures of the greater tuberosity must be surgically reduced and fixed if reduction of the dislocation does not reduce the fracture too.

The fragment is approached through a split in the deltoid and its reduction is achieved by judicious use of hooks while the arm is abducted and rotated. A wire loop is used to fix the fracture. Other internal fixation devices are too large, and cause late subacromial impingement. The arm is kept in a sling for three weeks for the internal fixation is not rigid; early active movement may displace the fragment. At three weeks graduated active and passive mobilization is begun (Fig. 13.9).

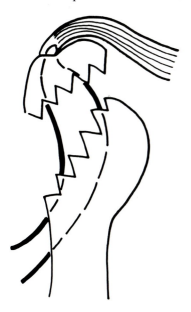

*Fig. 13.9* Open reduction and wire-loop fixation for displaced two-part fracture of greater tuberosity.

233

# Shoulder injuries

Similar fractures of the lesser tuberosity occur. They should be dealt with according to the same principles, for late malunion of the lesser tuberosity causes as much late impingement as a similar degree of malunion of the greater tuberosity.

Three-part fractures are seen on occasion. The principles of treatment are the same as those for two-part fractures: reduce the dislocation; if the fragments remain displaced after the reduction reduce and fix them operatively. Perfect reduction is less readily achieved. Late residual pain and stiffness is commoner than in two-part fractures.

In displaced four-part fractures the humeral articular surface is devascularized by fractures of both tuberosities and the surgical neck of the humerus. The incidence of late humeral head necrosis after this injury is very high. The only hope of achieving any sort of useful shoulder function is to replace the dead articular surface with a prosthetic one and to attach the rotator cuff to the prosthesis by, for example, the Neer technique.

## 13.10.3 COMMENT

To return to any sport which involves vigorous shoulder movement after a two- or three-part fracture requires anatomical reduction. The attending doctor should ensure that this has been achieved before active rehabilitation of the shoulder is allowed. Open reduction and internal fixation, although producing scars, leave by far the best shaped humeral head and the best chance of full recovery.

Curiously, the incidence of recurrence of dislocation is much lower after fracture-dislocation than after dislocation. This is presumably because the increased soft-tissue reaction to the bony damage stabilizes the shoulder. Of course it is also due to the fact that the muscles of the rotator cuff are necessarily intact after the episode.

## 13.11 Clavicle fractures and sternoclavicular dislocations

A heavy fall on to the outstretched hand or arm often fractures the clavicle. Usually the bone breaks quite cleanly in the middle third. Less frequently the outer third breaks. Medial third fractures are quite rare. Dislocation of the sternoclavicular joint, either anteriorly or sometimes posteriorly, may occasionally occur after the same sort of fall.

## 13.11.1 DIAGNOSIS

Local pain, swelling and bruising suggest the diagnosis. Radiographs in two planes are diagnostic.

Middle-third fractures are rarely associated with denervation or vascular blockade in the arm. However, it is incumbent on the attending doctor to seek these complications and to initiate treatment if they are found. Compound fractures are also rare. The combination of complication and compounding is not as rare as one would surmise for both are manifestations of a common feature, extreme violence.

Lateral-third fractures may be associated with acromioclavicular disruption and complete instability of the lateral fragment due to rupture of coracoclavicular ligaments.

Sternoclavicular dislocation may be complicated by compression of the trachea if the medial end of the clavicle is displaced posteriorly. This may simply cause a tickly cough, or it may produce severe respiratory embarrassment.

## 13.11.2 TREATMENT

The vast majority of middle-third fractures heal in spite of the treatment they receive. The process takes four to six weeks and during this time analgesics and a sling are all that are required. A degree of malunion is inevitable with this regime. The advantage is that there is little late stiffness, which is usually produced by tight bandages and slings, not by the fracture. The traditional yoke devices for bracing back the shoulders are ineffective at best. At worst they cause ischaemia of the arm and brachial plexus palsies.

The vain may demand perfect reduction, for malunion produces a bony lump at the site of the fracture. Reduction can only be achieved without operation by recumbency. The patient is instructed to lie flat on his back with no pillow until the fracture is stable after two or three weeks.

Severe displacement of the fracture exists when the fragments remain some distance from each other. The non-union rate for such fractures is high: internal fixation is justified. The fracture is approached through a skin cleavage-line over its prominence. A thick-threaded pin is passed laterally through the lateral fragment and is brought out through the skin near the acromioclavicular joint. The fracture is reduced and the pin is passed medially into the medial fragment until firmly impacted. The pin is cut off flush with the skin over the lateral fragment. Gentle active and passive shoulder movement is begun early and the pin is removed when the fracture is united radiologically.

Lateral-third fractures are treated on the same principles. However those associated with displacement of the acromioclavicular joint should all be opened and fixed, for late non-union and acromioclavicular instability is extremely common otherwise. The threaded pin should

235

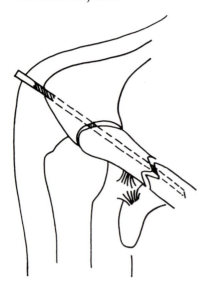

Fig. 13.10 Reduction and fixation of lateral third clavicle fracture associated with instability of the acromioclavicular joint and rupture of the conoid and trapezoid coracoclavicular ligaments.

transfix the acromion and the reduced acromioclavicular joint so as to stabilize the joint as well as the fracture (Fig. 13.10).

The surgeon may be tempted to simply excise the lateral fragment for displaced lateral-third fractures. This temptation should be resisted strenuously. Late untreatable acromioclavicular instability is the inevitable result.

Vascular and neurological complications are dealt with on their merits. Arteriography is required to localize the arterial lesion before arterial surgery. This need only be considered when limb circulation is so poor that permanent damage is considered likely. The artery may be approached via the fracture. The clavicle is internally fixed by means of a threaded pin after restoration of arterial patency. Post-ganglionic brachial plexus palsies should be identified by electrophysiological tests. Normal conduction velocities in numb areas imply preganglionic, inoperable lesions. Diminized or absent potentials in numb areas imply post-ganglionic, surgically remedial lesions. The best chance of surgical salvage occurs in the first week, and patients with such lesions should be explored via the fracture promptly.

Medial-third fractures are almost never badly displaced or complicated. They heal rapidly with a sling and analgesics.

Most sternoclavicular dislocations reduce easily and become stable after a few weeks. Some, however, require operative reduction. This may be an emergency procedure on those cases associated with respiratory obstruction. Rarely the unreduced dislocation goes unnoticed: late symptoms are rare. Most sportsmen return to full activity blithely unaware of the displacement. A few get late discomfort from the established dislocation. The medial end of the clavicle may be excised for this. There is no functional penalty after the procedure.

## 13.12  Injuries of the upper arm

Blows or excessive pressure on the dorsum of the upper arm can contuse the radial nerve and produce a wrist and finger drop. Fractures of the shaft of the humerus are generally treated by a 'U' plaster of Paris support and a 'collar and cuff' sling. The weight of the arm itself provides sufficient traction and non-union can be produced by applying excessive distraction, as by the 'hanging' cast where the forearm is encased in plaster to provide extra traction weight.

## 13.13  Impingement syndrome

Many sportsmen and women complain of post-traumatic pain in the shoulder brought on by movement and relieved by rest. In a large proportion the pain occurs during the mid-range of movement, and eases as the extremes are approached, giving the condition its alternative name, the 'painful arc syndrome'. The pain is due to impingement of elements of the rotator cuff beneath elements of the coracoacromial arch during joint excursion. It is an almost universal complaint, for most people have had some degree of painful subcoracoacromial impingement at some time in their lives. In most the pain is due to an acute lesion, and the symptoms rapidly subside. In a few severe chronic impingement takes place: symptoms may severely curtail the athlete's potential (Kessel and Watson, 1977).

### 13.13.1  DIAGNOSIS

Other chronic painful disorders should be excluded. These include cervical spondylosis, acromioclavicular degeneration and recurrent glenohumeral subluxation. In none of these is there the characteristic mid-range pain. The combination of mid-range pain with full active excursion is virtually pathognomonic of rotator cuff impingement. Local tenderness over one or other of the tuberosities confirms the diagnosis. The impinging structures should be identified for only then can a reliable prognosis be given and can rational treatment be instituted.

In the young athlete the commonest impingement syndrome affects the posterior part of the rotator cuff: it is nipped between the greater tuberosity and the angle of the acromion. During the abduction and external rotation sudden severe pain momentarily interrupts the movement. Symptoms usually follow an unexpectedly vigorous movement, such as throwing when the ball slips out of the hand. There is exquisite tenderness over the posterior part of the rotator cuff just distal to the angle of the acromion. Radiographs are normal. These patients usually respond rapidly to treatment and recovery is quick, complete and permanent.

The older sportsman may be prone to bouts of impingement symptoms after strenuous sport. Examination reveals tenderness over the tuberosities of the humerus, and there is often swelling and tenderness of the acromioclavicular joint. Radiographs usually show enlargement of the tuberosities and degenerative changes in the humeral head and in the acromioclavicular joint. There may be narrowing of the space between the humeral head and the acromion.

Exploration of these has revealed that symptoms are due to impingement and degeneration of the rotator cuff. Impingement occurs against a variety of structures, the common ones being the anterior end of the acromion, a hypertrophic coracoacromial ligament, an enlarged degenerate acromioclavicular joint, an incomplete congenital coracoclavicular bar and a combination of these. The cuff frays, thins and eventually ruptures as a result of the impingement. The long head of the biceps tendon shares in this process, and may rupture during an acute phase drawing attention to the degenerative process for the first time.

Acute calcific tendonitis must be excluded. The possibility of bicipital tendon dislocation from an abnormal, shallow groove must be considered. The depth of the groove can be seen on an axial radiograph.

## 13.13.2 TREATMENT

Patients with acute posterior forms of the impingement syndrome respond rapidly and reliably to a single injection of locally active steroid placed in the area of greatest tenderness. Of course this is extremely painful: the steroid should be mixed with local anaesthetic. On no account should the steroid injection be repeated. It is likely that repeated steroid injections lead to rupture of the rotator cuff. During the recovery phase following the injection the shoulder should be kept mobile and strong within the limits of pain. Local heat supplied by a lamp or diathermy eases symptoms. This phase of recovery takes two to four weeks usually.

The acute-on-chronic lesions seen in the older sportsman respond much less reliably and rapidly. It is worth differentiating between those patients whose symptoms arise from the subscapularis region primarily and those where the supraspinatus is chiefly involved. This is because it has been found that the response to treatment depends, amongst other things, on the site of the source of the symptoms: subscapularis lesions often respond to one injection of local steroids, supraspinatis lesions very rarely do. Thus it is worth injecting the tender area with local steroid if the tenderness is confined to the region of the lesser tuberosity. Success is heralded by gradual lessening of symptoms over the days and weeks which follow. The injection should not be repeated, whether successful or not. If symptoms recur then other methods of treatment should be instituted.

A course of local heat and mobilization is sometimes effective. Systemic non-steroid anti-inflammatory drugs are often useful too. Ketoprofen is an example. These drugs should be given in full dosage for at least a month to be effective.

Many patients who sustain repeated acute-on-chronic impingement injuries learn to live with the affliction: when severe, local head and systemic anti-inflammatory drugs get the patient back on to the sports-field. However, some find the symptoms intolerable. Operative decompression should be considered in these cases, as well as in those whose symptoms worsen with each attack in spite of non-operative treatment.

The details of the operation depend on the impinging structures and on the severity of the resultant degeneration. The commonest variety is impingement of the anterior part of the cuff beneath a swollen degenerate acromioclavicular joint. The outer end of the clavicle and the osteophytes on the deep surface of the acromion are excised. The coracoacromial ligament is removed via a split in the deltoid. The rotator cuff is inspected and repaired if necessary. The details of the repair depend on the size and position of the defect. Small tears are simply approximated by tough sutures. Large tears need transfer of muscle bellies across the humeral head before snug approximation can be achieved.

The surgeon should be aware of the potential pitfalls of the procedure: it is possible to remove too much of the outer end of the clavicle, releasing the attachment of the coracoclavicular ligaments, thereby destabilizing the articulation between clavicle and scapula. It is also possible to remove too little, rendering ineffective the excision arthroplasty. Failure to inspect the cuff carefully by fully rotating the arm may lead to persistent symptoms from unrecognized cuff rupture (Fig. 13.11).

Rehabilitation following surgical decompression should be energetic provided that the cuff was found to be intact. Once the postoperative pain begins to subside a programme of active and passive exercises generally restores function within a matter of weeks. The surgical approach is designed to allow this, and delay invites stiffness to become established, unnecessarily prolonging return to full activities.

# Shoulder injuries

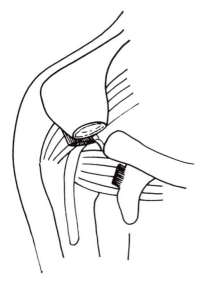

Fig. 13.11 Decompression of the rotator cuff by excision arthroplasty of the acromioclavicular joint and excision of the coracoacromial ligament. The cuff is well exposed by retraction of the edges of the sulcus between the anterior belly of the deltoid muscle and the middle belly.

Cuff repair necessitates rest of the repaired tissue for three weeks after the operation. Strictly passive movement may be possible in the co-operative sportsman, but active movement should be prevented. The help of a skilled physiotherapist is essential for this to be effective. If such help is not available it is wiser to forbid all movement for three weeks: overenthusiastic unskilled supervision may tear the repair before it is healed. Graduated active and passive mobilization is begun at three weeks.

## References

Bankart, A. S. B. (1983) The pathology and treatment of recurrent dislocation of the shoulder joint. *Br. J. Surg.*, **26**, 23.

Boyd, H. (1972) Recurrent posterior dislocation of the shoulder. *J. Bone Joint Surg.*, **54B**, 379.

Kessel, L. and Watson, M. (1977) The painful arc syndrome. *J. Bone Joint Surg.*, **59B**, 166.

Lombardo, S. J., Kerlan, R. K., Jobe, F. W. *et al.* (1976) The modified Bristow procedure for recurrent dislocation of the shoulder. *J. Bone Joint Surg.*, **58A**, 256.

Neer, C. S. (1970) Displaced proximal humeral fractures. Parts I and II. *J. Bone Joint Surg.*, **52A**, 1077.

Reeves, B. (1966) Arthrography of the shoulder. *J. Bone Joint Surg.*, **48B**, 424.

Weaver, J. K. and Dunn, H. K. (1972) Treatment of acromioclavicular injuries especially complete acromioclavicular separation. *J. Bone Joint Surg.*, **54A**, 1187.

# 14 Elbow and forearm injuries

## JOHN CHALLIS

Injuries to the elbow and forearm region are seen in a variety of both contact and non-contact sports. They are best considered under two main groups: trauma and overuse. The first arises as a result of a single episode of severe force, either extrinsically or intrinsically, and the second are a result of repeated stresses (see Table 14.1).

Most injuries caused by a single episode of extrinsic trauma, usually a fall or a collision, differ little from those sustained in non-sporting accidents. It is in this group that most fractures and dislocations occur. The consequences of mis-management of such an injury may be permanent pain and stiffness and for this reason it is important that they are treated by an orthopaedic surgeon.

The overall incidence of acute elbow injuries in sportsmen is low (Galasko et al., 1982) but it is a common site of overuse injuries in sports involving throwing (Reilly, 1981) and rackets (Sanderson, 1981). Such injuries may result in prolonged disability and inability to continue sports. In children and adolescents permanent damage can result from alteration in the normal pattern of ossificiation in the elbow (Pappas, 1982).

*Table 14.1* Two main groups of injury

| Trauma | extrinsic | : | fall or collision |
|---|---|---|---|
| | intrinsic | : | sudden excessive force from within athlete |
| Overuse | repeated stress | | |

## 14.1 Contributory factors

Factors which contribute to injury to the elbow or forearm may be general or local (Table 14.2). If the sport is not matched to the physique of the

# Elbow and forearm injuries

*Table 14.2* Factors contributing to injury

| General | Local |
| --- | --- |
| Wrong build for sport | Deformity of elbow, congenital or acquired |
| ? Excessive joint laxity | |
| ? Abnormal use of joints | Pre-existing pathological condition in the elbow |
| Inadequate fitness and training | |
| Excessive/inappropriate training | |
| Incorrect technique | |

sportsman then there is an increased likelihood of injury. The muscle fibre type which predominates in any individual is an inherited characteristic. The explosive muscular forces required, for example, in shot putting would be produced by muscles having a predominance of type II fibres, such fibres being well adapted for vigorous efforts of short duration. An individual with a predominance of type I muscle fibres, however much he trains, will never be able to obtain the same performance and would be more liable to injury and therefore would be advised to take up a sport not demanding such muscular strength.

It is common experience that knees which hyperextend are more vulnerable to injury. Whether the same applies to the elbow joint is not known. Osteoarthritis is commoner in lax joints (Ansell, 1972) and repeated impingement of the olecranon against the coranoid fossa could be a factor in its development. Whether or not repeated use of a non-weight bearing joint for weight bearing as, for example, in gymnastics predisposes to injury is also unknown.

Injury predisposition in the unfit, poorly trained and ill-equipped applies to the elbow and forearm as well as other joints, and the importance of pre-exercise stretching and limbering up cannot be over-stressed.

Excessive or inappropriate training, especially in the skeletally immature, can result in permanent damage. There is increased pressure upon children and adolescents to compete at sport. While such competition is healthy and a part of education, over-ambitious parents and coaches may be responsible for creating overuse injuries. 'Little leaguers' elbow' occurring in the young baseball players as a result of the repetitive stresses of throwing has been recognized in North America for over 20 years (Brogdon and Crow, 1960; Tullos and King, 1972).

In throwing and racquet sports correct technique is all-important. Incorrect technique, poor performance and the increased incidence of injury are interrelated.

Deformity at the elbow, either congenital or acquired, and pre-existing disease, will increase the risk of injury.

## 14.2   Relevant anatomy

The humero-ulnar joint is such that:

(1) There is inherent bony stability.
(2) In full extension there is 10–15° of valgus which disappears on flexion of the elbow or pronation of the forearm.
(3) In full extension the tip of the olecranon lies within the olecranon fossa, being separated from it only by synovium.

The humero-radial joint is a very shallow ball and socket and is inherently unstable, but provides valgus stress resistance to compressive loads across the joint.

It has been shown that the anterior oblique component of the medial colateral ligament is the mainstay of elbow joint stability, and has two components (Fig. 14.1). The posterior oblique part inserts into the medial side of the ulna, is tight in flexion and its division does not significantly alter elbow stability; the anterior oblique part inserts into the medial side of the coronoid, is tight throughout flexion and extension and its section produces marked valgus instability (Schwab et al., 1980). Together with the common flexor origin it is the main structure resisting medial tension stresses arising within the elbow joint during a fall on the outstretched arm (see Section 14.3).

Functionally the lateral collateral ligament arising from the lateral epicondyle and inserting only into the annular ligament does not provide stability as none of its fibres insert directly into either the radius or ulna.

## 14.3   Mechanics of injury

The elbow and forearm are part of a chain of levers running from the shoulder to the fingers. In movement of the arm the links of this chain are used in combination rather than isolation. Injury occurs when the stress upon the limb produces a strain which is greater than the tissue (capsule, ligament, tendon, bone or cartilage) can withstand.

During a fall or collision large amounts of energy are generated. There are many ways in which this energy may be absorbed: muscle contraction, elastic strain in ligaments and bone and absorption by protective clothing or padded surfaces (Frankel and Burstein, 1970). Of these mechanisms involuntary co-ordinated muscle action between flexors and

243

Elbow and forearm injuries

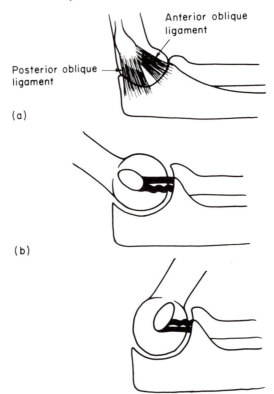

Fig. 14.1 The medial collateral ligament. (a) The two parts of the medial collateral ligament. (b) Diagram showing the two functional components of the anterior oblique ligament which remain taut throughout flexion and extension (after Schwab *et al.*, 1980)

extensors holding the elbow in an elastic position of slight flexion upon impact is of great importance (Carlsoo and Johansson, 1962). When muscle co-ordination is lost there is an increased chance of injury, hence the importance of training and fitness.

Which structures are injured as a result of sudden severe force depends upon the direction and magnitude of the force, the anatomical structure limiting movement (Table 14.3), and the angle of the elbow and position

Table 14.3 Factors limiting movement at the elbow

| | |
|---|---|
| (a) | Muscle tone |
| (b) | Tension in capsule/ligaments |
| (c) | Soft tissue apposition in flexion |
| (d) | Bony impingement in extension |

of the forearm at the time of the injury. In children and adolescents the actively growing epiphyseal plate is often the weakest point and avulsion of the epiphysis may occur.

The most common force is a combination of axial compression and valgus angulation as a result of a fall onto the outstretched arm. A variety of structures – soft tissue, bone or epiphyseal plate – may be injured (Fig. 14.2).

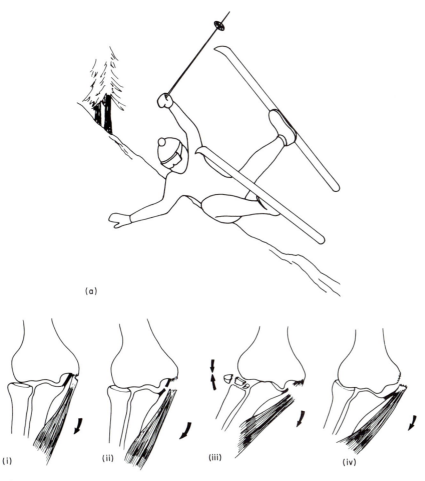

(a)

(i)  (ii)  (iii)  (iv)

(b)

*Fig. 14.2* (a) Axial compression and valgus angulation following a fall. (b) A variety of structures (soft tissue, bone, epiphyseal) may be injured. (i) Tear in common flexor origin; (ii) muscle tear plus tear in medial collateral ligament; (iii) soft tissue injury as in (ii) plus bony injury (fracture of radial head) due to lateral compression; (iv) in a child, avulsion of the medial epicondyle.

## Elbow and forearm injuries

In the analysis of overuse injuries in the elbow and forearm it is valuable to understand the mechanisms of throwing and hitting. The mechanism varies in different sports but the basic pattern can be divided into three main phases: wind-up, acceleration, and follow through (Table 14.4).

*Table 14.4* The throwing mechanism

(1) Wind-up
> Shoulder externally rotated
> Elbow flexed 45°, flexor and extensor tone balanced
> Wrist in extension

(2) Acceleration
> (i) Shoulder and elbow brought forward
> Forearm and hand left behind
> Medial side of elbow stressed
> (ii) Shoulder goes from external to internal rotation
> Medial side of elbow stressed
> Wrist flexes

(3) Follow through
> Forearm pronates
> Elbow extends

Strong static contraction of biceps and triceps occur in the wind-up phase (Tullos and King, 1973). A very large tensile stress is imparted to the medial side of the elbow during the acceleration stage. The medial collateral ligament together with the flexor musculature absorbs this stress. At the same time there is a large compressive stress upon the lateral side of the elbow between the radial head and capitellum (Fig. 14.3).

In follow through the triceps mechanism contracts to extend the elbow and great forces are developed along the course of the extensor mechanism and the forearm pronators and anterior joint capsule (Fig. 14.4).

Thus, for throwing, injuries can be classified into those resulting in medial tension, lateral compression and extensor overload – anteriorly and posteriorly (Slocum, 1968; Pappas, 1982). Similar mechanisms can be evaluated for the golf swing, the tennis backhand and the shot putt and discus thrower. Of course, the stress imposed will vary according to the speed of throwing or hitting and the weight of the object thrown or struck. Also movements of the arm are assisted by movements of the trunk and legs. It has been calculated, for example, that in throwing the torque created by rotation of the hip and trunk is more than 50% of that accountable by the elbow (Toyoshima *et al.*, 1974).

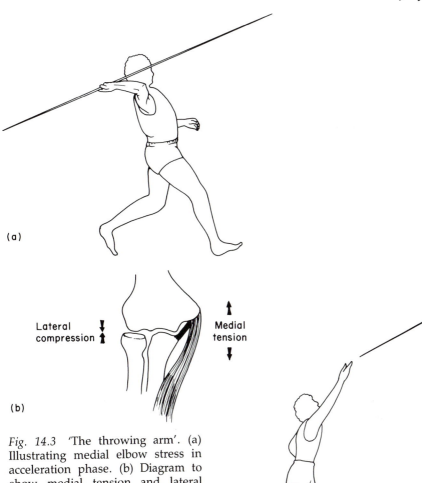

(a)

Lateral
compression

Medial
tension

(b)

Fig. 14.3 'The throwing arm'. (a)
Illustrating medial elbow stress in
acceleration phase. (b) Diagram to
show medial tension and lateral
compression.

(a)

Fig. 14.4 'The throwing arm'. (a)
Elbow extension in follow through
phase. (b) Diagram to show tension
in anterior capsule (AC) and triceps
tendon (TT) and compression at tip
of olecranon (o).

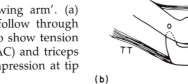

AC

o

TT

(b)

247

# Elbow and forearm injuries

## 14.4 Diagnosis

Diagnosis should answer the following questions:

(1) Which anatomical structures are involved? (Skin fascia, muscle, tendon, capsule, ligament, cartilage, synovium and bone.)
(2) What is the pathology? (Contusion, laceration, sprain – partial or complete, fracture or dislocation.)
(3) Are there any complications? (Neural or vascular.)

In order to answer these questions, a history and physical examination is necessary, sometimes supplemented by X-ray examination.

In making the diagnosis the extent to which painful conditions of the elbow may be due to referred pain should be taken into account and the patient should be examined from neck to fingers.

### 14.4.1 FEATURES IN THE HISTORY

In cases of trauma the number of structures damaged is usually proportional to the severity of the injury. The exact mechanism of the injury may be difficult to identify but nearly always it is possible to determine whether the injury was direct or indirect.

Direct injuries may cause fracture or dislocation but there will also be severe damage to overlying fascia, fat and skin. Indirect forces may impose very large stresses on the elbow causing ligament rupture with dislocation or fracture. In overuse injury, inquiry should be made as to any change in techniques or equipment.

### 14.4.2 FEATURES ON EXAMINATION

The examination should proceed in an orderly fashion as indicated in Table 14.5. The analysis by the degree, direction and strength of movements active and passive and resisted causing pain is termed 'selective tension' (Cyriax, 1982) and is very helpful in diagnosing the particular tissues from which the symptoms arise.

### 14.4.3 X-RAYS

Standard, anteroposterior, lateral and oblique X-rays will identify nearly all fractures and dislocations. Stress X-rays under a general anaesthetic may confirm complete lateral or medial ligament tears. In children, confusion between fractures and centres of ossification can be resolved by taking an X-ray of the uninjured elbow in the same position as the injured one.

248

*Table 14.5*  Features in examination of the elbow

| | | |
|---|---|---|
| (1) | Quick assessment of neck and shoulder | |
| (2) | Look: | deformity<br>swelling<br>colour of fingers and nails |
| (3) | Feel: | relationship of bony points<br>local tenderness<br>temperature of skin distally<br>capillary return nail beds (distal pulses)<br>crepitus (e.g. tenosynovitis) |
| (4) | Move: | active and passive and resisted movements |

Abnormal soft tissue shadows sometimes help in diagnosis. The fat pad in the olecranon fossa does not normally show up on an X-ray but when the joint is distended with blood or synovial fluid it may appear as a dorsal translucency (Fig. 14.5).

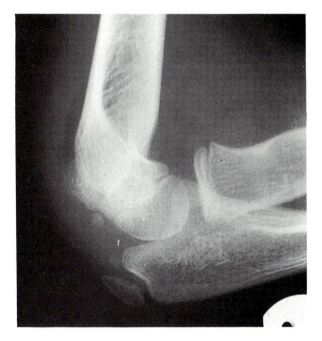

*Fig. 14.5*  The fat pad sign. The presence of the dorsal fat pad shown on this X-ray indicates distension of the joint by synovial fluid or blood and should stimulate the search for fracture.

# Elbow and forearm injuries

Arthroscopy and arthrography have not yet attained the popularity in the diagnosis of elbow disorders as they have in the knee.

## 14.5 Treatment

The aims of treatment in injuries to the elbow and forearm are no different to those in sporting injuries elsewhere and are summarized in Table 14.6. It is convenient to think in terms of first aid, definitive treatment and prevention. Who does what depends upon the place of injury and severity (see Table 14.7). First aid must involve a decision as to whether the sportsman should continue participation after the injury or be referred for definitive treatment. Whichever decision is made consideration should always be given to prevention. A summary of the various forms of treatment available is made in Table 14.8.

*Table 14.6* Aims of treatment in sports injuries to elbow and forearm

---

(1)  Reduce haemorrhage by:
      ice
      compression
      elevation

(2)  Allow healing with:
      minimal scar
      minimal loss of power
      minimal loss of movement

(3)  Return to sport only when:
      full power
      full movement
      full extensibility

(4)  Prevent recurrence by:
      analysing technique
      training and fitness

---

## 14.6 Acute traumatic conditions – elbow and forearm

### 14.6.1 SKIN

Penetrating wounds to the elbow are uncommon and may involve major blood vessels or nerves. Circulation, sensation and motor power should always be assessed.

*Table 14.7*  Treatment of sports injuries – who does what?

|  | *Where?* | *Who?* |
|---|---|---|
| First aid | Place of injury | Lay personnel (St John's coach)<br>? Physiotherapist<br>? Doctor |
| Definitive treatment | GP surgery<br>A & E Department<br>Sports clinic<br>Fracture clinic | Doctor<br>Doctor<br>Doctor/physiotherapist<br>Orthopaedic surgeon |
| Prevention | Training area<br>GP surgery<br>Sports clinic | Coach<br>Doctor<br>Doctor/physiotherapist/coach |

*Table 14.8*  Treatment of sports injuries – methods available

|  | *Trauma* | *Overuse* |
|---|---|---|
| Non-invasive | Dress abrasions | Adjust techniques of throwing, hitting, etc. |
|  | Ice strains and sprains | Adjust training programme |
|  | Elevate limb | Adjust equipment |
|  | Splint fractures | Ice |
|  | Tetanus prophylaxis | Ultrasound |
|  | ? Antibiotics | Interferential |
|  | Analgesics | Diapulse |
|  |  | Laser |
| Invasive | Treat vascular emergencies | Steroid injections |
|  | Aspirate haemarthrosis | Soft tissue operations e.g. tennis elbow |
|  | Debride contaminated wounds |  |
|  | Suture clean wounds | Bony operations e.g. removal of ulnar traction spur |
|  | Repair ruptured tendons |  |
|  | Repair ruptured ligaments |  |
|  | Reduce fractures:<br>  closed<br>  open and fixation |  |

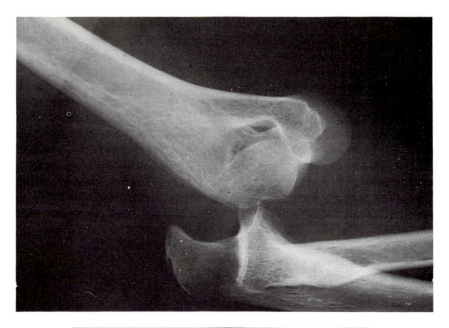

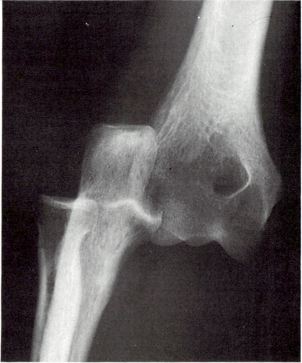

*Fig. 14.6* Radiographs showing posterolateral dislocation of the elbow. Think of the soft tissues!

## 14.6.2 MUSCLE TENDON UNIT

Injury can occur at any point along the musculotendinous unit. *Partial* tears of muscle bellies or junctions of muscle and tendon are common in the biceps, brachialis and forearm flexors in sports involving lifting, hitting and pulling. In prevention of such injuries it is important that stretching and limbering up precede vigorous exercise.

In these injuries characteristically there is pain on resisted movement and tenderness localized to the damaged area. Treatment is by ice and elevation followed by progressive mobilization.

*Complete* ruptures of the musculotendinous unit most commonly occur in the long head of the biceps tendon, but can also occur distally (Dobbie, 1941). The latter is usually the result of lifting very heavy loads or from contraction of the muscle against unexpected resistance. There is weakness of flexion and supination and swelling proximal to the tendon insertion. The best treatment is by surgical repair, the safest procedure probably being that of reinserting the tendon into that of the brachialis (Meherrin and Kilgore, 1960) and accepting the weakness or supination.

Rupture or avulsion of the triceps tendon is extremely rare. As loss of active extension of the elbow results, surgical repair should be undertaken. Avulsion of epiphyses may occur following violent muscle contraction in children; the commonest site is that of avulsion of the medial epicondyle and this is considered below.

## 14.6.3 CAPSULE AND LIGAMENTS

*Partial tears* of the ligaments are more common on the medial side. They result from a tension force in the medial ligament arising usually from a fall onto the outstretched arm (see Fig. 14.2). There is localized tenderness over the ligament and pain on stressing it but the joint remains stable. Treatment is by ice followed by early active movement. Immobilization of the joint is to be discouraged as this may lead to stiffness. The undamaged ligament fibres splint those that are torn so that healing can take place without loss of function.

*Complete* capsular and ligamentous tears are usually associated with dislocation and this most commonly occurs posterolaterally (see Fig. 14.6). There is considerable pain, swelling and deformity and the relationship of the bony landmarks are altered. It is mandatory to check whether or not there is any associated vascular or neural complications. It is also important to exclude an associated fracture by appropriate radiographs. The dislocation should be reduced under either regional or general anaesthetic as soon as possible. Following reduction a firm wool and crepe bandage with the elbow flexed at 90° is preferred to plaster. Gentle

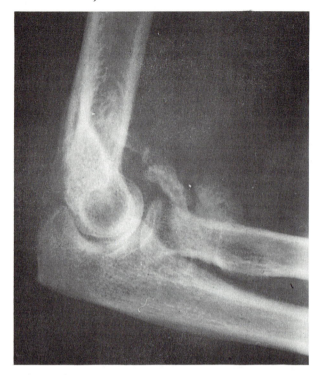

*Fig. 14.7* Radiograph showing myositis ossifications in brachialis following forced passive movements of the elbow.

active exercises can be started at two weeks and gradually increased. Under no circumstances should passive movements be allowed as this prejudices recovery and may lead to myositis ossificans (see Fig. 14.7). When muscle power, joint movements and muscle extensibility have been restored return to sport can be allowed.

An elbow dislocation should be treated by an orthopaedic surgeon. The condition of 'pulled elbow', most commonly seen in infants, is occasionally seen in children following sports injuries where there may be sudden traction applied to the arm. There is sudden pain in the elbow and the forearm is held in pronation. Attempted passive supination causes pain. It is believed that the condition is caused by a subluxation of the radial head in the annular ligament. Nearly always dramatic recovery follows the manipulation of the forearm into supination with the elbow flexed to 90° and pressure applied laterally over the radial head.

## 14.6.4  SYNOVIUM

Synovitis of the elbow most commonly results from a contusion but may be caused by an intra-articular nipping of a synovial fringe or impingement of bone against synovium as for example in the olecranon fossa.

There is boggy swelling and movements are generally restricted. Radiologically the fat pad sign may be visible. Treatment is by rest initially followed by progressive movements supervised by the physiotherapist. Non-steroidal anti-inflammatory drugs should be prescribed but intra-articular steroid injection should be avoided as this may cause damage to articular cartilage.

## 14.6.5  BLOOD VESSELS

Bleeding into the elbow joint occurs after either a ligamentous or bony injury. In contrast to the synovitis a haemarthrosis develops within minutes of the injury. There is pain and swelling and loss of movement and there may be deformity. The treatment of a haemarthrosis is that of its cause. A tense haemarthrosis can be aspirated by introducing a needle into the lateral aspect of the joint. This should be carried out in sterile conditions so as to minimize the risk of infection.

## 14.6.6  ISCHAEMIA

Two types of ischaemia may result from an injury to the elbow: firstly that due to abrupt cessation of blood flow through the brachial artery and secondly that caused by a progressive rise in compartmental tissue tension within the forearm (Eadie, 1979).

At the elbow the brachial artery lies midway between the humeral epicondyles being separated from the joint by the anterior capsule and the brachialis tendon. It divides into radial and ulnar arteries just below the joint line and there is an extensive arterial anastomosis around the elbow joint.

The deep fascia of the forearm is a dense tissue which forms an envelope for the flexor muscles of the forearm. It is attached to the humeral epicondyles, giving origin to the muscles arising from them, and is bound to the posterior border of the ulna. The lacertus fibrosis arises from the medial border of the biceps tendon, blends with it and below is continuous with the flexor retinaculum of the wrist.

In fracture or dislocations – particularly the supracondylar fracture in the child – the brachial artery may be damaged. It may be lacerated, contused or compressed. This leads to arterial occlusion (Type I ischaemia). There will be absence of peripheral pulses below the elbow,

255

## Elbow and forearm injuries

pain in the ischaemic forearm muscles, pallor of the limb and eventually anaesthesia and paralysis. If arterial circulation is not restored then there will be gangrene or massive muscle fibrosis. Occlusion of the brachial artery requires urgent surgical treatment and is best carried out by a surgeon with expertise in vascular surgery.

Compartmental ischaemia (Type II ischaemia) is caused by a rise in the tissue tension depriving muscle and nerve of blood supply. It may lead to the fibrosis of the muscle and contracture as originally described by Volkmann (see Fig. 14.8). It occurs most commonly when there is increased swelling due to bleeding, but can occur when there is a rise in the tissue volume due to excessive muscle activity as an overuse injury in athletes (Bennett, 1959; Bird and McCoy, 1983).

Because of the extensive arterial anastomosis around the elbow it is often this type of ischaemia which occurs even after acute occlusion of the brachial artery. It may not become apparent until several hours after the injury and for this reason all patients who have had major trauma to the elbow with extensive swelling should remain in hospital for a period of 72 hours until the danger of such a closed compartment syndrome has passed.

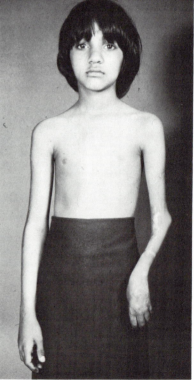

*Fig. 14.8* Volkmann's ischaemic contracture of the forearm.

256

The features of such a syndrome will be pain in the forearm flexor muscles, inability to extend the fingers and increased pain if the fingers are passively extended. The distal pulses may be normal. Treatment is by urgent decompression by fasciotomy. The treatment of the associated elbow injury takes second place.

## 14.6.7 NERVES

The three major nerves to the upper limb (median, ulnar and radial) may all be involved in injury to the elbow. Damage to nerves by penetrating injuries is rare. Such injuries require urgent surgical exploration, and it is important that diagnosis is not missed at the time of injury.

Nerves are more commonly damaged as a result of fractures, dislocations or contusions. The ulnar nerve, as it passes behind the medial epicondyle in close relationship to the medial collateral ligament, is most prone to injury, either by direct blows or by traction as a result of the dislocation.

The physical signs will be that of loss of sensation over the ulnar nerve distribution together with weakness of the intrinsic muscles of the hand. The median nerve is less commonly involved but the posterior interosseous branch of the radial nerve can be damaged in fractures of the upper forearm as it lies very close to bone as it winds around the radial neck. Damage to this nerve leads to wrist drop.

In most cases of nerve injury the continuity of the nerve remains intact and the outlook for recovery is generally good. Surgical exploration is usually only necessary when a nerve becomes entrapped in a fracture or within the elbow joint following dislocation.

An ulnar neuritis may arise as a result of entrapment within the cubital tunnel following repeated throwing (Godshall and Hansen, 1971). Stretching of the ulnar nerve with an associated neuropathy may occur many years after a supracondylar fracture as a result of growth disturbance causing cubitus varus.

## 14.6.8 EPIPHYSEAL AND BONE INJURIES

All such injuries are caused by severe forces applied either directly or indirectly. They present with a painful swollen deformed joint. The circulation to the limb must always be checked as well as the integrity of the major nerves.

The management of such injuries and their complications is the province of the orthopaedic surgeon and there are many excellent accounts of this in standard orthopaedic texts. Only an outline is given here. The subject of stress fractures will be dealt with in Section 14.7 on overuse injuries.

### 14.6.9  CHILDREN'S FRACTURES

Fracture patterns in children differ from those of adults because of the presence of bony epiphyses around the elbow; knowledge of these is essential for successful management.

A supracondylar fracture occurs most commonly as an extension type of injury when the small distal fragment is driven backwards and laterally (Fig. 14.9). The vulnerability of the brachial artery has been referred to above and it is essential that all injuries in which such arterial damage may occur are managed in hospital where a close watch can be kept on the circulation to the limb to avoid the catastrophe of ischaemic contracture (Fig. 14.8).

At the scene of the accident no attempt should be made to move the elbow. Attempting to do this may prejudice the circulation to the limb. As the injured patient will require a general anaesthetic, nothing should be given by mouth.

Avulsion of the medial epicondyle and its attached common flexor origin in isolation is a result of sudden muscle contraction. It may occur in combination with fractures of the olecranon, radial neck or lateral condyle following a valgus stress to the elbow.

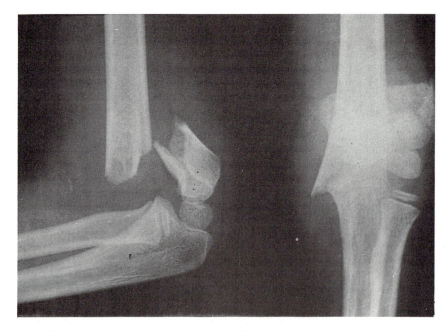

*Fig. 14.9*  Radiograph of a supracondylar fracture in a child of six.

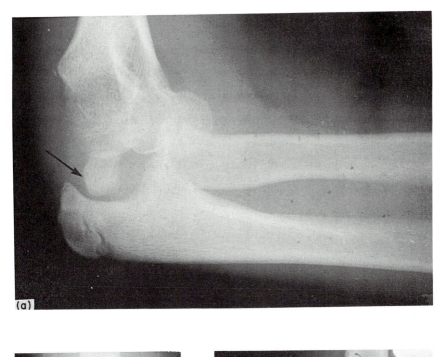

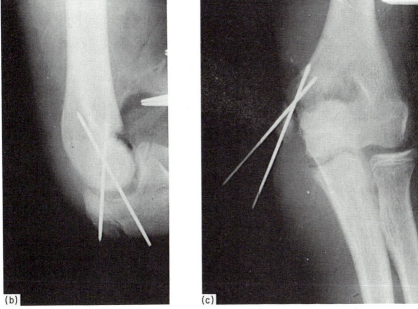

*Fig. 14.10* (a) Radiograph showing entrapment of the medial epicondyle (arrow) in the dislocated joint. (b) and (c) Open reduction is mandatory.

259

## Elbow and forearm injuries

Major avulsions of the medial epicondyle should be treated surgically in order to restore the position of the fragment. Occasionally such a fragment may become entrapped in a dislocated joint and open reduction is therefore mandatory (Fig. 14.10).

When there is a minor degree of displacement of the medial epicondyle then treatment is debatable. There is no doubt that conservative management accepting the minor degree of displacement gives good results (Wilson, 1960). It can be argued, however, that even minor degrees of displacement of the medial epicondyle by virtue of the attachments of the medial collateral ligament will create relative ligamentous laxity on the inner side of the elbow (Schwab et al., 1980). Probably the best treatment is to evaluate the medial collateral ligament using gravity stress X-rays (Fig. 14.11) and if there is significant opening up of the elbow on the medial side then undertake an open reduction and internal fixation.

X ray plate

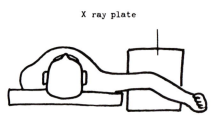

*Fig. 14.11* Gravity stress X-ray of the elbow (after Swab *et al.*, 1980).

Fractures of the radial neck in children usually follow falls when a valgus stress is applied to the joint resulting in compression in the lateral compartment. The displacement of the radial head may need open reduction (Fig. 14.12).

Lateral condylar fractures are, like radial neck fractures, a result of a valgus stress applied to the elbow. These fractures may fail to unite and a progressive cubitus valgus may occur (Fig. 14.13).

Olecranon fractures may occur following a fall onto the hand with the elbow flexed. The tension in the triceps may avulse the olecranon and lead to loss of continuity of the extensor mechanism. Treatment is by surgical reattachment of the olecranon.

Fractures involving the elbow joint in children and adolescents are potentially very serious as they may lead to serious growth disturbances and joint incongruity if mismanaged. Forearm fractures in children and adolescents are no more frequent in sports than in other forms of trauma. The presence of an intact periosteal bridge between the fracture ends makes for stable reduction in most of these fractures which can therefore

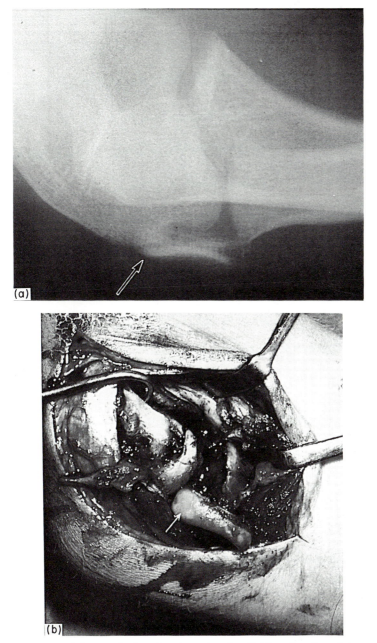

*Fig. 14.12* (a) Radiograph showing fracture of radial head and neck in a child. The radial head is displaced through 90° (arrow). (b) At operation the radial head is lying separate from the rest of the joint, it must be replaced anatomically.

# Elbow and forearm injuries

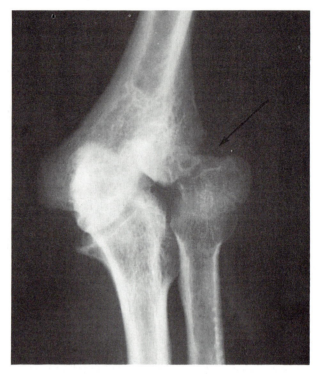

*Fig. 14.13* Radiograph showing cubitus valgus following non-union in a fracture of the lateral humeral condyle (arrow) in a child.

be treated conservatively (Fig. 14.14) in contrast to forearm fractures in adults, most of which require operative treatment. (Fig. 14.16).

### 14.6.10  ADULT FRACTURES

Supracondylar fractures may occur as a result of axial compression and can therefore frequently involve the elbow joint. The capitellum and trochlear may be separated producing a 'T' or 'Y' shaped fracture. There may be isolated fracture of the lateral condyle with associated rotation of the capitellum through 90°. Such injuries are occasionally not diagnosed and may result in serious loss of flexion due to mechanical block (Fig. 14.15).

Avulsion fractures of the olecranon will lead to loss of active extension of the elbow and produce local pain, swelling and possibly a palpable gap. Fractures of the radial head may give rise to loose bodies in the elbow joint which will produce locking.

With the exception of comminuted radial head fractures, which are best

262

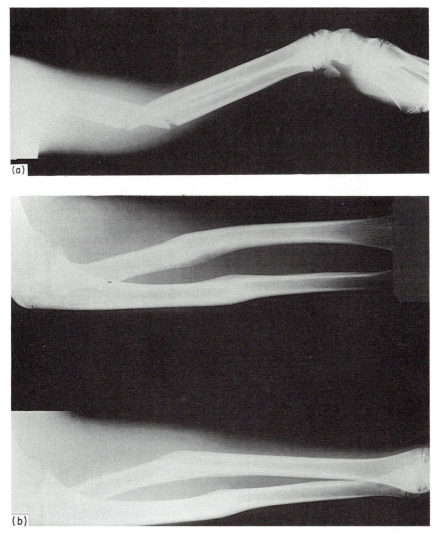

*Fig. 14.14*   Fracture forearm bones in a child. (a) Fresh fracture midshaft radius and ulna; although there is considerable angulation the periosteal tube ensheathing bone is only partially disrupted. (b) The united fracture showing moulding of bone taking place.

treated by excision, all other intra-articular adult fractures should be treated by open reduction and internal fixation so as to restore anatomical congruity of the joint.

Sometimes as a result of injury an osteochondral fracture occurs. These are more commonly on the convex surface of the capitellum and are

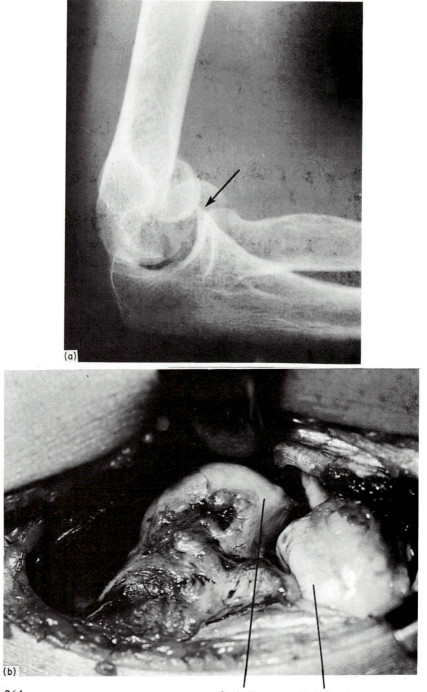

(a)

(b)

Capitellum     Radial head

analogous to the osteochondral fracture involving the femoral condyles of the knee. The osteochondral fragment may become a loose body and cause locking of the joint. Opinion differs as to the best treatment but if this fracture is diagnosed early then it is probably reasonable to replace and fix the osteochondral fragment. In the late case, and if the fragment has completely separated, then it is best removed and the resulting defect to the capitellum allowed to fill in with fibrous tissue.

Forearm fractures in adults follow severe direct or indirect trauma and are in general difficult to manage conservatively and require open reduction and internal fixation. When there is a displaced fracture of one forearm bone, particular care should be made to detect an associated dislocation of either the superior or inferior radio-ulnar joint (Fig. 14.16).

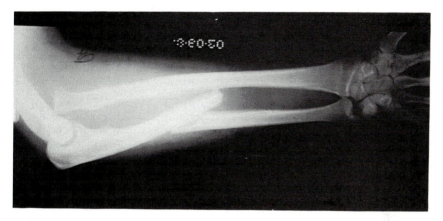

*Fig. 14.16* Monteggia fracture dislocation in adult. Ulnar shaft intact, but dislocate radial head and isolated fracture of the ulnar shaft. This nearly always needs open reduction and internal fixation. (Compare the child's forearm fracture in Fig. 14.14.)

## 14.7 Overuse injuries to elbow and forearm

The throwing mechanism has been described in some detail (p. 246) and it has been noted that in throwing, considerable tensile stresses occur on the medial side of the elbow whilst on the lateral side compressive stresses develop.

In other mechanisms, however, for example golf swing and the tennis backhand, these forces may be reversed and for the purposes of discus-

---

*Fig. 14.15* (a) Radiograph of adult with malunion of a fracture of the capitellum showing block to flexion (arrow). (b) The appearance at operation.

# Elbow and forearm injuries

sion therefore it is easier to describe overuse injuries on the basis of where the pain is felt rather than than using the mechanical classification of Slocum (1968). It must be appreciated, however, that pathological changes in the tissues may not always correspond to the site of the pain.

In taking the history it is helpful to have some knowledge of the techniques involved in the particular sport which may involve hitting or throwing. It is important to enquire not only about the site, quality, time of onset and duration of pain but also to elicit a history of locking or stiffness. It is sometimes helpful in overuse injuries to examine the sportsman immediately after the activity that provokes the symptoms.

In all the overuse injuries changes may occur sequentially in the musculotendinous unit, joint ligaments and capsule, the articular cartilage and bone and, in the child or adolescent, the epiphyses. It is important in diagnosis to determine which structures are involved.

## 14.7.1  MEDIAL ELBOW PAIN

Pain on the inner side of the elbow is common in sports involving overhead throws such as javelin and baseball and in racket sports. It is usually the acceleration phase of throwing that is the mechanism responsible (see Fig. 14.3 and Table 14.4). Pain is felt in the region of the medial epicondyle and common flexor origin and may radiate to the front of the forearm. Local tenderness may be felt over the same distribution. There is pain on resisted active flexion of the wrist with the elbow extended. Pain which is brought on by passive valgus stress applied to the elbow indicates damage to the ulnar collateral ligament.

The elastic musculotendinous unit is a structure which guards the relatively inelastic ligaments and capsule. Partial tears in the flexor muscles and pronator teres can develop and are manifest by local tenderness and pain on resisted movements. Sometimes there is swelling of the forearm which limits complete extension of the elbow and presents as a closed compartment syndrome (see the section below on pain in the anterior aspect of the forearm).

Repeated stresses in the child and adolescent's elbow may lead to secondary changes in the epiphyses which will effect subsequent ossification (Adams, 1965; Pappas, 1982). Although there may be several factors in the aetiology of the osteochondroses – ischaemia, trauma or a growth disorder – it seems that in general, articular epiphyses fail as a result of compression and non-articular epiphyses (apophyses) as a result of traction (Douglas and Rang, 1981). Continuing stresses may lead to partial separation of the medial epicondyle with relative lengthening of the medial collateral ligament (Schwab et al., 1980) and sometimes there is traumatic ulnar neuropathy (Godshall and Hansen, 1971). As the medial

266

epicondyle is extra-articular permanent irreversible changes in the joint do not occur, however, the compression stresses in the lateral side of the joint may lead to a crushing type of osteochondritis with fragmentation of the capitellum and loose body formation (Fig. 4.18).

Repeated stresses to the medial collateral ligament may lead to partial ligamentous tears and secondary traction spurs on the ulna in relation to the anterior oblique band of the medial collateral ligament. Compression stress within the lateral compartment may lead to osteochondral fractures in the capitellum and eventually osteoarthritis (Slocum, 1968; Tullos and King, 1973; De Haven and Evarts, 1973; Kerlan et al., 1975).

The treatment of conditions presenting with pain in the medial side of the elbow as a result of overuse depends upon accurate diagnosis. Prevention is most important. Expert coaching in order to master correct technique early in a sporting career is paramount. For example, in javelin throwing the round arm style must be avoided as this places enormous valgus stresses upon the joint (Fig. 14.17).

When the musculotendinous structures alone are involved, rest and ice application and gradual resumption of activity are usually adequate. Occasionally a local injection of steroid into the common flexor origin is helpful. Care must be taken to avoid injection into the medial collateral ligament as this will predispose to further injury.

Surgical release of the common flexor origin can sometimes relieve resistant cases of chronic medial elbow strain (e.g. golfer's elbow). Its use is not as effective as release of the common extensor origin for resistant cases of chronic lateral elbow stress (e.g. tennis elbow, see below) and this is probably because pain is arising as much from the stretched medial collateral ligament as from the flexor muscle origin. In undertaking such surgical release it is essential not to encroach upon the origin of the medial collateral ligament as this will certainly prejudice the stability of the elbow.

When changes have occurred in the bones of epiphyses the best advice that can be given is probably for the sportsman to give up the sport, but occasionally ulnar traction spurs – the stalactite lesion – can be excised (Slocum, 1968; Kerlan et al., 1975) and loose bodies causing joint locking must be removed.

The variety of pathological changes which may occur as a result of repeated medial stress are summarized in Table 14.9 and illustrated in Figs 18, 19 and 20.

14.7.2 LATERAL ELBOW PAIN

Lateral elbow pain may be experienced late in 'the throwing arm' as a result of secondary changes in the humeroradial joint resulting from

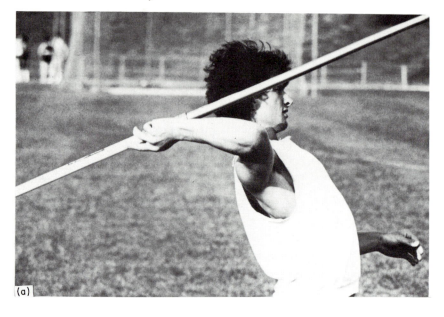

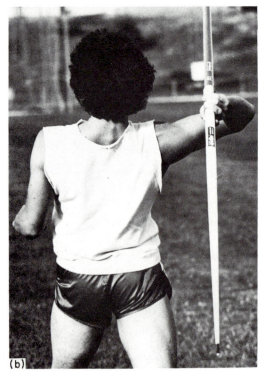

*Fig. 14.17* Different techniques of javelin throw. (a) This technique, the 'round arm' style, imposes a great stress on the medial side of the elbow. (b) In this technique, with the elbow straighter, there is much less stress on the inner side of the elbow. (Reproduced by kind permission of Vernon Turner and Nigel Stainton of the New River Sports Centre, Harringey.)

*Table 14.9*  Pathological changes in the elbow resulting from overuse

---

*Repeated medial tension*
Micro-tears at tenoperiosteal or musculotendinous junction of flexor muscles →
   fibrosis
Medial collateral ligament tears/stretching
→ avulsion of medial epicondyle (children)
→ ulnar traction spur ± loose bodies (adults)
Osteoarthritis

*Repeated lateral compression*
Osteochondritis of capitellum ± loose bodies (children)
Osteochondral fractures ± loose bodies (adults)
Osteoarthritis of lateral joint compartment

*Repeated extensor action*
Tears at tenoperiosteal or musculotendinous junction of triceps
Olecranon traction → olecranon spurs or stress fracture
Micro-tears at tenoperiosteal or musculotendinous junction of biceps and
   brachialis due to 'check rein' action of the flexors → fibrosis → contracture
Anterior capsular tears → fibrosis → coronoid traction spurs
Olecranon impingement → fracture tip of olecranon
                        → olecranon loose bodies
Osteoarthritis

---

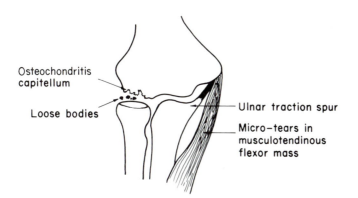

*Fig. 14.18*  Results of repeated medial stress to elbow. Diagram to show micro-tears in soft tissues on medial side of elbow, ulnar traction spur and osteochondritis of capitellum and loose bodies in later side of the joint.

compression stresses. It is, however, more commonly associated with lateral tensile forces which develop in backhand racket strokes and the leading arm in the golf swing and is familiarly known as 'tennis elbow'.
   Pain is characteristically felt over the lateral epicondyle and common

Elbow and forearm injuries

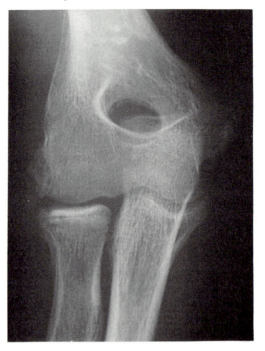

*Fig. 14.19*  Radiograph showing the results of repeated medial stress to the elbow in throwing in an adolescent. Note ulnar traction spur and osteochondritis of capitellum.

extensor origin and may spread to the forearm. There is local tenderness over the lateral epicondyle and common extensor origin and pain on resisted active extension of the wrist when the elbow is fully extended.

The exact aetiology and pathology are unknown although numerous pathological processes have been described: hypertrophy of synovial fringes, bursitis, degenerative changes in the annular ligament, and tears in the extensor origin. Certainly in cases in which surgery has been performed there is a high incidence of tears of the common extensor origin (Boyd and McLeod, 1973; Conrad and Hooper, 1973; Nirschl and Pettrone, 1979).

An entrapment neuropathy of the posterior interosseus nerve was postulated by Roles and Maudsley in 1972 but other reports, including electromyographic studies, have failed to substantiate this (Van Rossum *et al.*, 1978; Nirschl, 1980).

Priest investigated 2633 tennis players and found 31% had had elbow pain sometime in their careers. In 92% pain was felt laterally, most commonly over the lateral epicondyle. Age, weight, level of play, years of

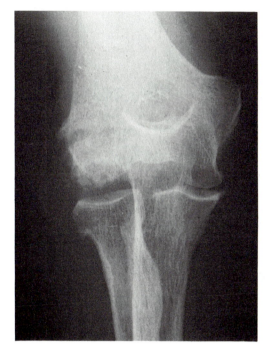

Fig. 14.20 Radiograph showing the results of repeated medical stress to the elbow in throwing in an adult. Note the ulnar traction spur and, in the lateral compartment, the loose bodies. Changes are a result of medial tension and lateral compression.

play and frequency of play were all found to be significantly greater in players with pain. The percentage of players with a history of elbow pain increased almost linearly from the age of 21 years to 55 years (Priest, 1982).

A number of factors contribute to the development other than those mentioned above and have been reviewed by Sanderson (1981). The common denominator is that of extensor overload which may result from faulty technique (Fig. 14.21) or inappropriate equipment.

Treatment should begin by an analysis of the technique of the sportsman. Correction of a faulty backhand stroke, relaxation of grip tension between strokes, alteration in the grip size, changing the type or the weight of the racket (Williams and Sperryn, 1976), and improving the power and extensibility of the forearm flexors by special exercises may help. Supports worn over the upper part of the forearm are sometimes beneficial.

In cases which prove to be resistant, local steroid injections into the site

271

# Elbow and forearm injuries

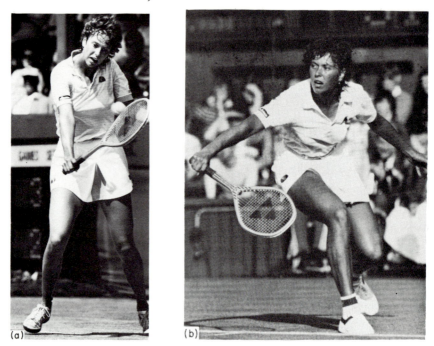

*Fig. 14.21* (a) A backhand volley. Player under pressure but demonstrating good balance. Note head of racquet held high and wrist dorsiflexed, failure to do this would produce considerable extensor overload. (b) A well executed backhand slice showing good weight transference onto leading leg and use of shoulder power to reduce extensor overload. (Reproduced by kind permission of Miss Jo Dury.)

of maximum tenderness can relieve symptoms. It is the author's practice never to give more than three such injections.

Manipulation of resistant tennis elbow by Mill's manoeuvre has its advocates (Wadsworth, 1982; Cyriax, 1982). The wrist must be fully flexed and the forearm pronated. From the position of elbow flexion the elbow is forcibly extended, the object being to break down scar tissue within the common extensor origin. It should not be carried out unless there is full extension present at the elbow. It can be carried out with or without a general anaesthetic and can be supplemented by deep frictions.

Patients who fail to improve with these conservative measures can be considered for surgery. As there is no established aetiology it is not possible to say which procedure is best. Many surgeons prefer a simple release of the common extensor origin but others include excision of part of the annular ligament (Boyd and McLeod, 1973), decompress the posterior interosseus nerve (Roles and Maudsley, 1978), or specifically expose the origin of extensor carpi radialis brevis to define an area of

272

degenerative change within the substance of the tendon (Nirschl and Pettrone, 1979).

The various methods available for treating 'tennis elbow' are summarized in Table 14.10.

*Table 14.10*  Methods available for the treatment of tennis elbow

Improvement of stroke technique
Relaxation of grip between strokes
Increase of forearm power, flexibility
    and endurance by special exercises
Alteration in racket grip size
Alteration in racket weight
'Alteration in type of racket frame
Alteration in racket string tension
Tennis elbow support
Local steroid injections
Surgery

### 14.7.3  POSTERIOR ELBOW PAIN

Pain in the back of the elbow occurs in sports demanding repetitive powerful elbow extension such as javelin throwing, shot putting, baseball pitching and weight lifting. Repeated overload of the extensor mechanism, usually in the follow through phase of throwing (see Fig. 14.4 and Table 10.4), may lead to a variety of lesions in both soft tissue and bone (see Table 14.9).

In injuries to the musculotendinous unit diagnosis and treatment are along the same lines for similar injuries elsewhere (see Section 14.7.1). In baseball pitchers, hypertrophy of the ulna and formation of olecranon spurs are common (Slocum, 1968; King, Belsford and Tullos, 1969). Such spurs may fracture and cause pain in a manner analogous to the ulnar traction spur. Surgical excision may then be required.

Olecranon stress fractures, although rare, should be suspected when there is a history of pain initially coming on after exercise, followed by pain accompanying exercise and then pain preventing exercise – the 'crescendo' of pain. There will be local bony tenderness. X-rays may not show the stress fracture initially but a bone scan will be strongly positive. Treatment is by rest followed by properly supervised resumption of training.

As well as lesions developing as a result of tension in the extensor mechanism, others may arise from impingement of the tip of the

273

## Elbow and forearm injuries

olecranon against the floor of the olecranon fossa when the elbow is forcibly extended (Fig. 14.22). This may result initially as a synovitis (the olecranon fossa is lined with synovium) but if repeated stress continues bone changes may occur at the tip of the olecranon (Fig. 14.22). These may progress and lead to loss of full extension of the elbow. Loose bodies may

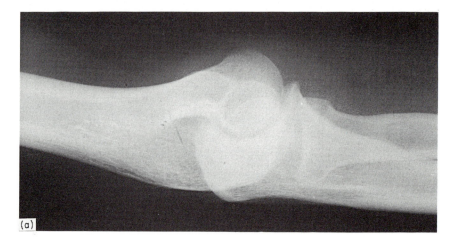

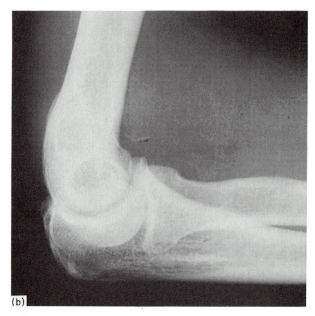

*Fig. 14.22* Lateral radiograph of javelin thrower's elbow showing impingement of tip of the olecranon in full extension. Note the ectopic bone at the olecranon tip shown in the radiograph with the elbow flexed (b).

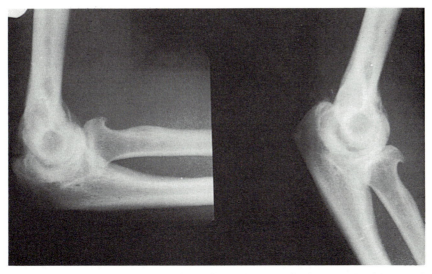

*Fig. 14.23* Lateral radiograph of an elbow showing the late result of repeated overuse–osteoarthritis. Note (1) The limited range of flexion and extension; (2) the ectopic bone at the tip of the olecranon; (3) traction spur on the coronoid process of the ulna.

form in the olecranon fossa and eventually osteoarthritis with permanent stiffness results (Fig. 14.23).

Such changes can occur in the elbows of baseball pitchers (Bennett, 1959; Slocum, 1968; Kerlan *et al.*, 1975; Pappas, 1982) and javelin throwers (Warris, 1946; Miller, 1960). Warris, in a radiological survey of seventeen Finnish javelin throwers, found that eleven had changes in the tip of the olecranon. These varied from mild irregularity to complete detachment of the tip and in one case an avulsion fracture of the entire olecranon had occurred.

Miller reported a top class javelin thrower who presented with pain felt in the elbow when it was forcibly extended and who had a fracture of the olecranon tip. Complete relief of her symptoms was obtained by excision of this bony fragment.

In discussing 'javelin throwers elbow' he distinguished two types: the first occurred in comparatively unskilled throwers, presented as pain in the medial side of the elbow and was invariably associated with the 'round arm' style of throwing (see Section 14.7.1); the second arises in more experienced throwers and is associated with impingement of the olecranon in full extension of the elbow as just described (see Fig. 14.22).

Treatment consists of rest in the acute stage followed by an analysis of

# Elbow and forearm injuries

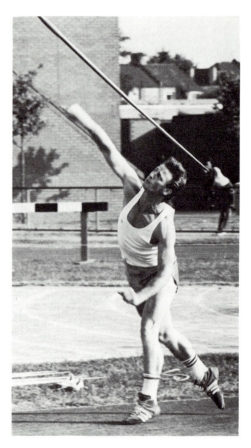

*Fig. 14.24* Note at the moment of release of the javelin (the follow through phase of throwing) the forcible extension of the elbow. It is not surprising symptoms arise from impingement of the tip of the olecranon in the olecranon fossa. Notice the pronated positions of the forearm which is said to reduce the amount of medial elbow stress and hence pain in inner side of the elbow felt so commonly in javelin throwers.

the throwing technique (Figs 14.17 and 14.24). When lesions occur at the top of the olecranon due to impingement, then surgery in the form of excision of the bony tip may help but the elbow can never be regarded as 'normal' and recurrence of symptoms demands retirement from the sport lest further damage be done.

When considering excision of the olecranon tip, the surgeon should be wary when a fixed flexion deformity exists at the elbow as this may be caused by contraction of the soft tissues anteriorly (see Section 14.7.4) and remain unaltered by surgery to the back of the elbow joint. Lateral tomograms with the elbow in full extension may help in diagnosis of olecranon impingement. The presence of a bony spur on the coronoid process shown in the lateral radiograph, however, is strong evidence that there is a fixed flexion due to contracture of the anterior soft tissues (Fig. 14.4).

### 14.7.4 ANTERIOR ELBOW PAIN

Pain in the front of the elbow may frequently arise in conjunction with pain posteriorly as described above because active extension of the elbow is always associated with synergistic action of both flexors and extensors.

The check rein action of the brachialis may result in tears at the musculotendinous junction and subsequent fibrosis leading to contracture. Similar changes may occur in the anterior capsule and may be associated with a traction spur of the coronoid process of the ulna which can be seen radiologically. In such an elbow there is likely to be a permanent fixed flexion contracture (Fig. 14.4).

### 14.7.5 ANTERIOR FOREARM PAIN

Pain in the front of the forearm is most commonly due to overuse in the musculotendinous unit. Pain felt proximally over the common flexor muscle belly and pronator teres has been referred to above in association with stress in the medial side of the elbow (see Section 14.7.1). Severe pain induced by athletic activity and felt in the flexor aspect of the forearm associated with inability to passively extend the fingers should alert the doctor to the possibility of an acute closed compartment syndrome (Bennett, 1959; Bird and McCoy, 1983). With Type II ischaemia (see page 256) a fasciotomy must be carried out without delay, unless there is rapid recovery following cessation of activity.

Pain felt more distally in front of the forearm is frequently caused by a tenosynovitis of the flexor tendons associated with repetitive wrist flexion. Treatment is along the usual lines with ice, rest and occasionally a steroid injection. Such an injection should be around the tendon and never into its substance.

### 14.7.6 POSTERIOR FOREARM PAIN

Posterior forearm pain is commonly due to a tenosynovitis of the extensor tendons. It occurs frequently in oarsmen and canoeists and the site of tenderness is usually felt over the dorsoradial aspect of the forearm. There may be crepitus and swelling. There is nearly always good response to rest and occasionally steroid injection. Surgical management by decompression of the bellies of abductor pollicis longus and extensor pollicis brevis has been described (Williams, 1977).

There is no doubt that prevention is of great importance in the treatment of overuse injuries around the elbow and forearm. Newcomers to a sport, be they children, adolescents or adults, should receive careful and conscientious guidance from the coach. Once bad habits are acquired

Elbow and forearm injuries

they are difficult to discard. Management of overuse injuries requires close co-operation between coach, physiotherapist, surgeon and sportsman.

## Acknowledgement

I should like to thank Mr Colin Bulbrook of the North Middlesex Hospital Photographic Department for his invaluable assistance with illustrations in this chapter.

## References

Adams, J. E. (1965) Injury to the throwing arm: a study of traumatic changes in elbow joints of boy baseball players. *Californian Med.*, **102**, 127.

Ansell, B. M. (1972) Hypermobility of joints, in *Modern Trends in Orthopaedics* (ed. A. Graham Apley), 6th edn, Butterworths, London.

Bennett, G. E. (1959) Elbow and shoulder lesions in baseball players. *Amer. J. Surg.*, **98**, 484.

Bird, C. B. and McCoy, J. W. (1983) Weight lifting as a cause of compartmental syndrome in the forearm. *J. Bone Joint Surg.*, **65A**, 406.

Boyd, H. B. and McLeod, A. C. (1973) Tennis elbow. *J. Bone Joint Surg.*, **55A**, 1183.

Brogdon, B. G. and Crow, N. E. (1960) Little leaguer's elbow. *Amer. J. Roentgenol.*, **83**, 671.

Carlsoo, S. and Johansson, O. (1962) Stabilisation of and load on elbow joint in some protective movements. *Acta Anatom. (Basel)*, **48**, 224.

Conrad, R. W. and Hooper, R. W. (1973) Tennis elbow: Its course, natural history, conservative and surgical management. *J. Bone Joint Surg.*, **55A**, 1177.

Cyriax, J. (1982) Diagnosis of soft tissue lesions, in *Textbook of Orthopaedic Medicine*, 8th edn, Baillière Tindall, London.

De Haven, K. E. and Evarts, C. M. (1973) Throwing injuries of the elbow in athletes. *Surg. Clin. N. Amer.*, **4(3)**, 801.

Dobbie, R. P. (1941) Avulsion of the lower biceps brachii tendon: analysis of 51 previously unreported cases. *Amer. J. Surg.*, **51**, 662.

Douglas, G. and Rang, M. (1981) The role of trauma in the pathogenesis of the osteochondroses. *Clin. Orthop. Rel. res.*, **158**, 28.

Eadie, D. G. A. (1979) Post-traumatic ischaemia, editorial. *J. Bone Joint Surg.*, **61B**, 265.

Frankel, V. H. and Burstein, A. H. (1970) *Orthopaedic Biomechanics*, Lea and Febiger, Philadelphia, pp. 84–89.

Galasko, C. S. B., Menon, T. J., Lemon, G. J. *et al.* (1982) University of Manchester Sports Injury Clinic. *Brit. J. Sports Med.*, **16(1)**, 23.

Godshall, R. W. and Hansen, C. A. (1971) Traumatic ulnar neuropathy in adolescent baseball pitchers. *J. Bone Joint Surg.*, **53A**, 359.

Katz, J. F. (1981) Non-articular osteochondroses. *Clin. Orthop.*, **158**, 70.

Kerlan, R. K., Frank, W. J., Blazina, M. E., *et al.* (1975) Throwing injuries of the shoulder and elbow in adults, in *Current Practice in Orthopaedic Surgery* (ed J. P. Alstrom), C. V. Mosby, St Louis.

278

# References

King, J. W., Belsford, H. J. and Tullos, H. S. (1969) Analysis of the pitching arm of the professional baseball pitcher. *Clin. Orthop.*, **67**, 116.

Meherrin, J. M. and Kilgore, E. S. (1960) The treatment of rupture of the distal biceps brachii tendon. *Amer. J. Surg.*, **99**, 636.

Miller, J. E. (1960) Javelin thrower's elbow. *J. Bone Joint Surg.*, **42B**, 788.

Nirschl, R. P. (1980) Correspondence. *J. Bone Joint Surg.*, **62A**, 314.

Nirschl, R. P. and Pettrone, F. A. (1979) Tennis elbow. The surgical treatment of medial epicondylitis. *J. Bone Joint Surg.*, **61A**, 832.

Pappas, A. M. (1982) Elbow problems associated with baseball during childhood and adolescence. *Clin. Orthop. Rel. Res. (Philadelphia)*, **164**, 30–41.

Priest, J. D. (1982) Elbow injuries in sport, *Minn. Med.*, **65**, 543.

Priest, J. D., Braden, V. and Gerberich, S. G. (1980) The elbow and tennis. Parts 1 and 2. *Phys. Sports Med.*, **8**, 77.

Reilly, T. (1981) Injuries in selected individual sports – the throws, in *Sports Fitness and Sports Injuries* (ed. T. Reilly) Faber and Faber, London and Boston, pp. 145–51.

Roles, N. C. and Maudsley, R. H. (1972) Radial tunnel syndrome: resistant tennis elbow as a nerve entrapment. *J. Bone Joint Surg.* [Br] **54**, 499–508.

Sanderson, F. H. (1981) Injuries in racket sports, in *Sports Fitness and Sports Injuries* (ed. T. Reilly), Faber and Faber, London and Boston, pp. 175–82.

Schwab, G. H., Bennett, J. B., Woods, G. W. and Tullos, H. S. (1980) Biomechanics of elbow instability: The role of the medial colateral ligament. *Clin. Orthop. Rel. Res. (Philadelphia)*, **146**, 42.

Slocum, D. B. (1968) Classification of elbow injuries from baseball pitching. *Texas Med.*, **64**, 48.

Smith, M. G. H. (1964) Osteochondritis of the humeral capitelum. *J. Bone Joint Surg.*, **46**, 50.

Toyoshima, S., Hoshikawa, T., Miyashita, M. and Oguri, T. (1974) Contribution of the body parts of throwing performance, in *International Series on Sports Sciences*, Vol. 1, Biomechanics IV (eds R. C. Nelson and C. A. Morehouse), University Park Press, Baltimore, pp. 169–174.

Tullos, H. S. and King, J. W. (1972) Lesions of pitching arm in adolescents. *J. Amer. Med. Assoc.*, **220**, 264.

Tullos, H. S. and King, J. W. (1973) Throwing mechanism in sport. *Orthop. Clin. N. Amer.*, **4(3)**, 709.

Van Rossum, J., Buruma, O. J. S., Kamphuisen, H. A. C. and Onvlee, G. J. (1978) Tennis elbow – a radial tunnel syndrome? *J. Bone Joint Surg.*, **60B**, 197.

Wadsworth, T. G. (1982) in *The Elbow* (ed. T. G. Wadsworth), Churchill Livingstone, Edinburgh.

Warris, W. R. (1946) Elbow injuries of javelin throwers. *Acta Chirurg. Scand. (Stockholm)*, **93**, 463.

Williams, J. G. P. (1977) Surgical management of traumatic noninfective tenosynovitis of the wrist extensors. *J. Bone Joint Surg.*, **59B**, 408.

Williams, J. G. P. and Sperryn, P. N. (1976) *Sports Medicine*, 2nd edn, Edward Arnold, London.

Wilson, J. N. (1960) Treatment of fractures of the medial epicondyle of the humerus. *J. Bone Joint Surg.*, **42B**, 778.

Woodward, A. H. and Bianco, A. J. (1975) Osteochondritis dessecans of the elbow. *Clin. Orthop. Rel. Res. (Philadelphia)*, **110**, 35.

# 15  *Hand and wrist injuries*

BASIL HELAL

There is a high incidence of injuries to the wrist and hand as British national insurance statistics illustrate. They comprise one third of the total of all injuries. The hand is, not surprisingly, very vulnerable because it plays a part in either the training or in the participation of every sport. It is the leading part and is part of a protective reflex on impact or in a fall. General statistical information on sports injury to the hand was not available, but in a prospective study of 200 patients attending our sports clinic 28% of all injuries involved the hand and a further 8% involved the wrist.

It is important to take a careful history which should include the environmental circumstances, the sport, the patient's occupation and hobbies (especially those involving music), the exact mode of injury, including factors such as the position of the hand at the time of injury, and handedness. Any history of previous injury, disease or operation is significant.

Examination should start with an observation as to the attitude in which the hand is held and whether there is deformity. The state of the skin and its appendages – that is the hair and nails – are examined. This includes swelling, colour, presence or absence of moisture, previous scars or signs of injury, blistering, or ulceration. Palpation should begin with the skin and warmth, moisture, elasticity and sensation tested. Palpation of structures deep to the skin must include muscles, arteries, tendon sheaths, joints and bones.

Movements both active and passive are then tested en masse and also those of individual joints. Integrity of motor power and then the general functional ability of the hand are assessed.

Examination of the hand and wrist is incomplete without examination of the remainder of the upper limb, the neck, shoulder and elbow joints, the key and pulp pinch, clench and power grip on small and large objects and the ability to grip a ball efficiently. Finally, the hand X-rays must be examined together with special views necessary to highlight difficult

281

# Hand and wrist injuries

areas. Tomograms, computerized scans, videotaped arthrography, scanning with technetium and other materials may also be required and finally vascular studies and nerve conduction tests may be helpful. The importance of an accurate initial record cannot be overemphasized from both a therapeutic prognosis and a medicolegal view point.

## 15.1   Problems at wrist level

A great variety of injuries occur at wrist level. Most of the injuries encountered in the context of sport do not involve a break of the skin. Open injuries with severance of tendons, major nerves and vessels are fortunately relatively rare and most of these are encountered in high speed sports such as various forms of motor cycling, motor racing, scrambling and power boat racing, where high velocity is in combination with broken metal and glass.

The bony injuries are most frequently due to contact collisions in those sports where impact of this type is usual, or to falls on to the outstretched hand. Commonly, the lower radius or radius and ulna are fractured and if displaced require reduction and usually plaster fixation. Carpal fractures, dislocations and minor subluxations about the wrist and carpus are easily missed.

Included in the differential diagnosis of pain of the ulnar side of the wrist are the following:

- Referred from neck or may be referred from ulnar entrapment or neuritis at elbow level.
- Due to damage to the ulnar collateral ligament.
- Subluxation of the ulnar head.
- Tendinitis of the flexor or extensor carpi ulnaris or bursitis related to these tendons.
- Recurrent subluxation of the extensor carpi ulnaris.
- Damage to the triangular fibrocartilage.
- Damage to the ulnar nerve at the wrist.
- Damage or subluxation of the pisiform.
- Damage to the hook of the hamate.
- Rarely due to ulnar arteritis or thrombosis.

In pain on the radial side of wrist the following must be considered:

- Tenosynovitis of the flexor carpi radialis or bursal inflammation related to these tendons.
- Tenosynovitis of the abductor longus and extensor brevis of thumb.
- Tenosynovitis of wrist extensors.

282

- Tenosynovitis of finger extensors.
- Injuries to the radial styloid.
- Injuries to the scaphoid and lunate.
- Dislocations and instability of the scaphoid and lunate, trapezio-scaphoid or trapezio-metacarpal joints.
- Avascular necrosis of radial carpal bones.
- Median nerve entrapment in the carpal tunnel.

## 15.2 Tendinitis, tenosynovitis and bursitis

In tendinitis and tenosynovitis local tenderness and crepitus on moving the affected tendons can be felt. Stretching the affected tendons will give rise to pain to pain, for example, in the thumb where there is abductor longus and extensor brevis involvement (de Quervain's disease) pain is felt on placing the thumb in the palm and deviating the wrist ulnarwards, as in Finkelstein's test.

Boxer's knuckle is a form of bursitis overlying the metacarpal head. Another form is due to intermetacarpal ligament stretching and instability associated with strapping which compresses the bases of the bones and distracts the heads when there is no synovial sheath (Sperryn, 1973).

## 15.3 Recurrent subluxation of the extensor carpi ulnaris

This is characterized by a painful recurrent snapping over the dorso-ulnar aspect of the wrist on supination (Burkhart, Wood and Linscheid, 1982). The instability is produced by an ulnar deviation, supination injury. These injuries have been described in soft ball, baseball, wrestling, weightlifting, golf, usually as an acute episode. If they do not resolve with rest then a surgical reconstruction of the roof of the sixth dorsal extensor compartment using a portion of flexor carpi ulnaris is carried out.

## 15.4 Median entrapment

Acute carpal tunnel compression in athletes usually follows tenosynovitis of the flexors and this has been seen on several occasions in inexperienced rowers. It is characterized by paraesthesiae felt in the radial three and a half digits and rarely by altered sensation. It usually abates with rest or splintage. A steroid injection into the carpal tunnel will accelerate the loss of symptoms. On only one occasion in a rower was it found necessary to decompress the carpal tunnel because of extremely severe pain and signs of total median knockout with paralysis of abduction and opposition of the thumb (Fig. 15.1).

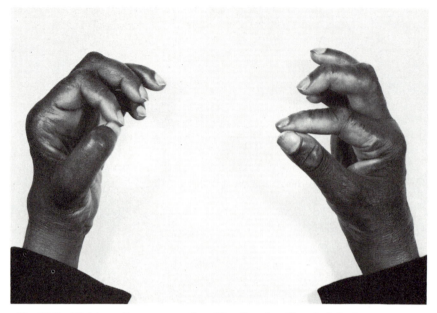

*Fig. 15.1*  Right median nerve palsy. The thumb will not abduct nor rotate.

## 15.5  Ulnar nerve

Four long-distance cyclists and one motor cyclist (scrambler) were seen with full motor paralysis of the ulnar nerve due to compression in the canal of Guyon, that is after the nerve has given off its sensory branch (Fig. 15.2) (Burke, 1981).

Direct trauma, especially in karate, has produced a full neuropraxia with sensory loss in the ulnar one and a half digits as well as paralysis of ulnar intrinsics resulting in clawing of the ulnar two fingers, weakness of abductor and adductors of the fingers and adduction of the thumb. (In Froment's sign the thumb on the affected side flexes at the inter-phalangeal joint to compensate. Later, wasting of the interossei and hypothenar muscles occurs (Fig. 15.3.) These will recover spontaneously if further trauma or compression is avoided. Sometimes suitably padding the handle bar hand grips with foam rubber is all that needs to be done.

284

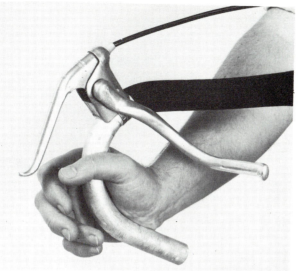

*Fig. 15.2* Mechanism of compression of motor branch of ulnar nerve by handle bar pressure.

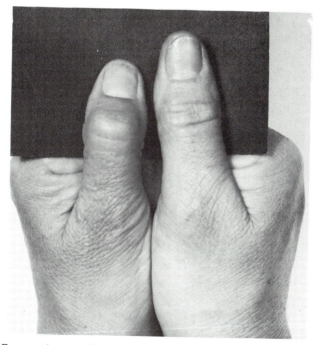

*Fig. 15.3* Froment's sign. The weakness of the adductor is compensated by use of the long flexor to the thumb on the left.

## 15.6 Ulnar collateral ligament of the wrist

This can be sprained or may be more rarely the site of acute calcification in the older sportsperson. Tests for gout and pseudogout should be carried out. Protection in a light splint may have to be continued for up to three months as these lesions are frequently slow to heal.

## 15.7 Ulnar head subluxation and styloid fracture

This can give rise to pain particularly on rotation of the wrist. Springing the ulnar head causes pain. Usually patience is rewarded by a loss of symptoms. Rarely is it necessary to excise an ulnar head but if this procedure has to take place then a stabilizing procedure using a loop of flexor carpi ulnaris round the distal stump is useful. A non-united ulnar styloid fracture sometimes gives rise to persistent pain. Excision of the loose fragment usually solves the problem.

## 15.8 Pisiform problems

Fractures and dislocations of the pisiform can occur in sport. A number of conditions relating to the pisiform and piso-triquetral joint have been encountered in the author's orthopaedic practice in the past sixteen years and are listed below. Several have occurred in athletes. As any of these conditions could occur in sportsmen their relative incidence is also listed.

| | |
|---|---|
| Fractures | 17 |
| Osteoarthrosis | 5 |
| Rheumatoid | 2 |
| Pre-pisiform bursae | 3 |
| Chondromalacia | 6 |
| Osteochondritis dissecans | 1 |
| Synovial chondromatosis | 1 |
| Intraosseous ganglion | 1 |
| Dislocations and subluxations | 8 |

Fractures usually of the crush type have been seen from the sports of karate and judo. Subtle instability can occur in racket handling games, especially those requiring a wristy action such as badminton or squash. There is pain on the ulnar and volar aspect at the base of the hypothenar eminence. Resisted ulnar deviation and flexion of the wrist aggravate the pain and there is point tenderness over the pisiform. Movement of the pisiform on the triquetral with the wrist flexed and ulnarwards deviated is attempted in a side to side and axial direction and normally no adventitious movement occurs. Four patients have been described with pain secondary to instability (Helal, 1978) and a further three have been encountered since the paper referred to above was published.

Persistent discomfort is best treated by excision of the pisiform, care being taken to avoid damage to the ulnar nerve which lies adjacent to the radial border of the bone.

### 15.9 Fracture of the hook of the hamate

The hook of the hamate gives attachment to the flexor retinaculum, piso-lunate ligament and two muscles, the short flexor digiti minimus and the opponens digiti minimus. The hook may be fractured by a direct blow as in a fall on to the base of the palm, in a karate 'chop', or by a blow from the handle of a golf or cricket bat in a mis-hit, especially if the ground is hit in the process of making a stroke or strike (Fig. 15.4) (Stark et al., 1977; Torisu, 1972).

Avulsion may possibly occur through powerful inco-ordinate contraction of the flexor carpi ulnaris via the pisiform and piso-lunate ligament. The patient complains of pain felt deep in the base of the hypothenar eminence and direct pressure or gripping is painful.

This fracture is sometimes difficult to display on a radiograph and an oblique view with the wrist radially deviated may demonstrate this best. The carpal tunnel view may not display the fracture due to overlap. A rare complication is an attrition rupture of the flexor profundus to the little finger which runs alongside the hook of the hamate within the carpal tunnel.

Persistently painful non-union is not uncommon and should be treated by excision of the detached fragment, care again being taken to avoid damage to the adjacent ulnar nerve motor branch.

### 15.10 Ulnar artery thrombosis

The hypothenar 'hammer' syndrome (Conn, Bergan and Bell, 1970) describes the effect of repetitive blows to the distal part of the ulnar artery against the hook of the hamate. This leads to pain on the ulnar side of the hand at the base of the palm which is ischaemic in nature. A Raynaud type of spasm of the vessels with pallor and blueness of the fingers occurs. This syndrome is seen particularly in karate and in those boxers who persistently punch with an open glove. The adjacent ulnar nerve can

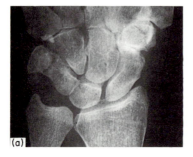

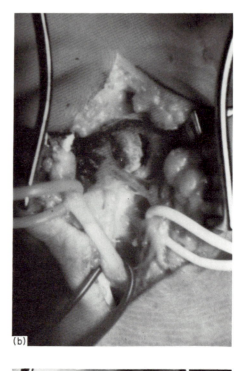

*Fig. 15.4* Fracture of the hook of the hamate. (a) Anteroposterior radiograph. (b) At operation the loose fragment is in close proximity to the ulnar nerve. (c) Lateral radiograph. (d) To show the size of the excised fragment.

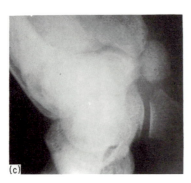

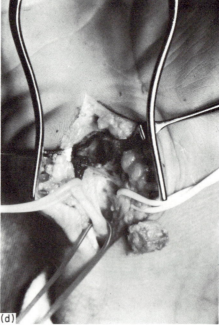

also be involved. The Allen test is carried out to see whether occlusion of the artery produces any serious ischaemic changes. This consists of obliterating both ulnar and radial arteries by finger pressure after clenching the hand to squeeze the blood out then releasing each in turn and watching the area of flush as blood enters the hand.

If the circulation to the hand is not at risk then simple resection will relieve symptoms. If this cannot be done without serious ischaemic changes resection and grafting is carried out.

## 15.11 Fractures

The most common of these is the fracture of the distal radius alone, commonly of a greenstick type in children or a Colles fracture in adults where it is combined with avulsion of the ulnar styloid. These fractures are dorsiflexion supination injuries produced by a fall on the outstretched hand or in player collisions in body contact sports, such as ice hockey, football or rugby.

Displaced fractures should be reduced and immobilized for three to four weeks in children and four to five weeks in adults. The radial styloid alone may be fractured and this is probably an ulnar deviation avulsion injury. If displaced, reduction followed by K wire fixation may be necessary to hold the reduction.

## 15.12 Fractures of the scaphoid

Diagnosis: pain on the radial side of the wrist aggravated by radial deviation and dorsiflexion; tenderness in the anatomical snuffbox. An X-ray may not show a fracture until two to three weeks have elapsed. In these fractures, the thumb should be included in the cast and the wrist should be in neutral or slightly flexed, not dorsiflexed as is often recommended for this increases the fracture gap.

Scaphoid fractures may fail to unite. This often depends on the vagaries of the blood supply. For the same reason the proximal pole may undergo an avascular necrosis if as happens in about 8% of people the blood supply is solely axial via the body of the bone.

A fracture may not be immediately detectable so suspicion alone should lead to treatment by a plaster cast which also holds the proximal phalanx of the thumb. Doubt as to the presence of fracture or avascular necrosis can be resolved by a technetium bone scan which, with the modern scanner, will locate the site very accurately (King and Turnbull, 1982).

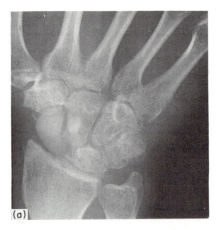

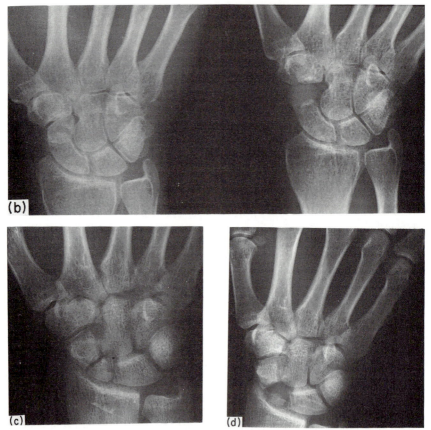

*Fig. 15.5* Scaphoid replacement. (a) Complete replacement of scaphoid. (b) Displaced distal pole fracture and its replacement by a universal small joint spacer (Biomet). (c) Non-union of proximal pole fracture. (d) Replacement of proximal pole by universal small joint spacer (Biomet).

290

Established non-union may require graft and screw fixation. The Herbert screw has proved a very satisfactory device for this purpose. Local necrosis may be treated by partial replacement of the scaphoid by a silicone elastomer ball spacer or a section of a Swanson silastic scaphoid (Fig. 15.5) (Helal, 1969). In more widespread necrosis it may be necessary to replace the whole scaphoid by a Swanson prosthesis.

Early resumption of sport in various types of rigid or soft silicone elastomer casts has been recommended, but this is not advised as most soft splints do not protect the part sufficiently well.

## 15.13   The unstable scaphoid

Two strong ligaments support the scaphoid: the volar radio-scapho-capitate ligament and the scapho-lunate ligament. These may be ruptured in the absence of any fracture or frank dislocation and the consequences are serious, producing early degenerative joint changes if they are not recognized.

The best X-ray view is one taken with the wrist supinated and the fist clenched when a gap greater than the normal 2 mm will appear between the scaphoid and lunate. This is the so-called Terry Thomas sign after the English actor and comedian who happened to have a large gap between his two upper central incisors (Fig. 15.6) (Frankel, 1977).

If discovered early the ligaments can be repaired. Alternatively the scaphoid can be stabilized by fusion to the lunate or to the trapezium (Watson, Goodman and Johnson, 1981). Many varieties of intercarpal instability have been described and both dorsal and volar intercalary segment instabilities have to be recognized to enable correct treatment to be instituted (Taleisnik, Malerich and Prietto, 1982; Linscheid et al., 1972).

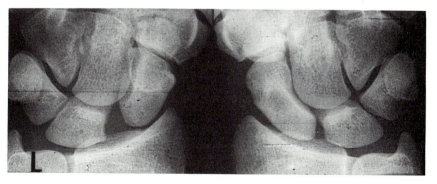

*Fig. 15.6*   The Terry Thomas sign of scapho-lunate dissociation.

## 15.14 Lunate dislocation, perilunate dislocation and transscaphoid periulnar dislocation

All these injuries may occur in the dorsi-flexion-supination injury to the hand. The study by Mayfield, Johnson and Kiloyne (1980) describes the mechanics of injury. All are serious and require urgent reduction. The inexperienced can easily miss these carpal injuries. As the displacements are almost always volar the median nerve and the tendinous contents of the carpal tunnel may be damaged. Closed reduction should always be tried and open reduction should follow if the former method fails. The lunate especially may lose its blood supply and undergo avascular necrosis.

## 15.15 Non-traumatic avascular necrosis of the lunate (Keinboch's disease)

This is a cause of wrist pain and may be associated with trauma or with a congenital variance of forearm bone length, namely a short ulna or long radius (Gelberman *et al.*, 1975). Treatment may consist of correction of bone length disparity in the early phases or replacement of the bone when bone collapse has occurred (Fig. 15.7).

## 15.16 Sprains about the wrist

There are a whole range of vague pains that are felt in the wrist commonly in young women for which no obvious pathology can be found. One is often driven to a full investigation including strain views, scans, computerized tomography and sometimes vascular studies and a search for more proximal referred causes. If all these draw a blank then reassurance and a light support for the wrist during exercise combined with simple analgesia such as aspirin will see them through the year or two that may elapse before symptoms abate.

It is important to exclude conditions such as osteoid osteoma, glomus tumours and bone infarctions due, for example, to diving which may be an unmentioned leisure sport indulged in by a serious athlete in some other field. Often minor clinically undetectable degrees of intercarpal instability are the cause for their vague pains and this is not uncommonly associated with a degree of generalized joint laxity.

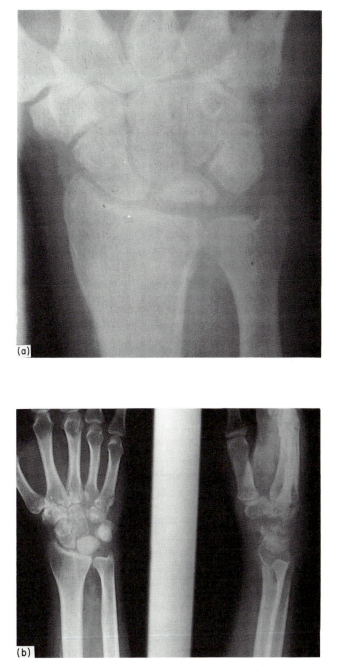

*Fig. 15.7* (a) Collapse of lunate in Keinboch's disease. (b) Replacement of lunate in Keinboch's disease.

Hand and wrist injuries

## 15.17   Skin abrasions: wounds and blistering

These must be managed correctly particularly when they have occurred on grassed pitches or in contaminated water. Cleansing should be thorough, antiseptic dressings applied and precautions taken against tetanus. With regard to tetanus immunization a ten year maximum period between active immunizations as described by Smith, Lawrence and Evans (1975) is probably too long and a five year maximum is preferred.

Human tetanus immunoglobulin should be given in the following circumstances:

(1) If five years or more have elapsed since previous active immunization.
(2) If the patient is uncertain about previous immunization or is unable to give a history.
(3) In veterinary and farm injuries.
(4) If injuries occurred on ground that had been fertilized with manure.
(5) In penetrating wounds (especially those involving muscle and bone).

Concurrent active immunization by toxoid is given into the contralateral limb. Antibiotic cover is given if the wound is badly contaminated and if there is delay between wounding and local antiseptic measures.

In dealing with wounds on the palmar aspect of the fingers and palm strong chemical irritants such as spirit or iodine should be avoided because even a small penetration of a digital flexor sheath will, if there is movement of the contained tendon, draw the irritant fluid into the flexor sheath and cause a severe and sometimes extensive damaging adhesive tenosynovitis. Mild detergent antiseptics such as chlorhexidine are best used.

Cuts should be closed by adhesive strips if they lie parallel to skin creases or Langers lines (the planes along which skin would split if sufficiently stressed) but sutured in areas where they have a tendency to gape. Wounds crossing joint flexor creases in the axis of the finger should be converted to Z plasties to avoid contractures (Fig. 15.8).

Blisters are common in rowers, water-skiers, sailors, weightlifters, gymnasts and in racket games. They should be evacuated by marginal incision or needle aspiration and the 'dome' retained as a 'dressing' and an elastoplast dressing can be placed over the area. Those involved in water sports should remember that the water may be heavily polluted and great care should be taken not to immerse raw areas and wounds.

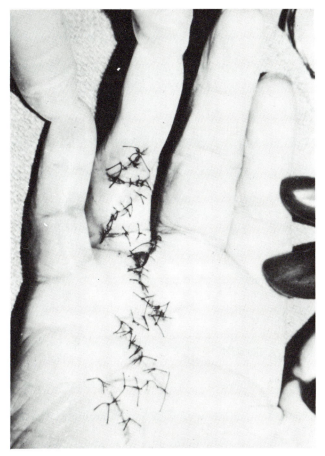

*Fig. 15.8* The contracture produced by a previously straight scar was overcome by converting this to a series of Z-plasties.

## 15.18 Frostbite

Low temperature injury is a very real hazard to the hand in water sports and in sailing and canoeing in cold climes, but most of all in snow sports, such as mountaineering and skiing in low temperatures (Fig. 15.9).

Skin that is frozen white should be warmed without delay in a bath at 42° if a dry heat facility is not available. Antibiotic cover is given. It should be remembered that mittens are warmer than gloves for they allow more movement of the fingers and repeated clenching of the hand aids the circulation. A thin pair of gloves worn inside mittens is useful if it is necessary to handle metal equipment such as ski bindings, or toboggan

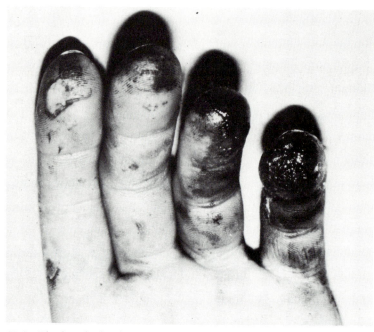

*Fig. 15.9* The hand of a ski mountaineer who was unconscious for ten minutes after a fall in which the mitten on this hand was torn off.

runners, for metal at −10° can produce cold burns and the skin will be lifted off the digit and left adhering to the object handled. Hands should be kept as dry as possible in very low temperatures.

Children's hands can suffer severe epiphyseal damage if allowed to freeze, with subsequent severe stunting of growth and abnormal growth patterns. The swollen blue hand of the child who has been playing out in the snow should be treated as for frostbite (Bigelow and Ritchie, 1963; Hakstian, 1972).

## 15.19  Traumatic amputation

If the amputated portion is preserved then it should be sutured back as a dressing. Although it may not survive it seems to promote healing (Fig. 15.10(a), (b) and (c)). Skin grafts from other areas should be avoided (Helal, 1981; Fig. 15.11). Normal sensation to the raw area will be restored as scar contracture draws normal skin over the apex of the pulp. Sensation and the quality of the skin (unique to the palm of the hand and sole of the foot) will always be poor if grafts from elsewhere are used. A

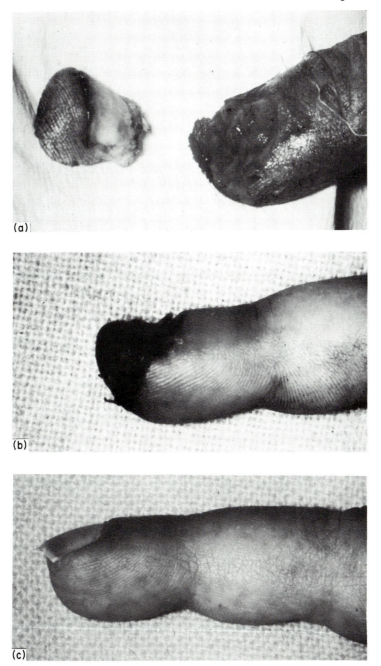

*Fig. 15.10* It is always worth 'reattaching' the part in apical finger injuries. (a) The injury. (b) Two weeks later. (c) Six months later.

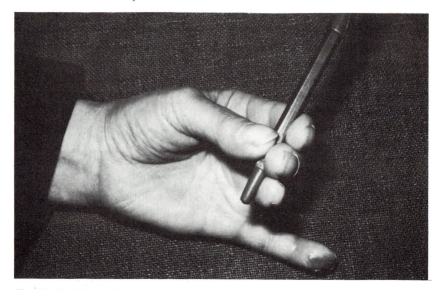

*Fig. 15.11* The subject is unwilling to bring the grafted pulp of the little finger into use – in effect he has mentally amputated this digit.

person is loath to employ a digit with abnormal sensation in a 'contact' area, thereby effectively producing a physiological amputation.

When cosmesis is important an advancement flap carefully preserving the nerve supply may be used. Occasionally with avulsion or degloving injuries it is necessary to use a full thickness graft in which case the groin flap is the best choice, for the skin is hairless, there is a good arterial supply, the hand can be comfortably taken to this site and the donor area can be closed immediately by end to end suture (Fig. 15.12).

If sensory loss is a great handicap, a sensory island flap may be used. Such a flap involves the transfer of skin with its nerve and blood supply from a non-essential area, such as the ulnar side of the ring or middle finger (Fig. 15.13).

### 15.20 Nail and nail bed injuries

Nails have an important role in protection of the finger tip and are also sensory amplifiers. A subungual haematoma should be drained by either a cutting needle spun between the finger and thumb to trephine the nail or by heating such a needle and burning a hole in the nail. Evacuating such a haematoma produces dramatic relief of pain and saves the nail bed from deformity (Fig. 15.14).

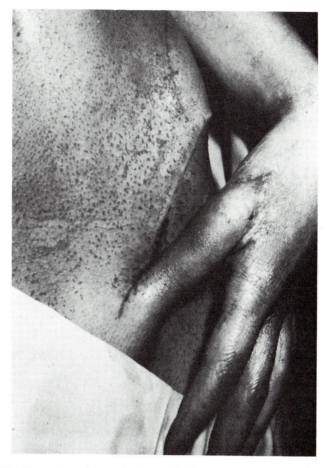

*Fig. 15.12* Illustrating the groin flap 'tubed' in this patient to reconstruct the thumb.

Scarring of the nail bed will result in partial detachment of the nail and depression or distortion of nail growth. These may sometimes be avoided by excising the bed down to the periosteum and applying a nail splint – rather like an artificial nail which will mould growth. Toe nail bed grafts will occasionally produce a reasonable result (Helal, 1981). The alternatives are ablation of nail growth when an artificial nail can be worn for cosmetic purposes.

Nail fold lacerations should be very accurately resutured otherwise permanent distortion will occur.

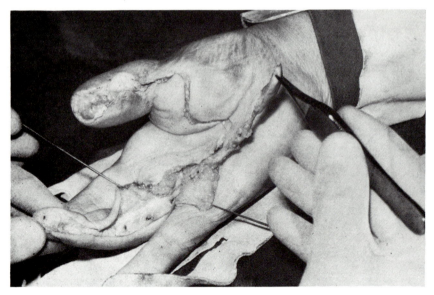

*Fig. 15.13*  A flap of skin with its nerve and blood supply is transferred from the ulnar side of the ring finger to the thumb. It is felt as the ring finger for about three months after which the brain learns to record the sensation as from the thumb.

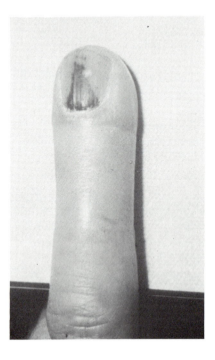

*Fig. 15.14* Subungual haematoma. The area near the trephine has been cleared of haematoma. A second trephine hole near the nail base would have completed the drainage.

300

## 15.21    The tendons of the hand

### 15.21.1    THE EXTENSORS

The extensor tendons are often injured. Tenosynovitis is common especially in rowers and in racket players. Rest is advised with the fingers and wrist supported in extension. Local and steroid infiltration around, but not into, the tendons is the next line of treatment and may be repeated three times at three-weekly intervals. Recurrent attacks or persistence of the symptoms may be successfully managed by division of the extensor retinacula. There is a price to pay for this in a degree of bowstringing of the tendons, but even when this occurs the patients retain excellent power.

In the thumb synovitis within the sheaths of abductor pollicis longus and extensor pollicis brevis overlying the radial styloid (de Quervain's disease), which fails to respond to the conservative measures outlined, is surgically decompressed. Care is taken to avoid damage to the dorsal sensory branch of the radial nerve which crosses the radial styloid. It is also important to check that the duplicated or even triplicated tendons of these two muscles are not lying in a multi-compartmental sheath, all of which have to be decompressed if they are present. The more proximal form of paratendinitis (Williams, 1977) that does not respond to conservative measures may also have to have the fascia over the swollen long abductor and short extensor muscle bellies incised to decompress the underlying tendons.

Traumatic avulsion of the extensors can occur at two sites. From the dorsum of the base of the middle phalanx resulting in the bouttoniere deformity (Fig. 15.15) or from the dorsum of the base of the terminal phalanx producing a mallet deformity (Fig. 15.16). In either situation the tendon may be detached from the bone or carry away with it its bony insertion.

Other forms of mallet deformity are the impact type when an axial force pushes the cup-shaped base of the terminal phalanx onto the dome shape of the head of the middle phalanx, fracturing off a large fragment (Fig. 15.17). Early management should be by splintage in full extension or, in the case of the terminal phalanx, in hyperextension (Mikic and Helal, 1974; Fig. 15.18). If a large fragment of bone is detached from the base of the terminal phalanx then internal fixation is sometimes necessary (Fig. 15.19). In the child a pseudo-mallet deformity may be produced by displacement at the epiphyses at the base of the terminal phalanx. These injuries most frequently occur in ball catching games – cricket, baseball, rugby football and occasionally in football and volley ball. If the patient presents early then splintage is the treatment of choice. Patients

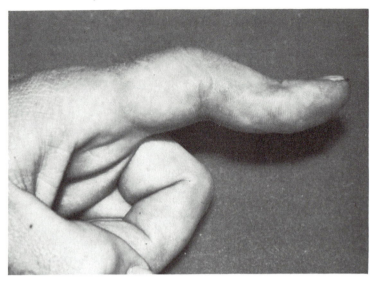

*Fig. 15.15* Boutonniere deformity which the French call 'le button-hole' deformity.

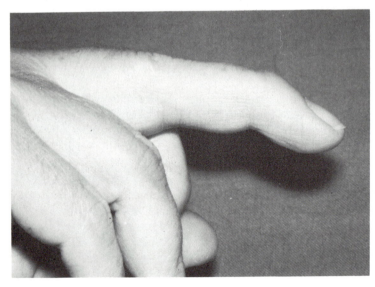

*Fig. 15.16* Mallet deformity.

presenting late with such injuries may require surgical reconstruction.

In the case of the bouttoniere deformity, refashioning the ruptured or avulsed middle slip of the extensor by using one of the two extensor slips to the terminal phalanx to prolong the middle slip, reattaching it to the

302

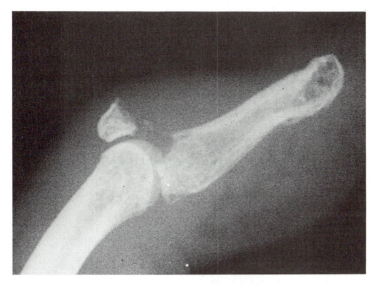

*Fig. 15.17*  Impact type.

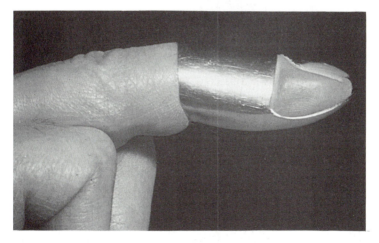

*Fig. 15.18*  The Oakley mallet splint allows free movement of the proximal joint.

middle phalanx with a lengthening of the remaining slip, as often happens, there is a hyperextension deformity of the terminal phalanx (Matev, 1969). This manoeuvre can produce a good result. It is important to achieve full passive mobility by lively extensor splintage before any surgical repair is contemplated.

Isolated rupture of the extensor pollicis longus can occur at the wrist (Helal, Chen and Iwegbu, 1982). Such a rupture has been seen in a pelota

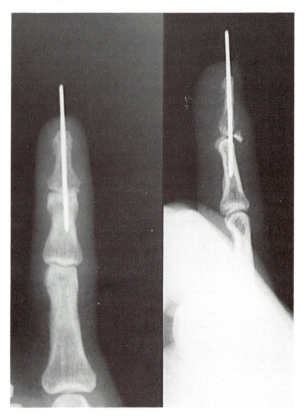

*Fig. 15.19*   Temporary internal fixation by a Kirschner wire.

player. Repair was effected by using the extensor indicis proprius as a transfer.

*(a)   Ganglia*

These frequently arise on the extensor surface and generally communicate with an adjacent joint. Excision, to be successful, must be complete and deroof that portion of the capsule through which they arise since the channel is usually a narrow one and acts as a valve trapping fluid in the ganglion.

15.21.2   THE FLEXOR TENDONS

*(a)   Tenosynovitis*

This occurs most frequently in rope handling by yachtsmen, tug of war teams, in gymnasts and in clothes pulling in rugby football and judo.

304

Measures such as temporary rest, oral anti-inflammatory agents or careful injection of steroid, avoiding entry into the substance of the tendon, are usually successful.

### (b)  Triggering

This can occur as the aftermath of repeated synovitis with thickening of the flexor sheaths usually at metacarpal head level. Alternatively, a nodule may form on the tendon due to superficial rupture of the spiral tendon fibres. Either cause is best treated by surgical decompression. This is common in fencers.

### (c)  Avulsion

This usually occurs at the insertion of the flexor profundus on the volar aspect of the base of the terminal phalanx (Leddy and Packer, 1977). It occurs most commonly in rugby football players and less frequently in judo when the clothes pulling flexed finger is jerked into extension. If the vincula remain intact and the sheath feels to contain the tendon, then splinting the fingers and wrist in flexion for three weeks is said to result in a satisfactory repair (Price, 1966). It is wise to explore these injuries. If this is carried out soon after injury, reattachment is usually straightforward. The profundus is anchored by the lumbrical and so cannot withdraw further than the palm. A fine rubber catheter fed carefully in retrograde fashion through the flexor sheath with minimal trauma to the stump of the tendon – usually found in the proximal part of the finger or distal palm – attached to the catheter by a suture, railroaded back and reattached to its insertion and then protected by Kleinert's rubber band technique will result in a satisfactory outcome (Fig. 15.20).

In the Kleinert banding technique, if the profundus is damaged in any of the ulnar three fingers the bands must include all three as there is a 'mass action' of profundus and the technique relies on the active relaxation of the flexor when the extensor tendons work against the elastic band (Fig. 15.21). To avoid stressing the flexors, the wrist is held in plaster in 30° of flexion. The patient is allowed active extension only and flexion is by recoil of the elastic bands. This ensures that any adhesions that form within the fibrous flexor sheath are long and will overcome by stretching. In the presence of a good superficialis function the risks of adhesions within the digital flexor sheath have to be weighed against the function required. Patients presenting later may require a tendon graft.

Usually stabilization of the terminal interphalangeal joint by tenodesis in the growing person or by arthrodesis in the adult is advisable but such a decision will depend on factors such as hand dominance, hobbies (especially musical ones and the degree of dexterity demanded by the subject's occupation.

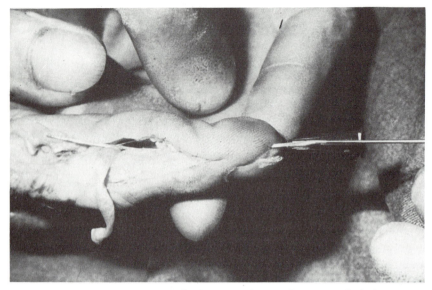

*Fig. 15.20* Reattachment of a flexor tendon to the terminal phalanx.

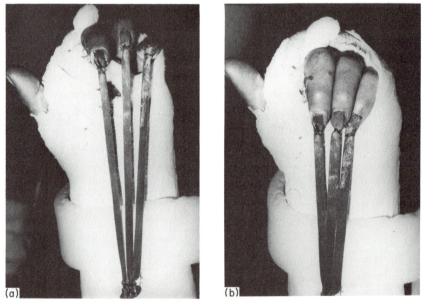

*Fig. 15.21* Kleinest bands. (a) Active extension. (b) Passive flexion.

## (d) Superficialis avulsion

Occasionally avulsion of this tendon from its insertion to the volar side of the base of the middle phalanx can occur. It will come to light if it embarrasses the action of the profundus by coiling in the palm or entrapping the profundus in the loop produced by its decussation. Normally flexion of the finger can be performed by the profundus. The test for a non-functioning superficialis in the ulnar three fingers is to ask the patient to flex the finger with the suspected injury whilst the others are held extended. They will fail to do this if the superficialis is not functioning. The index often has an independent action so in this finger ask the patient to pulp pinch against the thumb with the terminal joint extended. If the superficialis is not working then they can only do this with the terminal joint flexed.

## (e) Severed flexors

Yachting, power boating, accidents in sports vehicles, such as motor cycles, cars, planes and gliders, and water-skiers and divers can produce these injuries as well as the normal type of domestic accident with broken glass, tins, knives and power tools. Ideally, if the tendons are severed within the digital flexor sheaths both should be primarily repaired with minimal delay, preferably by someone with the appropriate skills and experience. Late or untidy injuries involving 0.5 cm or more of the flexor sheath may be best treated by a two-stage operation, the first stage being the insertion of a silicone elastomer tendon spacer from the finger tip to the palm. In the distal palm the superficialis and profundus are anastomosed (Paneva Holevich, 1969). The finger is kept passively mobile and ten weeks later the superficialis is detached at wrist level and taken into the palm, then attached to the tendon spacer which is withdrawn to the tip of the finger taking the tendon with it through the digital flexor sheath, where it is attached to the terminal phalanx. There is then only one anastomosis. This technique has produced above average functional results.

## (f) Flexor sheath ganglia

These are usually over the proximal half of the proximal phalanx, pea-sized, hard and painful. They respond well to needle rupture and rarely recur.

## 15.22 Nerve injuries

These are of two varieties. In the first there may be division of, or a severe traction on, the nerve which will not heal without surgical intervention.

307

# Hand and wrist injuries

The second type is called a neurapraxia; in this type the nerve conduction is temporarily 'knocked out'. Direct concussion or prolonged pressure will cause neurapraxis and this is the commonly encountered type of nerve lesion in sport.

The ulnar nerve is vulnerable at two sites: in its passage behind the medial epicondyle of the elbow and at the wrist where it can be damaged in the canal of Guyon which begins just behind the pisiform bone on the ulnar side at the base of the palm. Damage at elbow level results in weakness and clumsiness of the hand and, if severe and prolonged, wasting of the interossii and hypothenar muscles and weakness of thumb adduction. Sensory symptoms in the form of paraesthesia and numbness involve the ulnar one and half digits but can be altered by a digit radial and ulnarwards, depending on a pre-fixed or post-fixed situation. Damage within the canal of Guyon involves the motor branch alone and so is unaccompanied by sensory symptoms. This condition has been encountered in long distance cyclists and is also associated with other sports – judo, karate, gymnastics and wrestling.

The other major nerve that can be involved is the median where it takes passage through the carpal tunnel in company with the long finger flexors. Compression occurs because of inflammatory swelling of the synovium, which may be due to trauma or repetitive powerful finger flexions, for example in gymnasts. This usually responds to rest and the administration of anti-inflammatory agents or anti-prostaglandins, such as aspirin. Sometimes an injection of steroid into the carpal tunnel may be necessary and very rarely is surgical decompression warranted. This is achieved by division of the roof of the carpal tunnel which is formed by a strong fibrous layer, the flexor retinaculum.

## 15.22.1   TEN PIN BOWLER'S THUMB

This is caused by a neurapraxia of the ulnar digital branch which is caused by impingement of the edge of the hole into the which the bowler inserts his thumb in gripping the ball. Repeated damage causes an area of thickening and fibrosis with local tenderness and ulnar side paraesthesia (Minkow and Bassett, 1972). If rest and protection of the thumb do not result in a resolution of symptoms, surgical release of the nerve is carried out by dissecting off the thickened perineurium. This dissection or the repair of severed nerves and small vessels is facilitated by the use of the operating microscope (Figs 15.22 and 15.23).

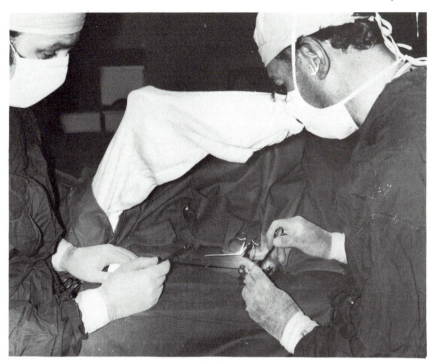

*Fig. 15.22*    The use of a microscope facilitates repair of nerves and small vessels.

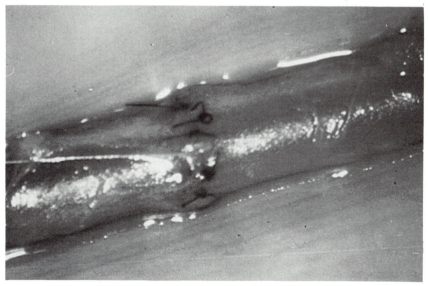

*Fig. 15.23*    This finger artery is 1 mm in diameter.

# Hand and wrist injuries

## 15.23   Joint injuries

These are particularly common in sports in which the ball is handled, thus they are commonly seen in cricket, basket ball, netball, boxing and rugby football. Thumb injuries are often seen in skiers. Instability or a fracture dislocation (Bennett fracture) of the carpometacarpal joint of the thumb has been seen in boxers and rugby footballers. The carpometacarpal joint of the little finger suffers fracture dislocation more rarely, but such damage has been seen in a rugger player and a boxer (Helal and Kavanagh, 1977). Immediate treatment is directed to rapid resolution of pain and swelling: elevation, cold pack, compression, ultrasound and Diapulse are all useful. Stable capsular injuries are tedious to patient and doctor alike. Several months may elapse before swelling and discomfort subside and active treatment, other than to encourage movement, is unrewarding. Occasionally surgical reinforcement is necessary. In the fracture dislocation accurate reduction and fixation is necessary.

### 15.23.1   INJURY TO THE THUMB METACARPOPHALANGEAL JOINT

Skiers in particular are prone to injury of the thumb (Gerber, Senn and Matter, 1981), especially in falls on artificial slopes. The thumb gets caught in the hollows of the plastic slope and the ulnar ligament of the metacarpophalangeal joint is torn (Fig. 15.24). A special glove webbed between the index and thumb has been devised to protect against this injury.

### 15.23.2   ACUTE DORSAL DISLOCATIONS OF THE FINGER JOINTS

This injury is rarely seen in athletes. Should it occur it has to be openly reduced as the volar plate folds into the joint and blocks reduction (Posner, 1977). According to McCue et al. (1970) the sport causing the most severe proximal joint injuries is football followed by baseball, lacrosse and basket ball. On the whole, early surgery is advised for disruptions with locking or important instability.

   Capsular and ligamentous injury resulting in instability are most serious on the radial sides of the digital joints, especially the proximal interphalangeal joint, and on the ulnar aspect of the thumb joints, especially the metacarpophalangeal joint. This is because in any action of the hand the thumb and fingers oppose each other, and the integrity of

310

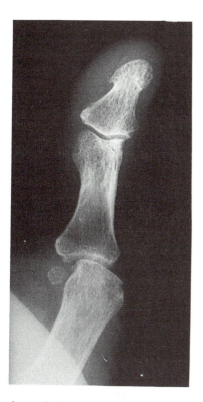

*Fig. 15.24* Rupture of the collateral ligament of a thumb metacarpophalangeal joint.

the radial side ligaments of the fingers and the ulnar side ligaments of the thumb resist displacement.

Experience has shown that conservative management of the finger interphalangeal joint and the thumb metacarpophalangeal joint ligaments provides the best results. The exception to this rule is the volar plate injury of the proximal interphalangeal joint, which must be surgically repaired if it is blocking flexion and producing a fixed swan-neck deformity of the finger (Fig. 15.25(a)–(d); Kristiansen, 1981). Thumb metacarpophalangeal joint ligament injuries settle remarkably well with conservative treatment. A degree of laxity is well tolerated. The exception is the crushed articular surface with subsequent chondrolysis which may require joint fusion. All dislocations (Fig. 15.26) should be reduced as soon as possible and movement started as soon as swelling has subsided.

## 15.23.3 INJURY TO JOINT SURFACES

Bony injury involving the joint is serious, for unless accurate reduction is carried out, pain and loss of movement will occur and degenerative changes will eventually take place. Therefore, fractures involving frag-

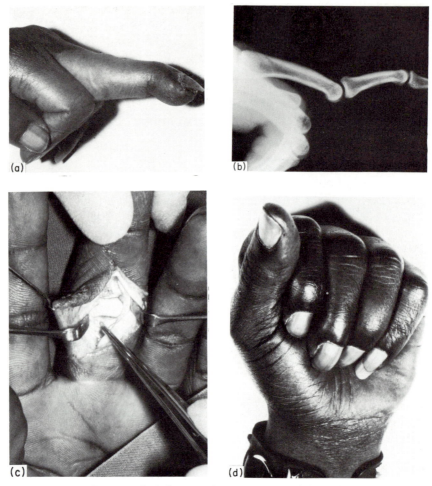

*Fig. 15.25* (a) Swan neck deformity due to rupture of the volar plate. (b) The radiographic appearance. (c) At operation showing the avulsed plate. (d) Restoration of function.

ment of bone with a ligament or condyle require very accurate reduction and fixation if joint movement is to be preserved. Late reconstruction of deviated digits and joints by osteotomies or replacements are not on the whole very satisfactory (Posner, 1977). Operative fixation of the fragments is essential because early movement is desirable to help remould surfaces and prevent stiffness. The completely disrupted joint surface may necessitate an arthroplasty or, in some circumstances, an arthrodesis. Fusion procedures are best confined to the terminal thumb and finger joints and arthroplasty to keep the others mobile. A professional

312

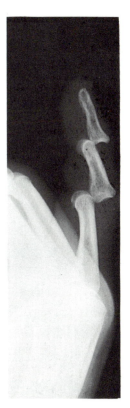

*Fig. 15.26* Dislocation of both interphalangeal joints.

goalkeeper was able to continue to play after the index proximal joint arthroplasty shown in Fig. 15.27.

## 15.24 Fractures of hand bones

It is important to be aware of rotational deformities which may easily be missed. The plane of the nails in relation to one another and the plane of flexion of the fingers, which should veer towards the scaphoid tubercle, should always be checked. Stress fractures can occur particularly at the bases of the proximal phalanges of the fingers, most commonly in gymnasts – the handstand injury (McCue *et al.*, 1970). Fractures may be inherently stable or unstable. It is desirable to maintain joint movement. Stable fractures can be splinted against an adjacent finger and both moved together.

Unstable fractures are best treated by internal fixation. There are many types of internal fixation (by small plates and screws or internal external fixation devices). Commonly, Kirschner wires are used under image

313

# Hand and wrist injuries

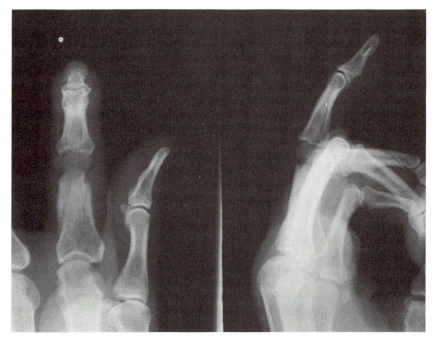

*Fig. 15.27* A silicone rubber arthroplasty of the proximal interphalangeal joint of an index finger.

intensifier control (Fig. 15.28). The ends of the wires are bent over and fixed together with acrylic cement. Compression can be provided by elastic band loops placed near the base of the protruding wires. The wires are introduced on the dorsoradial aspect of the digits and so do not interfere with adjacent digits. Adjacent digits can be managed in a similar fashion and movement, which is unimpeded, can be maintained. Epiphyseal injuries are easily missed in the young and an X-ray should always be taken in the 'sprained' finger in a child.

## 15.25 Conclusion

Too often, hand injuries have been considered to be a minor problem by athletes and their trainers. A ruined sports career or a lifetime's deformity or handicap is a high price to pay for this misconception. Hand injuries have to be dealt with by adequate expertise in suitable surroundings (Fig. 15.29). Flatt's wise statement bears repetition: 'Care must never be modified in response to non-medical considerations and there is no place for compromise in treatment' (Flatt, 1969). Our patients must be given the

314

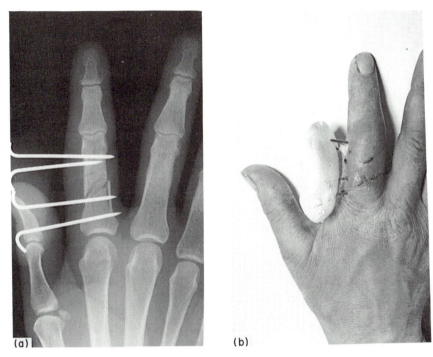

(a)                                       (b)

*Fig. 15.28*   Internal external fixation in a compound unstable fracture allowing early movement of the finger joints.

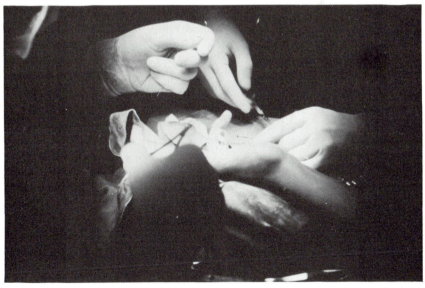

*Fig. 15.29*   Treatment of hand injuries requires expertise and good facilities.

# Hand and wrist injuries

best possible care and pressures of motivation by the injured persons, their parents, their trainers, their team or their national pride have to be resisted.

## References

Bigelow, D. R. and Ritchie, G. W. (1963) The effects of frostbite in childhood. *J. Bone Joint Surg.*, **45B**, 122.

Burke, E. R. (1981) Ulnar neuropathy in bicyclists. *Phys. Sportsmed.*, **9**, 53.

Burkhart, S. S., Wood, M. D. and Linscheid, R. L. (1982) Post-traumatic recurrent subluxation of the extensor carpi ulnaris tendon. *J. Hand Surg.*, **7**, 1.

Conn, J., Bergan, J. J. and Bell, J. L. (1970) Hypothenar hammer syndrome. Post traumatic digital ischaemia. *Surgery*, **68**, 1122.

Flatt, A. E. (1969) *Athletic Injuries to the Hand*, Symposium of Sports Medicine, C. V. Mosby, St Louis.

Frankel, V. H. (1977) The Terry Thomas sign. *Chir. Orthop.*, **129**, 321.

Gelberman, R. H., Salomon, P. B., Jurist, J. M. and Posch, J. L. (1975) Ulnar variance in Kienboch's disease. *J. Bone Joint Surg.*, **57A**, 674.

Gerber, C., Senn, E. and Matter, P. (1981) Skiers thumb. *Amer. J. Sports Med.*, **9**, 17.

Hakstian, R. W. (1972) Cold indirect digital epiphyseal necrosis in childhood. *Can. J. Surg.* **15**, 168.

Helal, B. (1969) Silicones in orthopaedic surgery, in *Recent Advances in Orthopaedic Surgery*, Vol. 5, J. & H. Churchill Ltd, London, pp. 91.

Helal, B. (1978) Racquet players pisiform. *The Hand*, **10**, 87.

Helal, B. (1981) Injuries to the finger tip, in *The Practice of Hand Surgery*, Blackwell Scientific Publications, Oxford, London, Edinburgh and Boston, pp. 23.

Helal, B. and Kavanagh, T. K. (1977) Unstable dorsal fracture dislocations of the fifth carpometacarpal joint. *Injury*, **9(2)**, 138.

Helal, B., Chen, S. C. and Iwegbu, G. (1982) Rupture of the extensor pollicis longus tendon in undisplaced Colles type of fracture. *The Hand*, **14**, 41.

King, J. B. and Turnbull, T. J. (1982) An early method of confirming scaphoid fracture. *J. Bone Joint Surg.*, **64B**, 250.

Kristiansen, B. (1981) Athletic injuries of the volar plate in the proximal interphalangeal finger joints. *Ital. J. Sports Traumatol.*, **23**, 57.

Leddy, J. P. and Packer, J. W. (1977) Avulsion of the profundus tendon insertion in athletes. *J. Hand Surg.*, **2**, 66.

Linscheid, R. L., Dobyns, J. H., Beabout, J. W. and Bryan, R. S. (1972) Traumatic instability of the wrist. *J. Bone Joint Surg.*, **54A**, 1612.

Matev, I. (1969) Bouttoniere deformity. *The Hand*, **1**, 90.

Mayfield, J. K., Johnson, R. P. and Kiloyne, R. K. (1980) Carpal dislocations. Pathomechanics and progressive perilunar instability. *J. Hand Surg.*, **5**, 226.

McCue, F. C., Honner, R., Johnson, M. D. and Gieck, J. H. (1970) Athletic injuries to the proximal interphalangeal joint requiring surgical treatment. *J. Bone Joint Surg.*, **52A**, 939.

Mikic, Z. and Helal, B. (1974) The treatment of the mallet finger by the Oakley splint. *The Hand*, **6(1)**, 76.

# References

Minkow, F. V. and Bassett, F. H. (1972) Bowlers thumb. *Clin. Orthop.*, **83**, 115.

Paneva Holevich, E. (1969) Two stage tenoplasty in injury of the flexor tendon of the hand. *J. Bone Joint Surg.*, **51A**, 21.

Posner, M. A. (1977) Injuries of the hand and wrist in athletes. *Orthop. Clin. N. Amer.*, **8(3)**, 563.

Price, E. C. U. (1966) Spontaneous repair of flexor tendons. *J. Bone Joint Surg.*, **48B**, 587.

Smith, J. W. G., Lawrence, D. R. and Evans, D. G. (1975) Tetanus immunisation. *Brit. Med. J.*, **23 August**, 453.

Sperryn, P. N. (1973) Traumatic bursitis in the boxer's hand. *Brit. J. Sports Med.*, **7**, 103.

Stark, H. H., Jobe, F. W., Boyes, J. H. and Ashworth, C. R. (1977) Fracture of the hook of the hamate in athletes. *J. Bone Joint Surg.*, **59A**, 575.

Taleisnik, J., Malerich, M. and Prietto, M. (1982) Palmar carpal instability secondary to dislocation of scaphoid and lunate. *J. Hand Surg.*, **7**, 606.

Torisu, T. (1972) Fracture of the hook of the hamate by a golf swing. *Clin. Orthop.*, **83**, 91.

Watson, H. K., Goodman, H. L. and Johnson, T. R. (1981) Limited wrist arthrodesis. Intercarpal and radiocarpal combinations. *J. Hand Surg.*, **6**, 223.

Williams, J. G. P. (1977) Surgical management of traumatic non-infective tenosynovitis of the wrist extensor. *J. Bone Joint Surg.*, **59B**, 408.

# 16   *Spinal injuries*

## JAMES ROBERTSON

Back pain is often described as the scourge of modern Western society for approximately 65% of the population will be absent from work at some stage in their career as a result (Hirsch, Johnson and Lewin, 1969). In a survey of an English suburban practice over a four year period Dillane, Fry and Kalton (1966) noted that 7.5% of the population at risk consulted their general practitioner with low back pain. The overall annual inception rate was 24.3 per thousand in males and 20.3 per thousand in females. In the majority of cases back pain settles within four to six weeks irrespective of the mode of treatment and less than 10% will need further advice. Statistics relating to sports people are, therefore, difficult to extract from the general population.

Many sports people accept a degree of back pain as par for the course and never seek advice. The high incidence in certain activities (butterfly swimming, gymnastics, javelin throwing, weightlifting and diving) are well recognized and may be associated with a hyperlordotic position in which certain of the manoeuvres are performed. Billings, Burry and Jones (1977), in reviewing one hundred men and women referred to a sports clinic, noted that the discomfort was severe enough for 65% to have lost time from work. After treatment 61% returned to their former sporting activities and standard, but 39% had to give up the sports activity (either partially or completely) as a direct result of the back injury. It is interesting to note that a high proportion of this group were injured not in competition, but in training, with 38% of the injuries occurring during weight training. Over half of those attending the clinic admitted no supervision of their training programmes and others had been concerned at the poor supervision and instruction especially when using weights as part of a training programme. Too often the young athlete walks across a room, sees the weights left out and just attempts what weight he can manage with potentially dire consequences.

Stripped of its muscles the spine has properties similar to a multi-jointed elastic rod. Secured at its base, the greatest vertical load it can stand without buckling is approximately 2 kg (Morris, Lucas and Bresler, 1961). Its stability is therefore dependent on the extrinsic support of the paraspinal and trunk musculature.

The major function of the pelvis and spine is to provide axial support to the trunk, but as well as structural strength there is the opposing need for flexibility allowing transmission of movement and locomotion. Its ancillary functions provide a shield to protect the spinal cord and major nerves whilst its overall shape and structure acts as a complex shock-absorber in reducing the jarring forces of heel strike and other movements being transmitted to the brain.

The vertebral column must not be thought of in isolation, but rather as part of a complex system by which momentum is relayed from one part of the body to another. Should any link in this system's mechanical properties be altered it would affect the pattern of transmission to the other components and, if continued, could lead to secondary structural or stress changes. Simple examples are an alteration in the height of a shoe or a tighter hamstring muscle thus altering pelvic tilt and, by so doing, modifying the spinal posture.

The anterior spinal structures are well designed to take compressive forces whilst the posterior structures are designed for tension (Fig. 16.1). In the major part of the spine the pathological changes are primarily in the anterior structures; Schmorl's nodes (herniation of the nucleus puposus through the vertebral end plate), endplate fractures and crush fractures of the vertebral body are probably all produced by compression. Below the level of the third lumbar vertebra there is a drastic change in the adult pattern of damage. Of 2500 clinical cases of disc protrusion studied by Spangfort (1972), 98% were either at the L4/5 or L5/S1 level. Friberg and Hirsch (1949) noted that in the lower lumbar spine it is invariably the

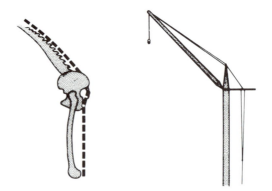

*Fig. 16.1* The hamstrings and spinal extensor muscles may combine in a similar manner to the reefing wires of a crane.

posterior arc of the disc that is damaged. The macroscopic and micro-scopic changes in disc degeneration have been well documented and reviewed by Farfan (1973) whilst Naylor (1971) has reviewed the bio-chemical and biophysical changes. Schmorl's nodes have a different pattern of distribution, being far more common in the upper lumbar region (Farfan, 1973) and rare in the sacrum (Farfan, Huberdean and Dubour, 1972). Reports of acute injuries indicate that discs rupture in tension, or tension and shear whilst the bodies fracture in compression (Schultz, 1974).

Similarly, in the posterior structures there is a different pattern of pathology above and below the L3 segment. Rissanen (1960), in a detailed study of postmortem material, demonstrated the anatomy and natural history of degenerative changes in the interspinous ligament. In patients over the age of twenty, 21% had established ruptures of which 92% were situated in the lowest two ligaments. The plane of rupture was caused by local mechanical factors and he postulated it followed Moore's law (Fig. 16.2). Roche and Rowe (1952), in a survey of 4200 skeletons, found 183 isthmal defects of which 94.6% occurred at the L4/5 and L5/S1 segments. This distribution of spondylolysis has been documented by many other authors.

RUPTURE OF INTERSPINOUS
LIGAMENT

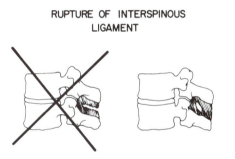

*Fig. 16.2*  The interspinous ligament ruptures in the plane shown in the right hand diagram, indicating a shearing force.

In normal subjects, when fully relaxed, lying, sitting or standing, there appears to be no electrical activity in the abdominal and posterior muscle groups although Nachemson (1966) recorded activity in the psoas muscle. When lying prone, flattening of the lumbar spine is controlled by the abdominal muscles with both the external and internal obliques taking part. Arching the lumbar spine is associated with activity in the posterior muscle groups with equal participation of multifidus and longissimus (Fig. 16.3). Standing, then flexing with return to neutral, exhibits only posterior muscle activity and when in the fully flexed position, with the subject relaxed, hands just off the floor, all trunk

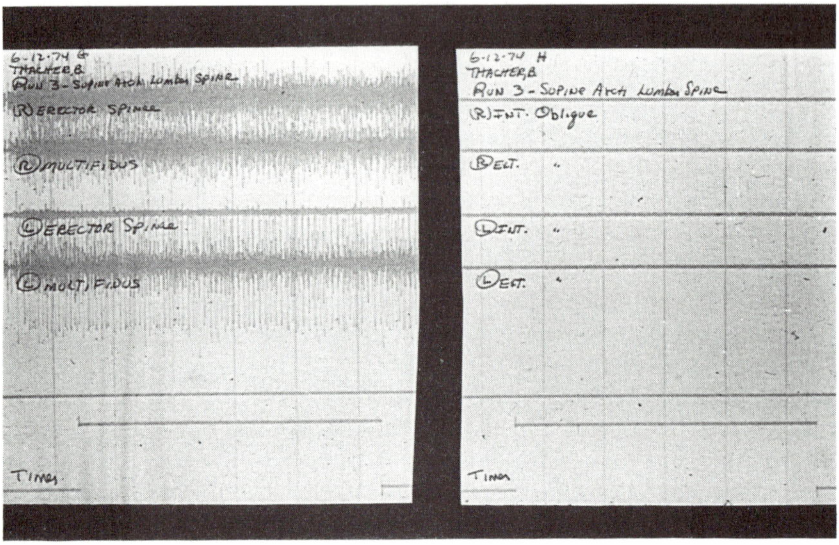

# Spinal injuries

*Fig. 16.3* The athlete is lying prone holding the lower back arched. Using fine wire intramuscular electrodes, electrical activity is recorded. The marked electrical activity in the multifidus and erector spinae is easily seen whilst the abdominal muscles (internal and external oblique) demonstrate no electrical activity.

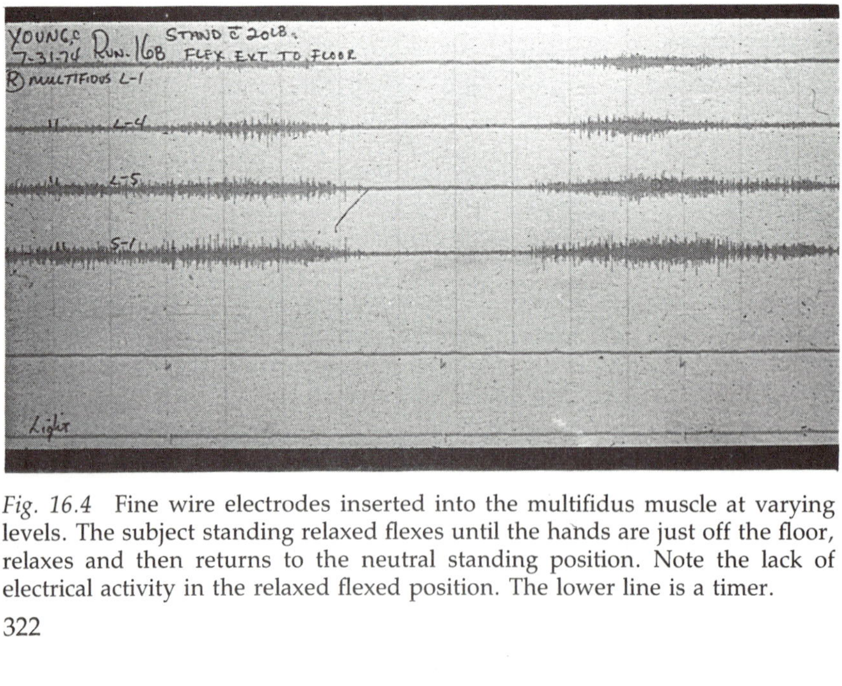

*Fig. 16.4* Fine wire electrodes inserted into the multifidus muscle at varying levels. The subject standing relaxed flexes until the hands are just off the floor, relaxes and then returns to the neutral standing position. Note the lack of electrical activity in the relaxed flexed position. The lower line is a timer.

muscle activity ceases (Fig. 16.4). However, when a 9 kg (20 lb) weight is held close to the chest, the abdominal muscles play a far more important role throughout the activity. From the standing position, extension begins with a short burst of posterior muscle activity, after which the abdominals are active as though paying out against gravity. The importance of the abdominal muscles cannot be overstressed and the enhancement of their activity by using a belt or corset is well recognized by weightlifters and power boat drivers (Waters and Morris, 1970). The abdominal muscles, acting individually or as a group perform a number of functions:

(1) By compressing the abdominal cavity they convert it into a semi-rigid cylinder of liquid and semi-solid material: with the diaphragm contracted (flattened and rigid), the rib cage can become fixed by the action of the intercostal and shoulder girdle muscles and with inspiration, act as a further semi-rigid cylinder filled with air (Fig. 16.5). Weight lifted by the arms is transmitted to the thoracic cage by the shoulder girdle muscles and then to the abdominal cylinder and pelvis, partially through the spinal column, but mainly through the rigid rib cage and abdominal cylinder. The rectus abdominis appears to act as a stabilizer, binding the rib cage to the pelvis and preventing pouching of the abdominal viscera. This is especially so in tall subjects or those with a long lumbar spine, with six lumbar vertebrae (Morris, Lucas and Bresler, 1961).

(2) By increasing the intra-abdominal pressure acting on the large expanse of the posterior abdominal wall, the shear forces occurring in the lower lumbar region are reduced (Robertson, 1975).

(3) With an increase in intra-abdominal pressure, venous blood is forced

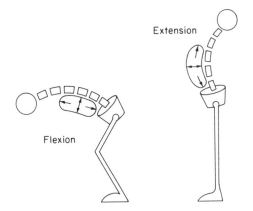

Fig. 16.5   The role of the air fluid cylinder created in the abdomino-thoracic cavity is demonstrated.

into Batson's plexus and into the vascular bone of the vertebral bodies, making them more turgid.

(4) When the abdominal muscles contract, tension in the interspinous and intertransverse ligaments is maintained via the thoracolumbar fascia (Fairbank and O'Brien, 1980).

(5) They are aided by the hamstring and other muscles in altering the pelvic angle (Robertson, 1975).

(6) They act as prime movers of the lumbar spine in lateral flexion and also in controlling other spinal movements.

Clyde Smith, a member of the Canadian medical staff at the 1976 Olympic Games, noted that whilst the athletes had strong extensor muscles of the spine and hip, the flexor muscles (especially those of the abdominal region) were often poorly developed. His article goes on to describe the techniques used by the Canadian team in advising and treating their athletes (Smith, 1977).

The anterior structures of the spine are supplied by the nerves of the anterior primary rami. The disc has never been shown to contain nerve fibres although the surrounding tissues are well supplied. Trauma to the main nerve produces pain in the segmental distribution of that nerve which is well localized and may be associated with sensory or motor changes in the limb.

The posterior spinal structures are supplied by the posterior primary rami through a network of nerves with fibres arising from many different levels and appearing not to cross the mid-line. This may explain the difficulty in localizing the anatomical pathology leading to such vague terms as lumbago, lumbo-fibrositis, etc. Pain can extend down the limb to the foot but is sclerodermal and poorly localized by the patient. There are no associated motor or sensory changes in the limb. Pedersen, Blunck and Gardener (1956), using the decerebrate cat, showed that mechanical stimulation of any of the posterior structures, whether it was joint, facet, ligament, periosteum or muscle, was followed by reflex spasm of the dorsal muscles mainly ipsilaterally. They also noted that hamstring spasm was present ipsilaterally and went on to say that other muscles, especially in the thigh and abdominal walls, also responded reflexly. Mooney and Robertson (1976) went on to demonstrate that irritation of a lower lumbar facet joint produced reflex spasm in the hamstring and may account for tight hamstring problems in some athletes.

To many sporting enthusiasts a degree of back pain is tolerated as a constant accompaniment to their activities, and over the years may result in radiological and structural changes to the disc or bony architecture of the spine. In the majority of cases the onset is caused by contusion, acute strain or chronic stress; the acute disc prolapse or other primary major

324

injury being the rarity. The words 'contusion', 'strain' and 'sprain' are often used, but in reference to the back it is difficult to identify the initiating pathology and most injuries are probably a combination of a number of factors. A sequence in contact sport may well be that the original injury is a muscle contusion produced by a direct blow. This results in local muscle spasm with further damage from stretching the unprotected injured muscle as the game continues.

## 16.1 Acute soft tissue injury

Whatever the initial cause, the primary treatment remains the same. Reduction in the overlying surface temperature, either by the application of ice or a coolant spray, helps to reduce the immediate pain and possibly advantageously alters the local vascular circulation. The injured area should be rested and an oral analgesic, possibly in association with an anti-inflammatory preparation, prescribed. There are practitioners who advocate the local injection of an anaesthetic agent with hyaluronidase and steroid, insisting that by using this technique they dampen the inflammatory process. The worry with such an approach is that by reducing protective pain in the acute stage the athlete feels fit to continue with the activity and may cause further extensive damage. The occasion may arise when this approach is justified, for example when an athlete has to compete in one further competition and accepts the risk.

Once the acute phase is over, in twenty-four to forty-eight hours, rehabilitation commences utilizing the physiotherapy facilities available. The basis of treatment is a combination of surface heat or ultrasound, often in combination with subliminal faradism and local massage. As the pain settles gradual slow stretching exercises of the muscles can be commenced and deep transverse friction applied to any local tender area. It is necessary to follow this with a full work-up programme aimed to get the player back on the field. During the early stages of this rehabilitation programme it is often worth continuing with an oral anti-inflammatory preparation, but it is not advised that this should continue for more than three to four weeks. It may be necessary in the early playing days to protect the back using local padding or a corset. It is not felt that the techniques of muscle stretching should be dealt with in detail in this chapter as they are well covered in the article by Smith (1977).

A local haematoma in the paraspinal area may become quite large, and occasionally encystment occurs resulting in a fluctuant mass marking the site of injury. In the majority of cases this will slowly be absorbed but can take a month or more. Whilst not limiting from a functional standpoint, it is usually of some concern to the athlete. Aspiration, using a sterile technique, followed by local compression, may accelerate the rate of absorption.

Damage to the psoas muscle lying anterior to the lumbar spine may be produced when its action in controlling the lumbar spine by contraction occurs at the same moment that the muscle is being fully stretched by an extended hip. Localized tenderness over the area of the transverse process with pain reproduced by extending the hip indicates the diagnosis. X-rays may demonstrate soft tissue loss in the normal contour of the psoas muscle or avulsion fractures from a number of the transverse processes. There have been a number of reports where, following a haematoma in the psoas muscle, pressure has been caused on the femoral nerve producing a temporary femoral nerve palsy. Treatment is as for any other muscular damage.

Direct trauma over the tips of the spinous processes may cause residual discomfort and can occasionally lead to a local periosteal reaction. The majority of these conditions settle following a single injection into the surrounding area of corticosteroid mixed with a local anaesthetic. Surface padding over the area may be necessary if repeated trauma occurs.

## 16.2   Recurrent and chronic soft tissue problems

These result from either an acute injury not being allowed to heal completely or following repetition of training or competition techniques that put abnormal stress on to an unprotected back. Many sports involve strong extension movements and the athlete concentrates on these muscles to the detriment of the stabilizing flexor muscles. The main area for concern is the abdominal musculature, where too often the only form of training is the curl-up or sit-up, performed at such speed that momentum is gained purely using the hip flexors and possibly rectus abdominus. These athletes tested for rotational power show marked weakness of their other abdominal wall muscles.

It is important to look at the total athlete, rather than examining the back in isolation when trying to diagnose and advise on these problems. Tight hamstrings, tight hip flexors and limited shoulder movement must be excluded. The athlete's footwear needs to be examined to make sure that it fits, gives the right support and that areas are not weakened or worn down. The way the foot hits the gound influences the rest of the balance of the body and this must not be excluded from the appraisal of the athlete's performance. Many a chronic back pain has settled following the insertion of a small raise into the shoe or by changing the counter using an insole. Observe the athlete dressed in the minimum of clothing going through the activity. In this way observation of the back musculature can be more easily seen (Fig. 16.6). Is the runner running in too hyperlordotic a position? Has the discus thrower tilted the back so that rotation due to partial spasm of one of the paravertebral muscles is occurring? Is the diver having to arch the back too far to obtain balance when entering the water? Stallard (1980) noted that the evolution of changing techniques in rowing had markedly increased the incidence of back pain in oarsmen and changes in techniques in other sports likewise can alter the pattern of chronic injury.

Having watched the athlete perform, the next step is to carry out a careful clinical examination. Assess the normal stance and range of

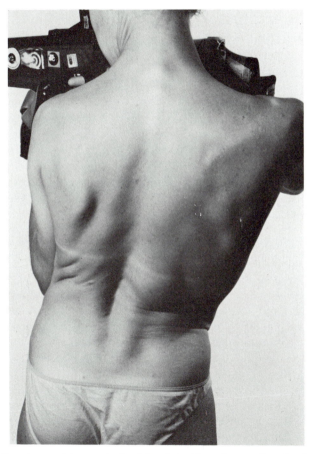

*Fig. 16.6* Sports requiring periods of fixed position also produce back problems. This top flight, small bore rifle shot was losing concentration as a result of low back pain. Modification of her standing position and an exercise programme markedly improved the symptoms.

movement, remembering that you are looking at an athlete. That which is acceptable as a range of movement to the general public may be far less than is necessary for the athlete to perform to the limits needed. Palpate extensively the relaxed muscles, remembering not just to include the paravertebral muscles but also the flank and abdominal muscles, for local areas of tenderness. These areas can be treated with ultrasound or occasionally can be used as trigger point for an injection of local anaesthetic and steroid. If any particular muscle group appears weak concentrate on building it up with training.

Treatment will be very dependent on the diagnosis made and should not end when the immediate relief of pain and spasm has been effected. Instruction in stretching the individual muscle groups and exercises to strengthen those muscles that are weak need to be given. A long-term programme, leading up to full competition should be discussed with the athlete and coach. Training techniques need to be reviewed and the athlete should be made more aware of the anatomy and mechanics of the spine. Education is not only important for the long-term prevention of future problems to the individual, but having so been instructed the athlete will become a missionary in discussing potential problems with other athletes in the locker room or warm-up areas.

The modern athlete often travels extensively and education should also extend to advise on how to cope when having to sit for long journeys, adapting the seat with the use of a pelvic or lumbar cushion if necessary, together with general advice on sleeping positions and adaptation to beds and mattresses.

## 16.3   The acute disc problem

Occasionally seen in the teenager, this is more often a condition presenting in the 20 to 40 year age group. Back pain with radiation to the legs should not immediately be thought of as a disc problem. Pain in the legs can also be experienced in facet and posterior structural damage as a referred-type phenomenon (Mooney and Robertson, 1976). Rarely an acute central disc herniation may occur following a vertical fall landing on the buttocks, or after lifting a heavy weight in the flexed position (Jackson et al., 1971). Should there be interference with urinary control this becomes an emergency and needs expert surgical help within twelve hours. The more common type of disc lesion is the lateral disc herniation, either presenting with peripheral leg pain radiating proximally or low back pain with or without leg pain. Clinically there may be loss of lumbar lordosis with reduction in the range of back movement and spasm, resulting in the classical pelvic lumbar tilt. Straight leg raising may be reduced with a positive Lasegue test, whilst neurological symptoms with sensory, motor or reflex changes may be present in the lower limbs.

Once the diagnosis has been made initial management is classically with bed rest. If straight leg raising is not limited to below 60° it may be that primary management should be with gentle mobilization using Maitland's techniques and a progressive exercise programme. The athlete does not take kindly to being told to take six week's bed rest and hankers for a more active treatment. Early epidural or caudal injections, using local anaesthetic and corticosteroid, may well be indicated. The role of manipulation in the acute disc is open to dispute, and there are many physicians who feel that it causes more damage than relieving symptoms. Traction similarly has its devotees, and in certain circumstances may be of help.

Should symptoms not settle with relatively conservative measures then the question of surgery is raised. The clinical diagnosis needs to be

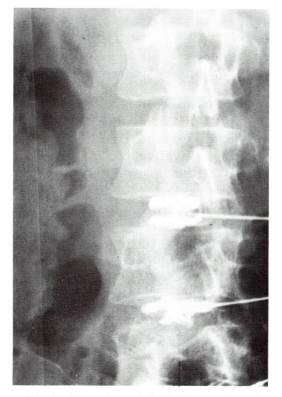

*Fig. 16.7* View of the lumbar spine on which discography is being performed. The superior disc demonstrates the 'hamburger' silhouette of a normal disc. The inferior disc is disrupted with dye draining out through a herniation.

supported by myelography, E.M.G.s or C.T. scans. Chemonucleolysis (a technique by which a proteolytic enzyme is introduced into the disc after discography under an image intensifier; Fig. 16.7) is appealing to the athlete as it does not leave a permanent scar. The enzyme softens the nucleus pulposis, allowing absorption by the body's normal mechanisms. This technique is indicated especially in those cases where primary pain is in the leg, and straight leg raising is limited to 60° or less and there is no neurological deficit. At present the technique is not advised in the teenage disc problem or in those patients with a known sensitivity to meat tenderizer. When open surgery is indicated simple removal of the disc through a Moore incision is preferable in the young athlete. Where degenerative changes are already occurring there may be indications for doing a wider laminectomy and decompressing the lateral gutters. With this latter technique some surgeons advise that the relevant vertebra should be fused with a lateral fusion. Whatever form of treatment is utilized it is necessary to instruct the patient in the recuperative stages with a detailed rehabilitation programme combined with regular outpatient check-ups.

### 16.4 Facet pain

This may occur as an acute incident or present a more chronic pattern of onset. Osteochondral fractures and stress fractures in the facet joint have been described. The classical story is that the athlete bends down to pick something up from the floor and suddenly locks, is in acute pain and is unable to move or only able to move with difficulty. This pattern probably represents a facet impingement or internal derangement within the facet joints, and is the ideal case for treatment by rotary manipulation. In the more chronic form the patient relates having low back pain, which is usually worse with rest but often relieved by movement. They also feel that the pain is increased by hyperextending the spine and partially relieved by flexing the spine with their knees tucked up towards their chest. They may demonstrate the so-called 'hitch' sign when returning to neutral from the fully flexed position. This is a short rotary movement of the upper body which occurs at the change from primary hip flexion to lumbar movement. In its more chronic form this may be demonstrated as a complete reversal of lumbar uncurling. In this group of conditions many cases are more adequately treated by the skilled manipulator than by the surgeon. If symptoms continue after a series of manipulations then an injection of steroid and lignocaine into the facet joint may prove successful (Mooney and Robertson, 1976; Fig. 16.8). Rarely do symptoms warrant local fusion.

330

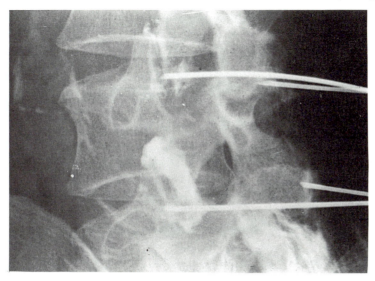

*Fig. 16.8*   Oblique view of the lower lumbar spine in which arthrography of the facet joints is being attempted. The lower joint is filled and dye is just starting to be injected into the superior joint.

## 16.5   The degenerative spine

The increasing age of the population has resulted in athletes continuing with active sport into what used to be termed the geriatric era. This has led to a greater number of older athletes appearing in clinics with complaints of degenerate back conditions. These may have arisen following acute injuries in the past, but the majority often present *de novo*. Aggrawal and colleagues (1979) discussed the role of sport in the production of degenerative changes in the spine and it would appear, together with other reviews, that its significance is still in dispute. Pain is usually situated in the lower back and rarely radiates to the legs unless there is associated foraminal or spinal stenosis. The only abnormal findings on examination may be minimal stiffness in the lower lumbar spine. With a full range of hip movement this could be easily overlooked. X-rays demonstrate changes from minor narrowing of the disc space, degenerative disease of the facet joints and interbody osteophytes, to gross changes at many levels.

The large majority of cases settle with slight modification to their activities and following general advice on muscle tone. A number obtain great relief from wearing a short abdominal support type of corset in which they can continue their activity. Rarely is surgery indicated, other than for local decompression of a nerve root which has not responded to epidural injections or for decompression of a local spinal stenosis. There is occasionally the indication for a fusion at the L4/5 level in the 40 year old female athlete with marked degenerative changes occurring just at this level. In the age groups who suffer from degenerative spinal conditions one must not forget the possibility of secondary neoplastic disease, and if there is any doubt as to the diagnosis a bone scan is indicated.

## 16.6   Minor fractures

Fractures of the transverse process and spinous process are not uncommon. They result from a direct blow or an avulsion-type injury and are only picked up on X-ray. The treatment is primarily that of the soft tissue injury with little note being taken of the fracture. Routine follow-up X-rays are not often performed, and it is accepted that a large number go on to asymptomatic non-union. A small proportion do continue to get discomfort round a pseudo-joint, and may settle following a local injection of corticosteroid and local anaesthetic. Very rarely may it be necessary to excise the distal portion surgically.

Compression fractures of the vertebral body are generally considered to be stable fractures. Many athletes are unaware that they have occurred and treat them just as though they were a normal soft tissue injury. Murray-Leslie *et al.* (1977), in a large review of veteran military parachutists, found that 21.7% had vertebral body collapse, most frequently at the T12 level, and of this number two-thirds were unaware that they had injured their back. He concluded that serious long-term disability from pain appeared to be uncommon amongst parachutists, despite the frequency of spinal trauma they had sustained.

## 16.7   Unstable fractures and fracture dislocations

Fortunately these are relatively infrequent injuries in the thoracic and lumbar spine. Violent trauma with severe localized back pain, with or without associated distal neurological deficiency, must raise the suspicion of these major injuries. The immediate management is all important, the aims being:

(1) To maintain respiratory and cardiovascular function; an adequate airway must be protected.
(2) To protect the spine, spinal cord and major nerves from further damage.
(3) To move the patient gently and quickly to appropriate hospital accommodation.

Unfortunately, a number of these accidents occur in situations where the participant's life has to be saved before being able to take more specific steps, e.g. in a motor injury where there is a fire problem, in mountaineering and in water sport accidents. Where life saving precautions are not necessary one should wait until adequate trained help is available to lift the injured person as a unit, maintaining the spinal position. Transport should be on a firm stretcher and, if possible, in the semi-prone or prone position with adequate maintenance of the airway.

Long-term care and rehabilitation ideally should be carried out in a unit specifically equipped to handle these complex problems. Steinbruck and Paeslack (1980) reviewed forty-one cases of paraplegia in their unit occurring as a result of sports injury. The main activities involved were horseback riding, mountaineering, skiing, gymnastics and motor sport. Gliding, parachuting and scuba diving accounted for the remainder. It is important to remember that in deep sea diving inadequate decompression, resulting in the so-called 'bends', may produce gas emboli in the small vessels of the spinal cord resulting in permanent spinal cord damage. One whole edition of *Paraplegia* (**18**, 1980) is devoted to major injuries of the back in sport.

It is to be remembered that even after such a major injury many athletes retain the wish to compete to the best of their ability, and it is essential that those sportspeople who are fit and well should help their unfortunate colleagues to achieve these aims.

## 16.8 Psychological assessment

The psychological magnification of back pain symptoms is well documented. Where the possibility is raised in relation to athletes the manager or coach should be brought into the discussion early. In the majority of cases the athlete is just hitting a 'low', possibly due to family or outside factors, and whilst most are easily dealt with by the coach, the help of a psychologist is occasionally necessary. Rarely the sportsperson is looking for an excuse, subconsciously, to opt out or reduce the level of activity. In these cases the physician will only meet failure unless the person's wish is realized.

## 16.9 Miscellaneous

Through the doors of a sports clinic may present any problem occurring in the population at large. Acute and chronic osteomyelitis, extradural and intradural tumours, ankylosing spondylitis and other polyarthropathies must not be overlooked. The sportsman presenting with vague back pain and morning stiffness should be screened with basic blood investigations, including HLA-B27 tissue typing, X-rays of the sacroiliac joints and, if available, bone scan and C.T. scan of the joints.

Major injuries of the thoracic cage have not been mentioned in this chapter. Stress fractures of the ribs, especially the lower ribs of weight-lifters and the first and second ribs of golfers and tennis players, may mimic back symptoms. Stress fractures of the first and second ribs primarily give referred pain to the arm, but local palpation will indicate tenderness over the rib. This may be demonstrated on an X-ray or, more likely, with a bone scan.

## 16.10 The growing child and teenager

Commercial and political interest for sporting excellence pressurize the young athlete more than ever before. Many youngsters spend three to four hours a day regularly training, especially in sports where peak performance appears to be achieved in the teens. There is early specialization, with the child going for medals rather than variety and a balanced pattern of activity. The young sportsperson trains easily and aggressively, without being aware of or interested in any pathological consequences. Oseid (1982) compared a group of 15 year old gymnasts in 1971 with a similar group in 1981, each with matched controls. The incidence of low back pain ranged from over 60% in the gymnasts to 22.5% in the controls. The paper reports that 44% of the 1971 group of gymnasts, when followed up long-term, appeared to have permanent back symptoms as against 2.5% of the controls. Kirby (1981) noted that a significant number of young gymnasts had low back symptoms, and felt that those with low back discomfort had greater toe touching ability and discussed the significance of this point. Schweiz (1975), after examining thirty female gymnasts aged six to sixteen years, found 30% complained of back pain but felt that fifteen, on clinical and radiological examination, were not fit for the sport, and that more careful examination and selection is necessary to protect the growing vertebrae of children from overuse damage. The problem is when to advise that enough is enough, for many top flight athletes whose spines radiologically show gross changes, turn in high class performances in event after event.

Doctors should be aware that recurrent damage to the juvenile spine may lead to abnormal growth patterns and should be trained to identify spinal deformity in its early stages, noting any compensatory patterns occurring in other parts of the spine. One should examine for tight hamstrings, tight shoulders and poor abdominal musculature, all of which may be associated with or responsible for spinal deformity. The doctor also has a role in monitoring injuries and trying to assess the factors responsible. Should a particular sport, or part of that sport, appear to be producing a crop of injuries then the pattern of play and techniques used need to be assessed and any changes brought to the notice of the governing body. Recent examples of this include the hyperlordotic rigid landing position adopted by young gymnasts alighting from apparatus and the mismatch of age and weight in contact sports at schools.

The growing spine should not be thought of as a smaller version of the mature adult column. The growth plates remain open, the spine is more flexible, the discs are relatively stronger than in adults, whilst the ligamentous structures are able to take greater strain than the bony members. The immaturity of the bony elements may raise difficulties when trying to interpret X-rays; variations in position mimic displacement, growth centres mimic fractures and variations of normal curvature may mimic spasm.

## 16.10.1  ACUTE TRAUMA

Young people recuperate from the effects of local soft tissue trauma, in general, faster than adults. Avulsion fractures of the transverse processes are not uncommon but fractures of the transverse processes and spinous processes caused by direct trauma are relatively rare. Enlargement of the spleen following glandular fever or other infections may occur in children and it can be ruptured by blunt trauma to the upper lumbar area.

The immediate care of more severe injuries follows the pattern as described for the adult spine. Holdsworth (1963) classified spinal injuries, whilst Hubbard (1974) has written an excellent article describing injuries of the spine in children and adolescents. He noted the three principal differences compared with adult injuries:

(1)  The relative benign clinical course in children.
(2)  The restoration of vertebral body height following fracture.
(3)  The potential development of spinal deformity.

The stable injuries in general were uncomplicated whilst the unstable injuries developed spinal deformity, a large percentage of which required bracing or surgery. Spontaneous intervertebral fusion was virtually never seen.

## 16.10.2  SPINAL DEFORMITY

The doctor and coach not only have a responsibility to the child for the management of the acute episode and pain, but should be capable of detecting early structural changes and potential hazards. The coach often sees the athlete stripped and should take the opportunity of actively observing the shape of the spine. Early detection may well prevent surgery.

## (a)  Scoliosis

Scoliosis is a descriptive term for lateral and rotary curvature of the spine. The normal child, when viewed from the back, has a straight spine with the head balanced over the sacrum. The child with scoliosis may remain balanced from this view because of the righting reflex stimulating the development of a compensation curve above or below the primary curve. Scoliosis may be subdivided into two primary groups:

(1) Non-structural: the scoliosis is mobile and can be fully corrected. This may be postural, compensatory to pelvic tilting (as in leg length discrepancy or hip problems), and occasionally, in sciatic scoliosis, secondary to a disc lesion.
(2) Structural: the scoliosis is rigid and cannot be fully corrected, either actively or passively. Because of rotation when the child bends forward, a posterior rib hump or prominence of the lumbar musculature is seen on the convex side of the curve (Fig. 16.9). These curves are usually progressive and, if noted early, advice from an orthopaedic surgeon is indicated as the child may well need bracing or could ultimately come to surgery.

## (b)  Kyphosis

Kyphosis is a descriptive term for posterior deviation of the spine in the sagittal plane beyond the normal limits (round shoulder appearance). The most common form is postural, especially during the adolescent growth spurt. It is more common in girls and may be associated with breast development making them self-conscious. The kyphosis is mobile and the individual can correct it.

Scheuermann's disease was originally described by Scheuermann in 1920 as a fixed kyphosis developing at puberty, the final diagnosis only being made after X-ray examination. The classical kyphosis includes at least three adjacent vertebrae with wedging of five degrees or more in each vertebra. Scheuermann's disease now seems to be used to describe any X-ray in which there is evidence of mechanical damage to the anterior epiphyseal ring or anterior part of the vertebral body in the growing child (Fig. 16.10).

The aetiology of Scheuermann's kyphosis is unknown and, whilst mechanical factors may be implicated, others feel that it could either be caused by local vascular changes or be part of a juvenile osteoporosis.

336

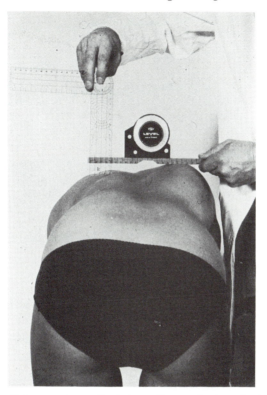

*Fig. 16.9* The rib hump of a scoliosis is easily noted when the individual flexes forward. This demonstrates a technique of measuring the height of the hump.

Refior and Zenker (1970) noted changes in the spine with 50% of young competitive sportsmen, whilst the frequency in the control population was only 30%. Querg (1958) examined fifty-nine rowers and found 51% with radiological changes of the spine diagnosed as Scheuermann's disease. Of 139 children in competitive alpine sport, 44% had changes similar to those described by Mathie (1977), whilst Boron, Galaj and Lasek (1978) found that twenty-five of the gymnasts from the Polish national team all demonstrated well developed Scheuermann's disease of the spine.

The characteristic sequence of events usually starts around the age of ten years, often with bad posture and increased thoracic kyphosis. At first this kyphosis is mobile but later it becomes fixed. Pain is reported in about one-third of the patients, whereas others talk about vague back stiffness. A number of the youngsters will be noted to have tight hamstrings (the so-called 'pseudo Lasegue phenomena'). Radiographic changes vary from minor irregularities of the anterior growth plate and Schmorl's

337

Spinal injuries

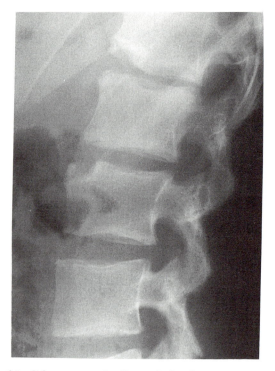

*Fig. 16.10* Is this Scheuermann's disease? Or does it represent a different pathology following damage to the disc?

nodes to severe vertebral wedging with later secondary repair and osteophyte formation. In the majority of cases, treatment by exercise alone is all that is necessary. More severe cases require exercises in conjunction with the wearing of a hyperextension type brace for up to three years.

Other forms of kyphosis include congenital, paralytic, post-traumatic, inflammatory (usually due to tuberculosis, but it can occur with other forms of osteomyelitis) and kyphosis related to a tumour (eosinophilic granuloma and neurofibromatosis).

*(c) Hyperlordosis*

This occurs in the lumbar spine and may be associated with a compensatory long thoracic kyphosis. The majority are postural and are present only when the child is standing. It may represent a transient overgrowth syndrome, the bony elements outstripping the ligaments and tendons during the second growth spurt. The association of tight lumbodorsal fascia and tight hamstrings with weak abdominal muscles leads to a posterior decompensation of the torso over the pelvis. In the more rigid variety an underlying bony disorder, for example spondylolisthesis or a deficiency in the posterior structures of the lower lumbar region, should be excluded.

### (d) Spondylolisthesis

This is a term used to describe the slipping of one vertebral body on an adjacent vertebral body. The degree of slip ranges from Grade 1, where there is a slip of 25% of the superior vertebral body over the vertebral body below, to Grade 4, where the superior vertebral body is lying directly anterior to the vertebral body or sacrum below. The classification of spondylolisthesis normally referred to is that described by Newman and Stone (1963).

*Group 1: congenital spondylolisthesis* There is a forward slip of the last lumbar vertebra on the upper sacrum at the lumbosacral junction. This is secondary to a congenital sacral defect with poor development of the sacral facets. There may be elongation or an actual break of the neural arch of the last lumbar vertebra. Symptoms usually present during the second growth spurt, with low back pain often radiating to the legs. The hamstrings may be so tight that, when lying prone, lifting the leg from the bench causes the buttock to hitch up from the couch.

*Group 2: spondylolytic spondylolisthesis* The slip is secondary to a break in the pars interarticularis (Fig. 16.11). Wiltse, Widell and Jackson (1975) felt that the defect in the pars interarticularis is a product of two factors: an inherent dysplasia and a fatigue fracture through this weakened pars interarticularis. The majority of authors are of the opinion that the repetitive stress which leads to the actual fracture is probably a hyperex-

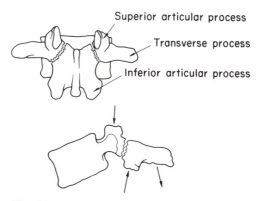

Fig. 16.11   Spondylolytic spondylolisthesis.

tension movement, although one or two have raised the possibility that it can also occur with flexion. The defect is not present at birth and the incidence tends to arise around the early teens. There is considerable interest in this particular defect in relation to sports medicine. Ferguson, McMaster and Stanitski (1974) drew attention to the high incidence in college football linesmen. Semon and Spengler (1981) found no difference with the position played and no significant difference in the time off sport, comparing those with low back pain and a defect with those without a defect. He therefore felt that a radiological defect should not discourage participation in sport. Mutoh (1977) noticed the increased incidence in butterfly swimmers, Wakabayashi (1977) in weightlifters and judo, and Rossi (1978) in high jumpers who practised the Fosbury flop, and also in divers and weightlifters.

Akimoto (1979) examined 1966 Japanese schoolboys aged eight to seventeen years. They were subdivided into 1186 boys undertaking rigorous athletic training and a non-athletic group of 780 boys. In 350 of the athletes radiological examinations were repeated from one to seven years. Initial examination showed that 120 athletes (10.3%) compared with 25 non-athletes (3.3%) had spondylolysis. Amongst athletes the incidence gradually increased from 8% at the age of ten to eleven years, to 14.1% at the age of sixteen to seventeen years. In non-athletes there was no significant difference in incidence amongst age groups.

Radiologically, the transition from sclerosis to spondylolysis was noticed in serial follow-up studies. It would therefore appear that heavy athletic activity during the growing period increases the incidence of spondylolysis. Defects may be picked up prior to X-ray changes using a radioactive bone scan. Whilst it may not be seen on AP radiographs of the lumbar spine it is more often noted in the oblique views of the typical 'Scottie dog' profile, with a collar round the neck of the dog. Wiltse (1969) demonstrated that many cases with bilateral spondylolysis could be converted to spondylolisthesis if the lumbosacral joint was loaded at the time of X-ray, and recommended that weightbearing views should be taken.

A large number of adolescents with this defect are asymptomatic, but once symptoms arise they comprise low back pain, often with radiation to the leg, made worse by exercise, and they may exhibit evidence of tight hamstrings. Micheli, Hall and Miller (1980) reported a 90% good or excellent result in treating these patients with a modified Boston brace (Fig. 16.12). He allowed them to continue their sporting activities in this brace and noted that a number of them went on to produce bony union across the site of the isthmic stress fracture (Fig. 16.13). If symptoms continue in the teenage athlete, and serial X-rays demonstrate continuing slip, then surgical stabilization, either using a Buck procedure (1970),

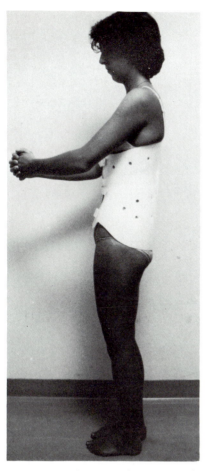

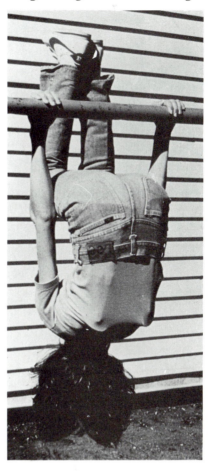

*Fig. 16.12* Flexion jacket – a modified Boston brace.

*Fig. 16.13* A patient in a Boston brace demonstrating her agility.

intertransverse fusion, or in the older age group an anterior fusion is indicated. After the age of skeletal maturity the isthmic defect is most likely not the cause of symptoms, and the underlying problem should be sought elsewhere. In a survey of pre-employment X-rays 5% were said to have demonstrated the defect without low back symptoms. A rare late problem is root pressure caused as a result of fibrous or bony overgrowth in relation to the defect.

*Group 3: traumatic spondylolisthesis* This is rare and usually follows a direct blow to the lumbar region or falling on the buttocks. Radiographs show the fracture running from the pars interarticularis into the pedicle (Fig.

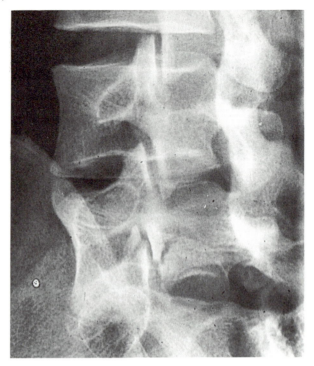

*Fig. 16.14* Oblique views of the lower lumbar, upper sacral spine in which there has been a fracture extending down into the pedicle. Note also the fracture of the superior facet of the sacrum. The patient had fallen from a horse.

16.14. The fracture heals with conservative management, consisting of mobilization in a plaster jacket for two to three months.

*Group 4: degenerative spondylolisthesis* This is not seen in patients under forty. There are marked osteoarthritic changes in the zygo-apophyseal joints, occurring usually at the fourth lumbar level, and it is three times more common in women than men. Neurological symptoms resulting from pressure on the fifth lumbar root, or less commonly the corda equina, may be seen in this group.

*Group 5: pathological spondylolisthesis* This is secondary to osteogenesis imperfecta, achondroplasia, Paget's disease, infection or neoplasm.

*(e) Disc pathology*

This is rare in children. De Orio and Bianco (1982) reported fifty cases seen at the Mayo Clinic over a twenty-six year period. Ten patients were injured during athletic activities, whilst a further seven followed falls from a height of approximately 1 metre or higher. Sciatica was present in 92% and 60% had low back pain.

## References

Aggrawal, N. D., Kaur, R., Kumar, S. and Mathur, D. N. (1979) A study of the changes in the spine of weight-lifters and other athletes. *Brit. J. Sports Med.*, **13**, 58–61.

Akimoto, T. (1979) Etiology of spondylolysis with reference to athletic activities during the growth period. *Orthopaedics [Jpn]*, **30**, 638–46.

Billings, R. A., Burry, H. C. and Jones R. (1977) Low back injury in sport. *Rheumatol. Rehabil.*, **16**, 236.

Boron, Z., Galaj, Z. and Lasek, W. (1978) Stress lesions in gymnasts. *Pol. Przegl Radiol.*, **42**, 205–9.

Buck, J. E. (1970) The repair of the defect in spondylolisthesis. *J. Bone Joint Surg.*, **52B**, 432–37.

De Orio, J. K. and Bianco, A. J. (1982) Lumbar disc excision in children and adolescents. *J. Bone Joint Surg.*, **64A**, 991–95.

Dillane, J. B., Fry, J. and Kalton, G. (1966) Acute back syndrome – a study from general practice. *Brit. Med. J.*, **2**, 82.

Fairbank, J. C. T. and O'Brien, J. P. (1980) The abdominal cavity and thoraco lumbar fascia as stabilisers of the lumbar spine in patients with low back pain. *I. Mech. E. Publications*, **82**, 83–85.

Farfan, H. F. (1973) *Mechanical Disorder of the Low Back*. Lea and Febiger, Philadelphia.

Farfan, H. F., Huberdean, R. M. and Dubour, H. I. (1972) Lumbar invertebral disc degeneration: the influence of geometrical features on the pattern of disc degeneration – a post mortem study. *J. Bone Joint Surg. [Am]*., **54**, 492.

Ferguson, R. J., McMaster, J. H. and Stanitski, C. L. (1974) Low back pain in college football linesmen. *J. Sports Med.*, **2**, 63–69.

Friberg, S. and Hirsch, C. (1949) Anatomical and clinical studies on the lumbar disc degeneration. *Acta Orthop. Scand.*, **19**, 222.

Hirsch, C., Jonsson, B. and Lewin, T. (1969) Low back symptoms in a Swedish female population. *Clin. Orthop.*, **63**, 171.

Holdsworth, F. (1963) Fracture, dislocations and fracture dislocations of the spine. *J. Bone Joint Surg.*, **45B**, 6–20.

Hubbard, D. (1974) Injuries of the spine in children and adolescents. *Clin. Orthop.*, **100**, 56–65.

Jackson, F. E., Sazima, H. J., Pratt, R. A. and Back, J. B. (1971) Weight lifting injuries. *J. Amer. Coll. Health Assoc.*, **19**, 187–89.

Kirby, R. L. (1981) Flexibility and musculo-skeletal symptomatology in female gymnasts and age matched controls. *Amer. J. Sports Med.*, **9**, 160–64.

Mathie, Z. (1977) *Orthop. Ihre Grenzgeb.*, **155**, 866–975.

Micheli, L. J., Hall, J. E. and Miller, C. O. (1980) Use of the modified Boston Brace for back injuries in athletes. *Amer. J. Sports Med.*, **8**, 351–56.

Mooney, V. and Robertson, J. A. (1976) The facet syndrome. *Clin. Orthop.*, **115**, 149.

Morris, J. M., Lucas, D. B. and Bresler, B. (1961) Role of the trunk in stability of the spine. *J. Bone Joint Surg. [Am.]*, **43A**, 327–52.

# Spinal injuries

Murray-Leslie, Lintott, D. J. and Wright, V. (1977) The spine in sport and military parachutists. *Ann. Rheum. Dis.*, **36**, 332–42.

Mutoh, Y. (1977) Low back pain in butterfliers. *Jap. J. Phys. Fit. Sports Med.*, **26**, 177–81.

Nachemson, A. (1966) Electromyographic study of the vertebral portion of the psoas muscle. *Acta Orthop. Scand.*, **37**, 177–90.

Naylor, A. (1971) The biochemical changes in the lumbar intervertebral disc in degenerative or nuclear prolapse. *Orthop. Clin. N. Amer.*, **2**, 2.

Newman, P. H. and Stone, K. H. (1963) The aetiology of spondylolisthesis. *J. Bone Joint Surg.*, **45B**, 39–59.

Pedersen, H. E., Blunck, C. F. J. and Gardener, E. (1956) The anatomy of the lumbosacral posterior rami and meningeal branches of spinal nerves. *J. Bone Joint Surg.*, **38A**, 1377.

Querg, H. (1958) Les resultats des examens radiologiques des rameurs juveniles. Kongressband des XII International Kongresses Krankreich, Sportmedizin, Moskau.

Refior, H. J. and Zenker, H. (1970) *Munch. Med. Wochenschr.*, **112**, 463.

Rissanen, P. M. (1960) The surgical anatomy and pathology of the supraspinous and interspinous ligaments of the lumbar spine with special reference to ligament ruptures. *Acta Orthop. Scand.*, Supplement, 46.

Roche, M. B. and Rowe, G. C. (1952) Incidence of separate new arch and coincident bone variations. *J. Bone Joint Surg.*, **34A**, 491.

Robertson, J. A. (1975) Dynamic control of the lumbar spine. *Ortho. Services USC*, Vol. 8.

Rossi, F. (1978) Spondylolysis, spondylolisthesis and sport. *J. Sports Med. Phys. Fit.*, **18**, 317–40.

Schultz, A. B. (1974) Mechanics of the human spine. *Appl. Mech. Rev. (ASME)*, 1487.

Schweiz, Z. (1975) *Sportmed.*, **23**, 189–93.

Semon, R. L. and Spengler, D. (1981) Significance of lumbar spondylolysis in college football players. *Spine*, **6**, 172–74.

Smith, C. F. (1977) The physical management of muscular low back pain in athletes. *Can. Med. Assoc. J.*, **117**, 632–35.

Spangfort, E. V. (1972) The lumbar disc herniation. A computer-aided analysis of 2504 operations. *Acta Orthop. Scand.* [suppl.], **142**, 1.

Stallard, M. C. (1980) Back ache in oarsmen. *Brit. J. Sports Med.*, **14**, 105–8.

Steinbruck, K. and Paeslack, V. (1980) Analysis of 139 spinal cord injuries due to accident in water sports. *Paraplegia*, **18**, 86–93.

Wakabayashi, W. (1977) Study of lumbar disorders in athletes with special reference to the posture taking weight lifting style. *Jap. J. Phys. Fit. Sports Med.*, **26**, 1–12.

Waters, R. L. and Morris, J. M. (1970) Effects of spinal supports on the electrical activity of the muscles of the trunk. *J. Bone Joint Surg. [Am.]*, **52A**, 51–60.

Wiltse, L. L. (1969) Spondylolisthesis classification and aetiology, in *American Academy of Orthopaedic Surgeons Symposium on the Spine*, Chapter 9, C. V. Mosby, St Louis.

Wiltse, L. L., Widell, E. H. and Jackson, D. W. (1975) Fatigue fracture: the basic lesion in isthmic spondylolisthesis. *J. Bone Joint Surg. [Am.]*, **57A**, 17–22.

# 17 *Pelvis, hip and thigh injuries*

JOHN KING and JAMES ROBERTSON

## 17.1 The pelvis

The pelvic ring and sacrum provide both for locomotion and protection of the contents of the lower abdomen and pelvic cavity. The major muscles of the abdomen are attached to the superior surface whilst the inferior and lateral surfaces give origin to many of the major muscles to the legs. Posteriorly, the sacrum and coccyx are joined to the hemi-pelvis on either side by the sacroiliac joints. These are plain synovial joints strongly reinforced above and behind by heavy ligaments and additionally strengthened by accessory ligaments, the sacrotuberous, the sacrospinous and iliolumbar ligaments. Each hemi-pelvis is composed of three bones, the ilium, ischium and pubis, which unite to form the acetabular component of the hip joint. Anteriorly the two pubic bones are united at the pubic symphysis which contains a fibrocartilaginous interpubic disc reinforced above by the superior pubic ligament and below by the arcuate pubic ligament. This disc is initially solid but with the passage of time a narrow fissure often occurs which may be synovialized, the result of degenerative changes.

Lesions will be discussed under the subheadings of contact (direct injury or extrinsic), non-contact (indirect injury or intrinsic), overuse and other conditions.

### 17.1.1 SOFT TISSUE INJURIES

*(a) Contact injury*

Where there is bone with little superficial soft tissue, for example over the anterior iliac crest, grazing and extensive superficial bruising are not uncommon. Extensive bruising in this area is often called the hip pointer (Fig. 17.1) which can be very painful. It needs immediate treatment with ice and pressure. Play can be resumed when comfort allows. When there is recurrent trauma local padding may be necessary to protect the area.

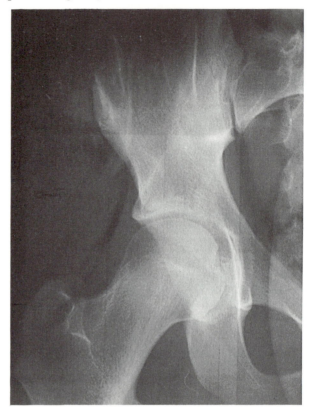

*Fig. 17.1* Injury to anterior iliac crest.

Other areas around the pelvis are well protected by deep layers of muscle, and blunt trauma in these regions can produce extensive bruising which only becomes apparent some days later and may be associated with a local haematoma and encystment. Direct trauma in the region of the greater trochanter can produce inflammation of the trochanteric bursa. This will normally settle with ultrasound, but should it become a problem then a local injection of steroid into the bursa may well relieve the problem.

### (b) Non-contact injury

Psoas muscle strains have been described in the chapter on the back. Other deeper muscles in the pelvis may occasionally be damaged and present with referred pain. Pace and Nagle (1976) described a variety of deep muscle trigger points primarily relating to the piriformis muscle, noting low back pain and hip pain with radiation down the back of the leg. In the female there is often an associated complaint of dyspareunia.

346

Pain and weakness on resisted abduction of the externally rotated thigh with tenderness and reproduction of the patient's complaints by digital pressure over the belly of the piriform muscle indicates the diagnosis. Local injection of the muscle belly relieves symptoms.

The origins of the internal and external oblique abdominal muscles from the rim of the pelvis may be strained. When this occurs it can be disabling as the abdominal stabilizers are used in nearly all activities. Local injections may help but the pain is often diffuse because of the length of origin and non-steroidal anti-inflammatories and rest may be needed.

## 17.1.2 BONY INJURIES

### (a) Contact injury

These occur by direct trauma to the pubis, ischium, ilium, sacrum or coccyx. The majority of these injuries are easily diagnosed on X-ray and can be treated conservatively. A 'hip pointer' may indicate damage to the iliac wing in the adult (Fig. 17.1) or to the iliac apophysis in the adolescent athlete (Lombardo, Retting and Kerland, 1983).

The injury to the coccyx usually takes the form of increasing the mobility of the proximal joint. The athlete usually complains of discomfort when sitting and the symptoms can be reproduced with bimanual palpation. The differential diagnosis is from referred pain at the lumbosacral articulation, but in the latter case there is no discomfort on bimanual palpation of the coccyx. Treatment involves manipulation, injection of steroid into the joint and, if these fail, excision of the coccyx. Radiographs are irrelevant.

### (b) Disruption of the pelvic ring

This is caused by excessive force and is usually seen in high speed trauma. The diagnosis and management of this condition are to be found in any major textbook of skeletal trauma. However, it is important to remember in these injuries that damage can occur to the contents of the pelvis. Bleeding can be catastrophic and on site resuscitation may be necessary. In the male, because of the close proximity of the urethra to the public symphysis, damage to the base of the bladder or urethra is not uncommon. Blood at the external urethral meatus of the penis is an indicator of this type of damage and a urological opinion should be obtained before contemplating catheterization.

### (c) Non-contact injury

*Avulsion fractures.* The peak incidence is in the second decade, the most common complaint being of pain, either acute or of several weeks' duration. Fernback and Wilkinson (1981) reviewed the findings in twenty patients with avulsion fractures of the pelvis and proximal femur. Lombardo, Retting and Kerland (1983) described nine patients with discontinuity of the anterior part of the iliac apophysis on radiographs. The avulsion may occur from the iliac crest, anterior superior iliac spine, anterior inferior iliac spine (Fig. 17.2), ischium, ischial apophysis (McMaster, 1945) and the lesser trochanter of the femur. The lesion is caused by the vigorous and unco-ordinated activity of muscle flexion in the muscles taking origin from the apophysis. There may be local tenderness in the region of the apophysis, whilst movements involving those muscles become painful and restricted. The radiographs demonstrate the apophyseal avulsion. Treatment consists of rest, in the acute severe cases, by bed rest and later by crutch ambulation. The prognosis is excellent, although radiographic deformity may persist. A

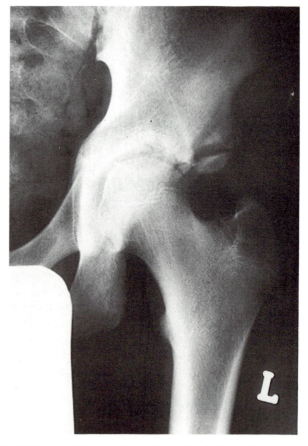

*Fig. 17.2*  Avulsion fracture of anterior inferior iliac spine.

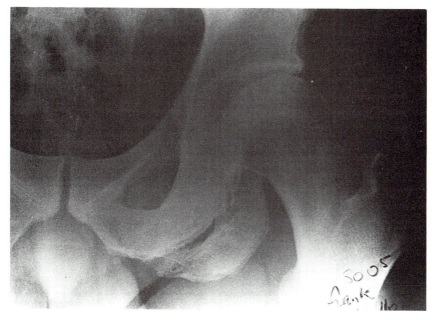

*Fig. 17.3*  Overgrowth of ischium following trauma.

rare complication is overgrowth of the apophysis, producing mechanical problems at a later stage (Fig. 17.3), and excision may be indicated. Painful fibrous non-union is a rare complication requiring surgery (Torg, 1982).

### (d) Overuse

*Stress fractures.* Devas (1975) covered this subject in depth and referred to lesions of the ischiopubic rami, the iliopubic rami and the femoral neck. Pavlov *et al.* (1982) collected a series of stress fractures of the inferior pubic rami, in which eleven of her twelve cases were distance runners, and with two exceptions the lesions occurred in women between the ages of nineteen and forty-eight. All cases presented with pain in the groin, buttock or thigh, the fractures were non-displaced and could easily be overlooked on initial radiographic examination. If doubt existed a radionuclide bone scan was diagnostic. On curtailment of running, symptoms disappeared. Mowat and Kay (1983) described a single case of a stress fracture in the ischium of a fourteen year old athlete.

*Periostitis.* The classical description of this refers to the so-called 'rider's bone' seen in horse riders following overuse of the adductor muscles in their riding position. This leads to a chronic periostitis of the adductor

# Pelvis, hip and thigh injuries

insertion on the lower pubis with radiological changes of calcification distal to the bone. In the majority of cases these are chance findings when the pelvis is being X-rayed for other causes, but occasionally it is genuinely associated with symptoms of discomfort in the groin. On examination, limited abduction of the hip is noted resulting from tight adductors. Gradual stretching of the adductors is indicated, but in the more chronic cases stretching under a general anaesthetic is occasionally beneficial. In soccer players a similar pattern of injury is referred to as the Gracilis syndrome. In the early stages semi-circular and oval radio-translucencies occur at the lower edge of the pubic bone at the origin of gracilis, adductor longus and adductor brevis musles. Stretching is the initial treatment followed by local injection of steroid, with or without a stretch under general anaesthesia.

## (e)  Osteitis pubis, sacroiliac joint stress and pelvic instability

Domisse (1960) talks of the pelvic symphysis being the hinge of the pelvis, indicating that any change in the mobility of this joint must, as a result of the ring structure of the pelvis, have an effect on the sacroiliac joint unless there has been an associated fracture. When the symptoms primarily arise from the pubic symphysis the player complains of discomfort in one or both groins, at first brought on by physical exertion and relieved by rest, with the periods of rest necessary for relief getting longer. Suprapubic and lower abdominal pain is not uncommon. Palpation over

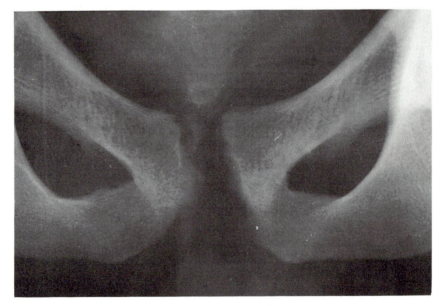

*Fig. 17.4*  Osteitis pubis.

the symphysis pubis may demonstrate discomfort or the symptoms can be reproduced by asking the player to do a scissor kick or other such manoeuvre. The changes on X-ray range from loss of definition at the margins of the symphysis in the early stages, followed by local osteoporosis, widening of the symphysis, periosteal reaction at the edge (Fig. 17.4), leading up to an unstable pelvis.

The width of the pubic symphysis is normally under 10 mm. 'Flamingo' views, in which the subject weightbears first on one leg then on the other leg whilst anterior posterior views of the symphysis are taken, are needed to diagnose pelvic instability syndrome. Comparison of the films will demonstrate the uppermost corner of one side of the symphysis being displaced superiorly as the player weightbears on the corresponding lower extremity. A difference in height of the superior pubic ramus on each side of more than 3 mm is abnormal (Fig. 17.5).

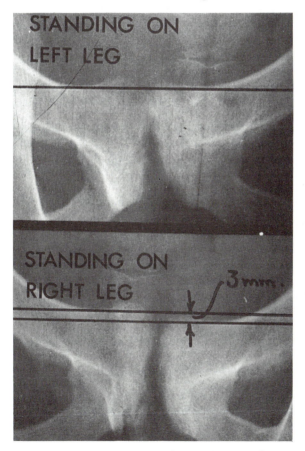

*Fig. 17.5* 'Flamingo' views of the pubic symphysis.

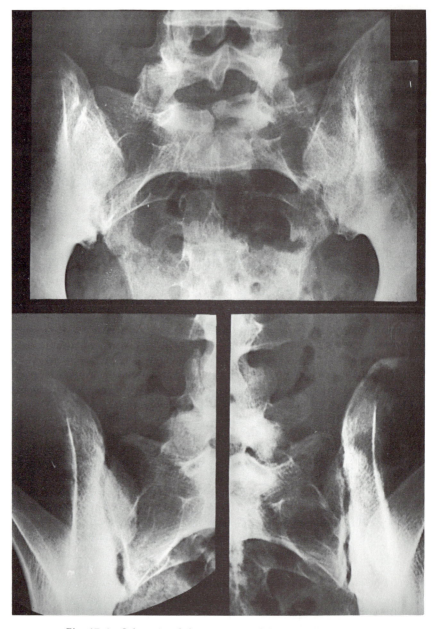

*Fig. 17.6* Sclerosis of the margins of the sacroiliac joints.

In the acute stage the athlete is advised to refrain from competing and instructed in doing abdominal muscle exercises. It may be worth putting a slight raise in one or other of the shoes on a trial basis. In the majority of cases with this type of regime, associated with general stretching of the adductor muscles, symptoms slowly subside. Injection of steroid into the pubic symphysis must be performed under general anaesthesia because of the pain. If a full abduction stretch is performed at the same time and a graduated return to sport imposed it is usually successful. Surgical fusion of the symphysis is still occasionally performed but the results do not appear to have been satisfactory, perhaps because the fusion takes about a year to become effective.

When symptoms primarily occur in the sacroiliac joint, discomfort is felt in the region of that joint with vague discomfort in the buttock generally. Stressing the joint by forced rotation using the fully flexed femur as a lever may reproduce the symptoms. X-rays will demonstrate sclerosis in the surrounding bone and loss of definition at the joint margin (Fig. 17.6). Early ankylosing spondylitis or other inflammatory conditions need to be excluded. Gentle manipulation and mobilization of the lower back and sacroiliac joint is indicated, together with a muscle building programme to strengthen the abdominals. Surgical fusion of a sacroiliac joint is rarely indicated but can be successful.

Increased sclerosis round the sacroiliac joint on one side has been noted in golfers. The relaxation of the symphysis in the child-bearing female and changes in relation to prostatic inflammation need to be excluded. Harris and Murray (1974) surveyed an entire professional soccer club and also a large number of controls. They noted an increased incidence of radiological changes in the symphysis pubis of those controls who had participated in active sport, but these changes were never as advanced as those seen in the soccer players. In this latter group of twenty-six professional soccer players, one third had instability of the symphysis, nineteen had marginal irregularity, seventeen had reactive sclerosis and there were thirteen with stress sclerosis in the iliac portion of one or both sacroiliac joints.

## 17.2 The hip

The hip joint is deeply seated and well protected by bulky overlying muscles. It is thus poorly amenable to palpation. It is stable because of the combination of its bone architecture, soft tissues (capsule and labrum) and the powerful muscles. It is not easily injured. It may be the site of a number of spontaneously occurring inflammatory lesions which may be revealed in sport, as well as some non-contact and overuse conditions. It is the only joint allowing rotation in the extended lower limb. Loss of rotation may be manifest by problems in the foot or knee as the rotation of the leg associated with pronation of the foot cannot be accommodated.

### 17.2.1 CONTACT INJURY

Fractures and dislocations are the most spectacular contact injuries; fortunately they are rare. They usually occur in sports with a risk of a blow to the front of the flexed knee (motor racing, horse riding). It is important to be aware of the risk and to recognize the diagnosis and its problems. Damage to the sciatic nerve can occur. Excessive handling may increase the risk of avascular necrosis of the femoral head. Painful loss of motion with shortening of the limb must be treated as a fracture or dislocation until proved otherwise. The patient must be gently transported to hospital. It is essential to check the integrity of the posterior cruciate ligament which is frequently injured at the same time.

Fractures may occur through the floor of the acetabulum after a fall directly onto the great trochanter or the trochanter itself may break. The management of fractures and dislocations is dealt with in standard texts. The sportsman may be capable of a very demanding rehabilitation program and often needs holding back rather than encouraging after dislocations of the hip.

### 17.2.2 NON-CONTACT INJURY

Avulsion injuries have been dealt with in the section on the pelvis. The greater trochanter may be the site of bursitis. It is more common in young female athletes and is associated with the ability to snap the edge of the tensor lata muscle over the greater trochanter. This gives the patient the impression that the hip is popping in and out of joint. The diagnosis is revealed by palpation over the trochanter during active flexion and internal rotation of the hip when the tendon snapping over the bone can be felt under the finger. Local injection is often enough. Ultrasound may help but surgical release may sometimes be necessary, removing the central area of the fascia in contact with the trochanter.

### 17.2.3 OVERUSE CONDITIONS

Stress fractures of the femoral neck do occur in normal bone. Pain comes on during activity, usually running, and becomes severe more and more quickly. There may eventually be rest pain. This region is not amenable to palpation and the diagnosis depends on special investigations. X-rays may be normal or show gradually increasing sclerosis across the femoral neck. The changes when the neck has completely given way are not dramatic as shown in Fig. 17.7 in which the neck gave up the struggle during the London marathon. If pain persists despite cessation of activities and the use of crutches, and a bone scan remains hot, an osteoid osteoma must be excluded by biopsy.

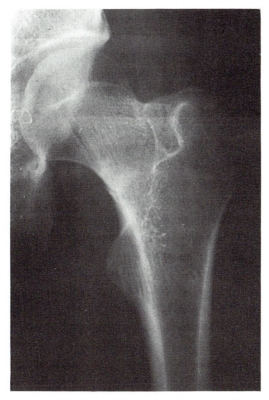

*Fig. 17.7*   Stress fracture of femoral neck.

## 17.2.4   OTHER CONDITIONS

The term 'irritable hip' is frequently confined to childhood but a similar condition may occur in adults. There is a limp with pain in the affected leg often poorly localized to the hip. There is not necessarily a history of injury and examination reveals varying degrees of loss of hip motion and discomfort. X-rays are usually normal and in the absence of systemic upset, treatment is simply bed rest until the pain goes. In more severe cases it is necessary to exclude infection by blood tests and aspiration of the joint. Injury may give the same clinical picture which is the consequence of a capsular strain.

## Pelvis, hip and thigh injuries

Perthe's disease is an idiopathic avascular necrosis of the femoral head occurring between the ages of three and ten, four times as common in boys as girls and bilateral in 10%. It presents as an irritable hip, perhaps with repeated episodes, and the diagnosis is confirmed on X-ray. Treatment is directed to preserving the shape of the head during revascularization and will vary from surgeon to surgeon but it is unlikely that any will allow sport during that time (Kemp, 1969; Wynne-Davis and Gormley, 1978).

Slipped upper femoral epiphysis occurs between ten and sixteen years of age, is twice as common in boys as girls and the majority show some bilateral change (Angel, 1983). The condition is seen in fat hypogonadal boys or thin rapidly growing teenagers of either sex. Acute slips are rare and very painful. They bring the child to the casualty department where there is usually enough clinical evidence and change on X-rays for the diagnosis to be clear. Far more common is the chronic slip in which the displacement is gradual but may represent a series of very small acute slips. The history is of pain felt down the front of the thigh towards the knee, which is often unjustly accused of being the cause. There is minimal shortening and the most obvious sign is loss of internal rotation. X-rays may be difficult to interpret and a lateral view must always be requested. Treatment is usually surgical in an attempt to stop further slip and diminish the risk of osteoarthritis in later life.

Some athletes will be found on examination to have very little rotation of the hip, although flexion and extension are normal. X-rays will show a rather domed femoral head which acts like an axle in a bearing, allowing rotation around the long axis of the neck only. This may be the result of a very small unnoticed slip in childhood (Murray and Jacobson, 1977). If a lot of pronation takes place in the foot producing excessive internal rotation of the tibia, the knee may become painful as the hip will not accommodate the internal rotation. Despite the cause being at the hip and the site of the pain the knee, it can only be stopped by preventing the pronation of the foot!

The iliopsoas bursa may be a problem. It may become distended and inflamed and cause hip pain. It overlies the front of the neck of the femur where there may be tenderness and passive abduction and extension may make the pain worse by stretching the tendon. These bursae may be very large (Warren, Kaye and Salvati, 1975) and three cases have recently been noted in which the presenting symptom was pain in the knee secondary to quadriceps insufficiency as a consequence of pressure on the femoral nerve from the bursa. Diagnosis was confirmed by ultrasound or arthrogram and excision of the bursa has alleviated the symptoms. Intensive rehabilitation is essential. Lyons and Peterson (1984) have recently described the iliopsoas tendon snapping over the

356

iliopectineal eminence stating that it is a common occurrence but usually asymptomatic.

## 17.3 The thigh

The mass of muscles which constitute the thigh control acceleration and deceleration of the body and support the knee. These muscles surround the femur and through them pass the nerves and blood vessels to the lower leg. The thigh combines the roles of power, control, support and protection. The long muscles in front of and behind the thigh cross two joints and the efficiency of their action on one joint depends on the position of the other. The quadriceps apparatus provides deceleration and, by paying out under load, absorbs energy and acts as a shock absorber. This action is essential as the kinetic energy absorbed in coming to a halt from running is of an order of magnitude greater than that needed to break the femur.

Pelvic ring problems, particularly those affecting the symphysis pubis present as pain in the thigh, especially in the adductor region, and are often confused with adductor strain. The pain from the hip joint is often perceived as pain in the front of the thigh.

The incidence of direct injuries is highest in the contact sports. Overuse injuries are seen in long distance runners and occasionally in professional footballers. Acute non-contact injuries are most frequently seen in sprinters.

### 17.3.1 CONTACT INJURY

Because of its position, the thigh is particularly susceptible to direct violence. One of the most common injuries is the surface 'burn', a consequence of sliding along a rough surface such as grass or artificial turf, or the road in cycling accidents. Extensive areas of the skin may be scraped, particularly over elevations such as the greater trochanter, lateral femoral condyle, or bulky muscles.

If these areas can be exposed and kept dry, healing is rapid. Frequently the necessity to play again too soon in professional sport or the work environment does not allow this, and secondary infection with further damage to the skin may occur and primary treatment is then an occlusive dressing of 'plastic skin' or adherent plastic sheet to allow healing without infection. Local antibacterial treatment will be necessary with frequent cleansing and changes of dressing if infection takes place.

A direct blow to the thigh muscle is very common, producing a haematoma which may be contained within the muscle fibres or leak out to be contained within the fibrous muscle sheath. This injury is called a Charley Horse in the USA and a dead leg in the UK. The history is clear. The examination reveals local tenderness and swelling. If the haematoma is outside the muscle and the sheath is torn there may be extensive bruising (Fig. 17.8).

The immediate management is ice, compression, elevation and rest. Overall, the role of ice remains debatable and it is difficult to give a physiological explanation as to its efficiency. Despite that there is ample day to day anecdotal evidence to suggest that there is at least an analgesic role and it is an indispensable part of any sports clinic. As pain and swelling diminish, active 'range of motion' exercises, perhaps after extensive icing, seem to promote the most rapid resolution. Any activity that leads to an increase in pain, swelling, local heat or loss of motion is excessive and must be diminished. Despite this, occasionally the haematoma forms a capsule and liquefies. Repeated aspiration may be adequate but frequently such cases will require excision of the lining of the cavity and its obliteration with stitches through and through into the muscles.

Another major complication of this muscle injury is abnormal bone formation within the muscle mass, myositis ossificans. This must not be confused with the ossification which occurs after a haematoma has stripped off periosteum (Fig. 17.9) and the new bone forms beneath it. In this case normal bone forming cells are going about their normal business (although the results can look alarming). Quite abnormal ossification takes place in myositis ossificans in that the bone appears to form away from the periosteum. The condition reveals itself by prolonged heat, swelling and tenderness. When it occurs there is no evidence that treatment with diphosphonates or calcitonin alters the course of the disease. If seen early it is important to stop all local treatment, particularly any form of stretching or manipulation.

Occasionally the ectopic ossification produces only mild symptoms. More frequently there is painful limitation of muscle excursion. In these cases it is necessary to wait for 'maturation' of the lesion with loss of both tenderness and local reaction. Radiologically the margins become smooth and the overall appearance homogenous; this usually takes at least six months to a year, at which time it is possible to excise the lesion if symptoms continue to be troublesome. By analogy with the formation of ectopic bone formation following total hip replacement it is possible indomethacin may allow greater range of motion after surgery, despite the fact that the calcification may recur on cessation of treatment. This point remains inconclusive. It is important that when surgery is performed it should be carried out through an adequate incision; excellent haemostasis is essential. The ossifying subperiosteal haematoma does

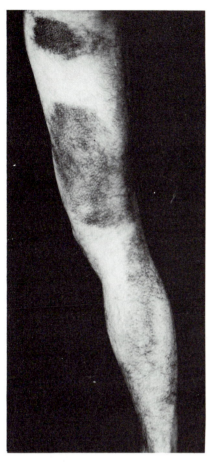

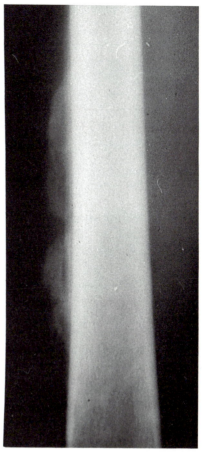

*Fig. 17.8* Extensive bruising following a direct blow to the thigh.

*Fig. 17.9* Ossification following a
subperiosteal haematoma.

not interfere with function and may be safely ignored once the initial
symptoms have gone.

The most dramatic contact injury is a fracture of the femur. There does
not necessarily always have to be contact. It has been seen in a young man
with normal bones twisting sharply on a squash court. There is immediate pain, collapse and deformity. The major consequence of this injury is
shock due to blood loss. Therefore early handling must be kept to a
minimum and should only consist of the patient's removal from continuing hazard. As a first aid measure the leg is stabilized by strapping it to the
intact one. Ideally a Thomas's splint is applied and one of these with an
open top ring should be available at all major sporting events. The injured
patient may then be gently transported to hospital.

## 17.3.2 NON-CONTACT INJURY

Injury occurs from tearing of the powerfully contracting muscles, when they themselves have suffered direct damage or their action is not co-ordinated. The extent of the injury depends upon the degree of muscle damage and the localization of resultant haematoma. The muscle itself may have a few fibres torn or may suffer complete separation. This may affect any of the muscles. There are two sites at which injury commonly occurs: it may be somewhere in the belly of the muscle or at its origin from the pelvis. In the adult a piece of bone may be avulsed and in childhood failure is more common through an area of cartilaginous growth, such as the iliac crest or origin of rectus femoris. These have been described already.

Non-contact muscle injuries have an increased incidence in those who are very muscular and lack a certain amount of extensibility. These injuries are also seen early in the new season when training is incomplete. They are seen late in an event, particularly football played on a heavy muddy pitch, where co-ordination is diminished because of tiredness. They are seen after failure of adequate warm-up even in a fully trained athlete. It is well recognized that a player who has received a heavy blow to a muscle group, perhaps with the temporary partial paralysis such as seen in a dead leg, may continue playing, lose co-ordination and sustain a more damaging spontaneous muscle injury – 'second injury syndrome' (King, 1983).

### (a) Hamstrings

Perhaps the most dramatic incident is the hamstring tear which causes a sprinter to pull up in the middle of a race. The demands on the muscle become too great and some fibres snap. The victim grasps the tender area which is often on the outer side. The short head of the biceps femoris has two motor points, one from the tibial and the other from the peroneal part of the sciatic nerve and this is implicated in the high incidence of tears to the muscle here (Burkett, 1975). It is essential to treat immediately with rest, ice, elevation and compression. The return to sprinting must be delayed until such time as the muscle can cope with the strains imposed on it. It is no use just allowing mobilization within the comfortable range and early resumption of training. Unless the muscle performance in terms of strength, extensibility and co-odination has been improved to above its previous best, recurrence of the injury takes place. This includes failure of technique where, for example, an abnormal foot alignment in the strike or stance phase may abnormally load the hamstring. There is no such thing as a chronic hamstring strain; it is an inadequately treated strain.

Complete tears are very rare and there are no guidelines as to the necessity for repair. Far more common is the incomplete tear. The frequent recurrences mentioned above produce scarred areas which eventually become obvious as nodules (often cystic) within the muscles. When this unnecessary sequence of events has taken place surgery has to be undertaken occasionally in an attempt to get rid of the scar or cyst. It is a last resort and too much must not be promised to the patient. It may be very difficult to identify the lesion in the muscle. Trillat (personal communication) showed a technique of electrically stimulating the muscle belly at surgery and noting the 'direction' of the twitch. When above the lesion it would go to the pelvis, when below to the knee! Despite being difficult to explain it has helped on occasions to find the lesion and may simply represent a conduction defect at the scar.

While sprinters seem to tear in the middle one-third of the muscles, athletes who fully flex the hip with the knee extended, such as hurdlers and steeple chasers in jumping, are more inclined to tear the hamstring much higher, actually at the origin of the hamstrings in the region of the ischial tuberosity. They often relate it to abnormal stretching for the next obstacle. The pain is well localized but therapy is not. This area is not readily available to ice, etc. Unless a large piece of bone is avulsed and widely separated there is no indication for operation.

Early return to sport must be forbidden as the pain may easily become persistent. If it does so local injections of hydrocortisone and lignocaine may help. Again surgery may be necessary as a last resort. Exploration may reveal a small partially separated area with granulation tissue within. This area is excised and there is no significant loss of strength. Occasionally it has been possible to confirm a local 'hole' on a C.A.T. scan, but apart from convincing the surgeon that an operation is necessary it has not made it any easier to identify the lesion at surgery. However, intervention at this site is more successful than that in the belly of the muscle and it is reasonable to be slightly more optimistic about the outcome.

## (b) Quadriceps

Tears here are less common. In the elderly there can be complete avulsion of the quadriceps tendon above the patella. This is a surgical emergency. The whole extensor mechanism function is lost and repair of the tendon is mandatory. More proximally the separate belly of rectus femoris may tear. This may be complete and sudden or there may be repeated partial tears until complete. The recurrent symptoms are a nuisance at each partial tear, needing a lay-off until the pain settles, but once the tear is complete symptoms disappear. As there is no detectable loss of function it is probable that the effect of the repair in the acute rupture is cosmetic rather than functional and it is difficult to recommend. Very rarely, vastus medialis obliquus (lower fibres of vastus medialis) tear from the medial retinaculum. The local bruising, tenderness and defect are diagnostic and repair is necessary to avoid patella imbalance symptoms.

### (c) Adductors

Injury in this region is less common than in other muscle groups but the consequences are of long standing and the differential diagnosis is always difficult. 'Groin strain' seems to cover most of the problems. It must be remembered that lesions of the symphysis pubis frequently cause pain radiating into the inner side of the thigh. Acute tears of the muscle bellies are very rare. Avulsions of the origin from the ischial and pubic rami occur. Treatment has already been discussed.

Genuine sprains of the adductor origins do occur. The diagnosis is made by exclusion of other lesions and the finding of persistent localized tenderness in the origins of the adductors with pain on stressing in abduction. Local injection may help but this condition is often refractory and injection with manipulation under anaesthetic with a blow from the side of the hand to the stretched muscle origin may be necessary. If this fails formal release of the painful portion of the adductor origin may have to be performed.

### 17.3.3 PREVENTION

Prevention falls into two obvious groups. The first and most important is the achievement of full flexibility before embarking upon activity. This is extensively discussed in Chapter 1 and its importance cannot be overemphasized. The second mode of prevention depends upon coaches and referees in that they should make themselves more aware of the risks that are identifiable in certain competitors. Those who are obviously particularly tired and at risk from poor co-ordination or those who have sustained an injury which has left them partially disabled should be removed from the competition as they represent a significant danger to themselves.

### 17.3.4 OVERUSE

Overuse injuries in the thigh are rare. They may appear common in the hamstring but nearly all of these conditions are a consequence of an inappropriately or inadequately treated acute lesion. Stress fractures of the shaft of the femur occur usually at the metaphysis. The presenting complaint is pain which occurs after activity. Classically, pain comes on sooner and sooner after the commencement of the activity as time goes on but severe rest pain is most unusual. Some aching pain after use is common. If the rest pain is an important feature suspect osteosarcoma. Three patients in the past year have presented in this way at The London Hospital.

Examination is difficult; the bone is well covered and the classical sign of local tenderness may be impossible to elicit. X-ray changes may be minimal with perhaps a slight bone condensation in the medulla and minimal subperiosteal reaction. In the very early stage there is usually no detectable change on X-ray. Radioisotope scanning here is very important in that it can reveal or confirm the lesion well before radiological changes take place. Differential diagnosis is a bone tumour and it is essential to bear this in mind. The common site is at the distal metaphysis and the radiological changes can be identical to a stress fracture (Fig. 17.10). It may on occasions be necessary to biopsy to be sure that the lesion is not a parosteal sarcoma. Such a biopsy *must* be done by an orthopaedic surgeon

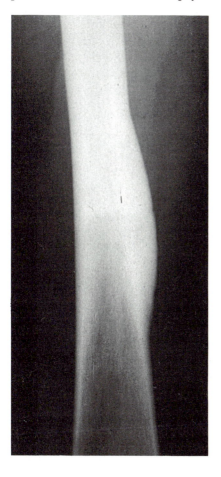

*Fig. 17.10* Osteoid osteoma of femur.

who knows which bit to take and examined by a pathologist experienced in bone tumours.

Once malignant disease is excluded the management is to allow the bone to heal and then stress it enough so that it increases in strength to cope with the imposed loads. The basic principle in the short-term, therefore, is diminution of activity to a pain-free level. If this can be achieved with reduced activity all is well and a graduated programme of increasing activity well within the limits of comfort can be commenced. If minimal activity still produces pain then some form of external support is necessary. In the distal femur a cast brace can be applied to support the limb. For the proximal femur non-weightbearing with crutches may be necessary.

Other overuse injuries occur in the thigh muscles but usually in their most distal part, i.e., the patella tendon, the insertions of the pesanserinus, semimembranosus and the iliotibial tract. These are dealt with in the chapter on the knee.

Enveloping fibrous sheaths contain the muscle bellies and very rarely may produce compartmental problems in overuse characterized by cramping pain on activity made worse by stretching the muscle passively. Treatment is release of the compartment (Mubarak and Hargens, 1981).

## References

Angel, J. C. (1983) *Clinical Orthopaedics*, Wright PSG, Bristol, London and Boston.

Burkett, L. N. (1975) Investigation into hamstring strains: the case of the hybrid muscle. *Amer. J. Sports Med.*, **3**, 5.

Devas, M. (1975) *Stress Fractures*, Churchill Livingstone, Edinburgh, London and New York.

Domisse, G. F. (1960) Diametric fractures of the pelvis. *J. Bone and Joint Surg.*, **42B**, 432.

Fernback, S. K. and Wilkinson, R. H. (1981) Avulsion injuries of the pelvis and proximal femur. *Amer. J. Radiol.*, **137**, 581.

Harris, N. H. and Murray, R. O. (1974) Lesions of the symphysis in athletes. *Brit. Med. J.*, **4**, 100, 211.

Kemp, H. B. S. (1969) MSc thesis, University of London.

King, J. B. (1983) Second injury syndrome. *Brit. J. Sports Med.*, **17**, 59.

Lombardo, S. J., Retting, A. C. and Kerland, R. K. (1983) Radiographic abnormalities of the iliac apophysis in adolescent athletes. *J. Bone Joint Surg.*, **65A**, 444.

Lyons, J. C. and Peterson, L. F. A. (1984) The snapping iliopsoas tendon. *Mayo Clin. Proc.*, **59**, 327.

McMaster, P. E. (1945) Epiphysitis of the ischial tuberosity. *J. Bone Joint Surg.*, **27**, 493.

Mowat, A. G. and Kay, V. J. (1983) Ischial stress fractures. *Brit. J. Sports Med.*, **17**, 94.

# References

Mubarak, S. J. and Hargens, A. R. (1981) *Compartment Syndromes and Volkmann's Contracture*, W. B. Saunders, Philadelphia, London, Toronto and Sydney.

Murray, R. O. and Jacobson, H. G. (1977) *The Radiology of Skeletal Disorders*, Churchill Livingstone, Edinburgh, London and New York.

Pace, J. B. and Nagle, D. (1976) Piriformis syndrome. *West. J. Med.*, **124**, 435.

Pavlov, H., Nelson, T. L., Warren, R. F. and Torg, J. S. (1982) Stress fractures of the pubic ramus. *J. Bone Joint Surg.*, **64A**, 1020.

Torg, J. S. (1982) *Year Book of Sports Medicine*, Year Book Medical Publishers Inc., Chicago and London, p. 235.

Warren, R., Kaye, J. J. and Salvati, E. A. (1975) Arthrographic demonstration of an enlarged iliopsoas bursa complicating osteoarthritis of the hip. *J. Bone Joint Surg.*, **57A**, 413.

Wynne-Davis, R. and Gormley, J. (1978) The aetiology of Perthe's disease *J. Bone Joint Surg.*, **60B**, 6.

# 18 Knee injuries

JOHN KING

The knee is in the middle of a series of levers which exert great forces on this link. Fortunately it is not constrained by the shape of its bones but depends for its stability, on the soft tissues within it (the cruciates and menisci), the soft tissues around it (the capsule and capsular ligaments), and the strength and co-ordination of the muscles that move it.

Despite these apparent safety features the knee remains the joint most susceptible to injury and injury occurs in a very broad spectrum of sports. Much of our information about these injuries (Nicholas and Minkoff, 1978) is generated by the high incidence in the commercialized, high profile American contact sports of football, ice hockey and baseball while Australian rules football promotes expertise on another continent. Out of the injuries in 47 sports documented at the National Sports Centre at Crystal Palace, complaints relating to the knee dominated in ten, varying from the expected such as rugby and cycling to the less expected, namely middle distance running and javelin throwing (Table 18.1).

The consequences of a knee injury seem to represent a greater hazard to continuing performance than those of any other common injury. The

Table 18.1 Sports in which the knee is the joint most commonly giving rise to complaint

| |
|---|
| Sprint |
| Middle distance |
| High jump |
| Javelin |
| Swimming (not defined by stroke) |
| Cycling |
| Soccer |
| Rugby |
| Hockey |
| Weight training |

# Knee injuries

injury records of a professional football club and of a good amateur team were studied over one year and in both cases 15% of the problems were at the knee. However, the time out of the game was 40% of the total time off for injury. Of the 90 players evaluated in that year the sporting careers of two were brought to a halt and both by injuries to the knee.

## 18.1 Functional anatomy

The knee consists of two joints: the tibiofemoral and the patellofemoral. The medial surface of the upper end of the tibia is basically flat, the lateral being slightly convex and sloping downwards and backwards. Lying on the articular surfaces are the menisci which create a shallow cupping effect.

The bones are held together by the ligaments, the cruciates inside the joint and the capsular ligaments outside it. The conventional view is that the cruciates control the anteroposterior gliding movements and the medial and lateral capsular ligaments resist the varus and valgus bending forces. The truth is far more complex than this. The principal motion of the joint is that of flexion but as the radius of curvature diminishes from front to back some gliding is imposed. In addition, because of the difference in length of the medial and lateral femoral condyles, there is also rotation. The control of this complex movement by the ligaments remains a subject of debate which is not appropriate to a book of this nature but it is important to remember that the ligaments are relatively weak and fail at loads lower than are regularly imposed on the joint during activity. They are protected by the coordinated action of the surrounding muscles either contracting or paying out. The menisci play an important role within the joint. It has been demonstrated that they transmit a significant proportion of the axial load but this work has been done in cadavers with older tissues than those encountered in the average athlete and a figure cannot yet be put on the amount of load transmitted in the younger knee (Seedhom, Dawson and Wright, 1974; Swanson, 1975). In addition to this, the menisci seem important in the thin layer lubrication of the joint, which depends on a thin film of synovial fluid remaining between the loaded articular cartilage surfaces. The duration of the action of this layer is greatly reduced in the meniscetomized knee. The biomechanics of the knee joint are indeed complex and the reader's attention is drawn to the appropriate sections of *Disorders of the Knee* by Helfet (1982).

## 18.2    Investigation of the injured knee

### 18.2.1    HISTORY

In the acutely injured knee it is often impossible to get a history other than by asking the player what he was trying to do. Occasionally an observer can describe what happened. In the chronically injured knee it is not unusual for the diagnosis to rest almost exclusively on the story both of the initiating injury and subsequent symptoms as often physical signs are scarce. Close enquiry into the exact nature of the injury may reveal the likely pattern of tissue damage. The position in which the knee gives way or the story of locking gives clues to the current pathology. Beware of the word 'locking'. It should mean that the knee can be flexed but not fully straightened but it has crept into 'lay' use and is used to describe anything from pain to stiffness. Facets of the history that are particularly useful in the diagnosis of a specific lesion are dealt with in the appropriate subsections.

### 18.2.2    EXAMINATION

In the acutely injured knee it is important to try and examine it immediately. The accurately localized tenderness of ligamentous strain or avulsion is rapidly lost and with that the increasing muscle spasm blocks the laxity that should be obvious in the very early acute state. If the injury is seen late enough for this to have happened then examination under anaesthesia may be necessary to complete the evaluation of the joint. Treatment should not be undertaken without a diagnosis. In the chronic lesion assessment must include muscle bulk and tone, the alignment of the limb, the presence of a fixed flexion deformity (remember that the absence of hyperextension, when present in the contralateral normal knee, is a fixed flexion deformity), the presence or absence of fluid in the joint, the anatomical localization of areas of tenderness and the stability of each component of the knee (see below).

### 18.2.3    RADIOLOGICAL ASSESSMENT

Routine anteroposterior and lateral views may be adequate. If a loose body is suspected then an intercondylar view is necessary. Radiographs for particular problems are described in the appropriate sections. Soft tissues may be outlined within the joint by the injection of air and a radio-opaque dye and lesions of the menisci and cruciates may be identified in skilled hands. C.T. scanning is sometimes useful to localize an obscure lesion (Fig. 18.1) but nuclear magnetic resonance remains a research tool.

369

# Knee injuries

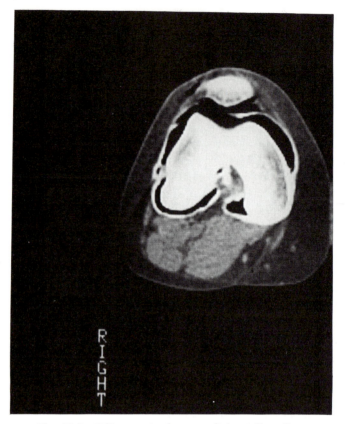

*Fig. 18.1*  C.T. scan to show medial patellar plica.

## 18.2.4  ARTHROSCOPY

The recent use of the arthroscope to visualize the contents of the knee and in the appropriate cases to operate within the knee has produced a great change in attitudes and to some extent controversy. There is no doubt that the interior of the joint can be seen better than ever before (Jackson and Dandy, 1976). The reduced morbidity of the operative procedures is still denied in some quarters but there is a growing body of evidence that the results are better in both the long- and short-term, and in experienced hands the recovery time from meniscectomy or removal of a loose body is greatly diminished (Dandy, 1978; Dandy, 1981; Tapper and Hoover, 1969; Dandy and Northmore-Ball, 1981; Northmore-Ball and Dandy, 1982). Arthroscopy in the acutely injured knee must be restricted to an expert. Fluid loss through a torn capsule may produce a secondary posterior compartment syndrome in the calf (Peek and Haynes, 1984).

## 18.3   The patellofemoral joint

The incidence of injury in this joint is frequently underestimated to the extent that it is only recognized after the failure of surgery directed to some other compartment of the joint. The syndrome of pain felt in the front of the joint, spontaneous in origin and often seen in young females, has by contrast in the past been blamed upon the patellofemoral joint whereas the pathology in these cases often involves some other structure and the pain in fact frequently has no definable pathological basis.

The somatotype and variations in the local anatomy are particularly important in the aetiology of problems in this area. Patella subluxation and instability are frequently seen in the knee which hyperextends, has some degree of tibial intorsion and has a laterally offset tibial tuberosity (alternatively referred to as an increased $Q$ angle or bayonet deformity). In addition, the patella may be unusually small or placed at a higher level than normal. This is traditionally called patella alta but Apley has recently made the plea that it be simply called 'high patella'. Likewise he suggests the term 'low patella' instead of 'patella baja', which may also cause some anterior knee pain. Some unilateral cases of high patella appear to be secondary to excessive elevation of one tibial tuberosity during the adolescent growth disturbance of Osgood–Schlatter disease. Generalized joint hypermobility is frequently implicated in problems in this region. While standard AP and lateral radiographs are useful, a skyline view of both the patellae on the same film with the knee flexed to about 30° (Fig. 18.2) can give more information about the position of the patella and occasionally films at 60° and 90° help.

The most clearly defined group of patellofemoral problems involve subluxation or dislocation. Congenital dislocation is rare. It is present

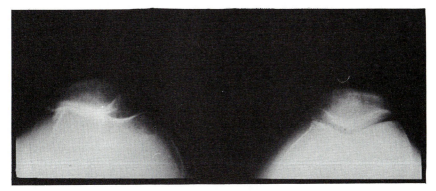

*Fig. 18.2* 30° Skyline views of patellae showing subluxation and early osteoarthritis on the left.

from birth and the patella never occupies its normal position. Habitual dislocation of the patellofemoral joint occurs each time the knee is bent. This unusual condition has the added problem that the repeated movement across the lateral condyle produces a secondary arthritis. Congenital dislocation is best left untreated. If habitual dislocation is producing a lot of pain and swelling then some form of stabilization is indicated, but usually it is necessary to transpose bone and this cannot be done before skeletal maturity (Hauser, 1938; Cox, 1976) because of the risk of premature anterior closure of the proximal tibial epiphysis. The consequence is severe recurvatum and the osteotomy to correct this is difficult. Major soft tissue realignment may see the patient through to maturity or beyond (Roux, 1888; Goldthwait, 1899; Galeazzi, 1922).

Traumatic dislocation is, as its name implies, due to injury. A hitherto normal patellofemoral joint is struck in such a way that the patella is forced off laterally. It may rarely reduce spontaneously but usually requires reduction under anaesthesia. The pathological anatomy is a tear of the medial retinaculum but this is very frequently associated with a chondral or osteochondral fracture. Unfortunately this latter problem is often missed and there is no doubt that many 'recurrent' problems are in fact caused by the loose body within the joint (Fig. 18.3). All traumatic dislocations should be arthroscoped and the joint washed out; occasionally a large fragment will merit fixation, ideally by the technique described

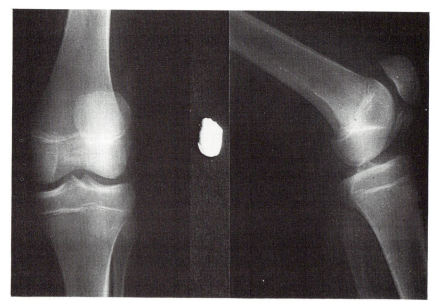

*Fig. 18.3*  The radiographs and actual loose body following patellar dislocation.

372

by Deacon (1981), for osteochondritis dissecans in which thin Kirschner wires are passed through the fragment, through the underlying bone and out into the soft tissues where the end of the wire can be felt left subcutaneously. The end within the joint is anchored by bending the terminal 3 or 4 mm to a right angle. The wires are pulled out through the skin at six weeks, obviating the need for a second arthrotomy. More controversial is the role of an immediate lateral retinacular relieving incision. The concept of weakening the lateral structures at the same time so that eventual tracking is symmetrical is appealing but not all traumatic dislocations go on to recurrent dislocation. It is advisable, therefore, to do a release only when the force which caused the patella to dislocate seems rather weak and suggests the possibility of a tendency for recurrent dislocation.

Recurrent dislocation may occur after a relatively minor injury in a knee with a predisposition, or after a major injury to a hitherto normal knee. On twisting the knee with the foot fixed and the twist in an inwards direction under load, the patella falls off laterally. This may be recognized by the patient but any variant of pain and giving way may be described. Clinically this is recognized mainly by apprehension on the part of the patient when an attempt is made to dislocate the patella laterally. It cannot be overstressed that pain in young women felt in the front of the knee is most commonly caused by a patella problem; the frequent diagnosis of 'cartilage trouble' is wrong. In Trillat's (personal communication) series of 6000 meniscectomies only seventeen were performed on women under the age of sixteen. The management of this condition is initially conservative and independent of age and if that fails then the type of surgery performed does depend on the age. Conservative treatment is an attempt to strengthen the vastus medialis obliquus muscle to pull the patella in a more medial track. This is difficult to do and usually involves terminal extension exercises. At The London Hospital for the last five years a method has been used in which the patient is laid bad side down on a couch with the bad knee resting on the edge of the couch. With the lower leg free and unsupported they do resisted extension exercises against the physiotherapist in an attempt to get increased proprioceptive input from the medial side, as the medial ligament is being stressed by gravity as well as the muscle activity.

When conservative treatment has failed some form of surgical intervention is indicated. As always the best is the least complex and it seems reasonable to start with a closed lateral retinacular release after further pathology has been excluded by arthroscopy. The early results of this procedure were reported in 1976 (Chen et al.) with a long term follow up in 1981 (Grange and King). Only 23% of patients were not improved and of those nearly half were immediate failures. The procedure has the added advantage that it is quite safe in the skeletally immature knee. In the immature skeleton, if the problem is complete patellar dislocation, then one of the soft tissue reconstructions of which there are many descriptions is indicated, but given the success of the lateral release these operations are becoming rare. In the mature skeleton with recurrent complete dislocation or an earlier failed release then a transposition of the tibial tuberosity is indicated. In the technique described by Trillat and ascribed to Elmslie (Cox, 1976), the tuberosity is elevated on an intact distal osteoperiosteal pedicle and the proximal end is swung medially, there being an osteoclasis at the distal end. It is secured by a screw and early mobilization is allowed. It may be that part of the effectiveness of this operation is due to the slight anterior transposition which results and thus reduces the need of formal anterior transposition (Maquet, 1976). The role of patellectomy in this condition remains debatable. It should never be done in the presence of maltracking as the remaining soft tissues will track the same way and cause symptoms. If the maltracking is corrected first then the symptoms often disappear. Patellectomy should be reserved for the severely damaged patella in which a lateral release has failed to help (Fig. 18.4).

Before leaving the section on the patellofemoral joint it is essential to discuss the syndrome of anterior knee pain (Table 18.2). Traditionally this has been attributed to softening, roughening or even loss of the articular cartilage on the back of the patella or occasionally on the front of the femoral condyle and it was this that gave rise to the much abused term

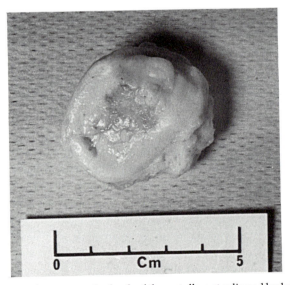

*Fig. 18.4*   Severe changes on the back of the patella not relieved by lateral release.

*Table 18.2*   Causes of the anterior knee pain syndrome

---

(1)   Loss or inadequacy of the patella articular cartilage
(2)   Patella subluxation
(3)   Anterior horn lesions of the menisci
(4)   Osteochondritis dissecans of femur or patella
(5)   Disease of the fat pad and/or alar folds
(6)   Parapatella shelf, medial or superomedial
(7)   Lesions of the patella ligament
(8)   Post-trauma

---

chondromalacia patella. This view has been challenged and Meachim (1971), has shown that these changes are probably age-related and independent of symptoms. There is no doubt that anterior knee pain is the final common pathway for symptoms from a variety of recognizable conditions and that in a significant proportion there is no proven cause.

A patella aetiology is suggested by the age of the girl (eleven to seventeen), discomfort on stairs, aching on sitting (the cinema sign), giving way on stairs and the indication by the patient of a vertical line of pain on the inner side of the patella. Examination may show apprehension on attempted lateral displacement of the patella. There may be pain on palpation of the medial or lateral articular surfaces when felt through the skin. The somatotype has already been described. The test of getting pain on quadriceps contraction with the examiner's hand pressing the patella down at its upper pole is almost always positive but its cause is obscure. Effusion is rare. The syndrome merges with that of patella subluxation in which there are more positive signs of maltracking. In the flexed knee the patellae may be in a slightly elevated and lateralized position, rather elegantly described as 'frog eye'. In addition to pain and apprehension there may be an abnormal amount of lateral excursion possible. During flexion/extension it may be possible to observe a sudden change in direction or tilt of the patella. This is an endless source of discussion and is well covered in *The Injured Adolescent Knee* by Kennedy (1979). Treatment overlaps extensively with that described for dislocation of the patella, see above, but varies from the nihilistic through conservative to minimal surgical intervention to the surgically aggressive (Pickett and Radin, 1983).

Anterior lesions of the menisci may be localized by tenderness specifically on the anterior joint line and may have an associated tenderness on the margin of the femoral condyle just above the joint line in the slightly flexed knee, this being the site of an elevated lesion just on the articular margin with anterior horn degeneration. Excision of the meniscal and marginal lesion gives relief.

# Knee injuries

Osteochondritis dissecans is usually thought of as a disease of the immature skeleton but Kennedy (1979) describes an incidence after closure of the epiphysis. It presents with spontaneous pain and is usually combined with a story of giving way, or at least apprehension, and a sense of unease about the knee. There may or may not be swelling. There is about a one in three risk of it being bilateral. Unless the fragment has separated, locking does not occur. On occasions in the fully flexed knee it may be possible to palpate an area of tenderness on the front of the femoral condyle. The child may walk with external rotation of the tibia and Wilson's sign may be positive, i.e. pain in the last 30° of extending the knee with the tibia internally rotated. When there are X-ray changes it is essential to exclude the rather frequent anomalies of growth which may mimic the changes of osteochondritis (Caffey, Madell and Royer, 1958). The aetiology remains obscure with advocates for a traumatic origin (Aicroth, 1971), as well as for ischaemia (Watson-Jones, 1952; Ficat, Arlet and Mazieres, 1975). In the relatively undisplaced fragment fixation is indicated (Deacon, 1981; Smillie, 1960). With displacement of any duration removal of the fragment and drilling of the subchondral bone with early continuous passive mobilization will give a good result, at least in the short term.

The existence of symptoms from the fat pad (Hoffa's disease) is denied by many, but it exists as a complaint of anterior knee pain with some episodes of giving way which are extremely painful. It is assumed to be caused by trapping of the hypertrophied pad within the joint or even an abnormality of the alar folds which may allow impingement. Examination reveals a little fullness on either side of the patella ligament. With the knee flexed the tenderness in this region is not marked, but with the examining fingers in the same place, as the knee is extended the tenderness becomes much worse. Management is to exclude other pathology by arthroscopy and then diminish the volume of the fat pad. Excision of as much as possible of the pad extrasynovially in the retropatella ligament recess, and closure of the space with a purse string suture allows early mobilization and relieves the symptoms.

There is little doubt that the medial plica (shelf) was overdiagnosed with the onset of arthroscopy, which allows observation of the distended joint and shows the normal anatomy for the first time. However, some patients have a definite sensation of pain and giving localized to this region and examination reveals a thick band which is felt on the inner side of the patella in extension and disappears under its medial aspect on flexion. The click as it does so is recognized by the patient. The diagnosis may be confirmed by C.T. scan (see Fig. 18.1). Treatment is to confirm a large plica which is inflamed and slips between the patella and femur during flexion/extension and which may be associated with a small area of granulation or erosion on the condylar margin. It is necessary to excise the majority of it under arthroscopic control as incision alone may lead to recurrent symptoms.

Lesions of the patella ligament are broadly divided into those of the ligament itself, usually in the adult, or of its insertion into the tibial tuberosity in the immature skeleton. There is pain in the ligament on active extension against resistance, such as jumping giving rise to the term jumper's knee or Sinding–Larsen–Johansson disease (Medlar and Lyne, 1978). The pathology in the adult may be inflammation of the tissue surrounding the patella ligament or a central cyst. There is local pain and tenderness in both cases and these are best distinguished on C.T. scan (Fig. 18.5). There is well localized tenderness with thickening of the ligament. In the immature skeleton the lesion is at the tibial tuberosity which is painful on activity, tender if hit in sport, painful on pressure and often obviously enlarged (Osgood, 1903; Schlatter, 1903). Treatment of the problem in the adult is surgical with removal of the lining of the tendon or excision of the cyst and closure with a purse string suture (Williams, 1976; Blazina, 1973). The ligament should be protected by a plaster cylinder for three weeks afterwards to diminish the risk of rupture. The immature lesion is best treated symptomatically with pro-

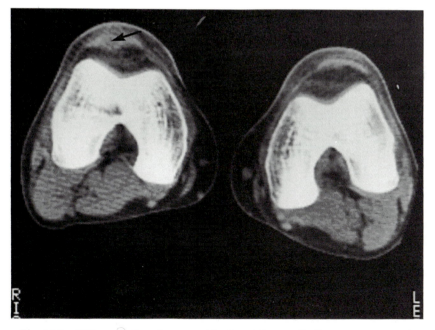

*Fig. 18.5*  C.T. scan showing a cyst in the right patella ligament, arrowed.

tection of the enlarged tuberosity with a guard during sport and a restriction of activity if the child cannot bear the pain. Parents often require reassurance as there is an obvious lump and X-ray may be necessary to put their mind at rest. Only a tiny proportion go on to separation of an ossicle within the tuberosity and there is no evidence that this is influenced by treatment. The need to immobilize these cases in a plaster cylinder is questionable. Very rarely symptoms persist to the extent that operation is necessary for a separated ossicle after skeletal maturity. This is found behind the patella ligament at its insertion into the tibia.

The knee may become painful after a blow on the front of the flexed knee and the symptoms are indistinguishable from those of spontaneous anterior knee pain. If there is no previous history and no maltracking the symptoms usually resolve within a year. When this is associated with pre-existing problems the pain is often persistent and treatment is directed to the underlying condition. The presence of a congenitally bipartite patella may prolong the symptoms and some may actually come to excision of the separate segment (Weaver, 1977). On considering the whole problem of anterior knee pain it is fortunate that the arthroscope enables the surgeon to distinguish more accurately between these varied conditions but it remains clear that a convincing explanation is not found in many of these cases despite the fact that a lateral retinacular release (or perhaps the arthroscopie) gives lasting relief.

Finally it must be remembered that anterior knee pain may be secondary. Any lesion that causes loss of the bulk of the quadriceps can produce this type of pain. The iliopsoas bursa at the front of the hip may enlarge so as to press on the femoral nerve and present with giving way of the knee. The rather nebulous anterior knee pain associated with a slipped upper femoral epiphysis must never be overlooked. The consequent shortening of the leg with fixed external rotation must never be missed as immediate treatment may diminish the long-term consequences of this condition.

## 18.4 The menisci

The load transmitting and thin layer lubrication functions of the menisci have already been referred to. The fibres within the meniscus run longitudinally and parallel to its capsular periphery. Thus the main resistance to stress is in this direction and as its shape is nearly circular and the extremities tied down, it can absorb and transmit the loads from the hemispherical femoral condyle to the tibia. It is for this reason that it is essential to preserve any intact peripheral longitudinal fibres and perhaps why the innocent looking transverse tear can produce such severe pain and degeneration. The consequence of this tear on thin layer lubrication has not been described. If a tear has taken place in a normal meniscus there is a suggestion of some, albeit small, degree of laxity in the joint. The degenerate meniscus can be damaged in the normal knee. The other type of meniscus more liable to injury is the discoid meniscus in which the tissue is excessive varying from a very large 'normal' shape to a complete disc and thought to be a genuine congenital malformation (Gray and Gardener, 1950; Kaplan, 1955).

## 18.4.1 MENISCAL LESIONS

There are two main groups of meniscal lesions separated on the whole by the age, mode of presentation, and the quality of the meniscal tissue. The majority of lesions occurring above the age of thirty-two consist of a tear in an already degenerating meniscus. The appearance of the tear is typical and consists of a horizontal split in the posterior half of the meniscus. The back end of one part, frequently the inferior, may become detached and a flap is then free to swing into the joint. It seems that this lesion is the consequence of shear and thus must originate as an intrasubstance tear which has been implicated as a cause of knee pain. If that is the case one must assume a secondary effect on another part of the joint as there are no pain fibres in the fibrocartilage. These lesions are most common on the medial side (as are all meniscal lesions in Europe with a ratio of 11:4). When seen in the lateral meniscus they are more often in the middle segment with a transverse element producing a blunt attenuated flap, often referred to as a 'parrot beak'. The anterior horn of the lateral meniscus may also be damaged by repeated axial load at the end of the 'lock-home' mechanism. Fibrillation and a small cyst are thus occasionally seen at this site. All the degenerative tears of the menisci may be associated with a cyst but it is rare on the medial side. On the lateral side it presents with a firm, often tender swelling at or below the joint line and may be noted on radiographs by a little dent just below the articular margin where it has been pushed into the bone by the tough capsule (Fig. 18.6).

Typically, the clinical presentation of the lesions above age thirty-two is one of spontaneous pain in the absence of a readily recognized traumatic episode. Pain is felt at and usually accurately localized to the lesion on full bending under load. It may occur at odd times, particularly on turning over in bed. Giving way is not a feature and effusion is unusual. True locking does not occur. The diagnosis is made on the basis of the history, local joint line tenderness and the absence of other signs typical of other conditions. In such cases an X-ray will probably show nothing other than perhaps the cyst referred to above. An arthrogram may reveal the

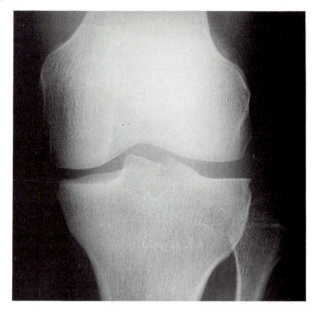

*Fig. 18.6*  Depression in subchondral bone from a meniscal cyst.

pathology. Some form of radiograph is mandatory before any form of operation is contemplated as there may be early osteoarthrosic changes which indicate that there will still be some symptoms after surgery. Conservative treatment with exercises and physiotherapy is unlikely to achieve anything as the lesion is mechanical, although good muscle control and tone always aid the surgeon. There is no doubt that the joint should be arthroscoped as this allows the lesion to be accurately identified and, in addition, the limited operation of simply removing the diseased area of the cartilage can be done with minimal damage to the rest of the joint. Management of the cyst is a different problem. After the degenerate lesion of the meniscus has been dealt with there remain three choices: doing nothing, excising the cyst or aspirating and injecting it with hydrocortisone. Large cysts should be excised but small tight tense cysts treated by aspiration and injection seem to do well although some do recur and will need operation. When the cyst is lax and an 'incidental' finding in the assessment of such a knee no action need be taken.

Despite the fact that it is a little less common, the other type of meniscal lesion is far better recognized, mainly because it is the consequence of a readily identifiable episode of trauma and occurs in players at the height of their aspirations. The history is of a twisting injury to the partially bent, loaded knee; something gives. The player may continue for some time but more usually is immediately disabled. Within a few hours the joint becomes swollen and it may not fully straighten. The probable mechanism is that the meniscus has become trapped between the two bone surfaces and the femur has acted as a blunt axe to split the meniscus in the line of its fibres at its posterior part. Trillat has devised a classification of these tears (Fig. 18.7). If the parts have returned to their normal position there will be full extension unless there has been a partial tear of the posteromedial capsule with enough oedema in the capsule in that region to produce a fixed deformity, even under anaesthesia.

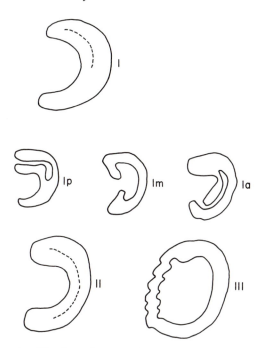

*Fig. 18.7* Trillat classification of meniscal injuries. I: The indisplaced initial split in the posterior horn. Ip: The split enters the joint posteriorly. Im: The split enters the joint in the mid portion. Ia: The split enters the joint anteriorly. II: The indisplaced split goes into the anterior segment. III: The intact free edge displaces into the joint.

The apparent fixed flexion of hamstring muscle spasm disappears under anaesthesia. The knee locked in fixed flexion from a tear displaced into the intercondylar space must be regarded as a surgical emergency. If untreated the knee will extend at the cost of an attrition rupture of the anterior cruciate ligament, the consequences of which are discussed later. When a mobile torn segment of meniscus slips in and out of the joint the history is of episodes of giving, with temporary locking released by a characteristic twisting extension movement with the sensation of something going back into place. In the early stages this is followed by an effusion but this feature diminishes with the passage of time. Examination in the acute stage, when there is a displaced portion, reveals a fixed flexion deformity, fluid in the joint and pain on attempting to extend the joint. There may be some joint line tenderness, but often at the back of the joint well away from the midline local tenderness typical of the more complex lesion involving the ligaments. In the knee in which the segment has returned to its normal position physical signs may be scarce. Apley (1947) has described the tests to distinguish a joint surface problem, producing pain on compression of the flexed knee, from a ligament problem, producing pain on distraction in the same position. McMurray's (1942) sign demands a painful click on rotation in flexion and can in fact lock the knee, both of which manoeuvres may alienate the patient. X-rays are normal but such a lesion can be expected to show on a double contrast arthrogram if the joint has been adequately manipulated so as to allow the dye into the split (Ireland, Trickey and Stoker, 1980; Fig. 18.8).

The management of the displaced segment is urgent and involves excision of the segment while ensuring that the remaining rim is stable (McGinty, Guess and Marvin, 1977). There can be no excuse for removing undamaged stable tissue. The management of the undisplaced tear is

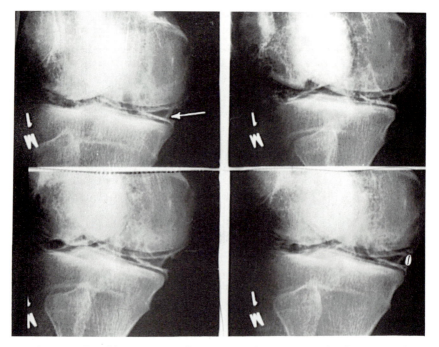

*Fig. 18.8* Double contrast arthrogram to show a vertical split, arrowed.

more difficult. If the injury is less than two weeks old and the split is within the peripheral one third of the meniscal substance it is probably justifiable to suture it back. The technique has become easier with special instruments (Henning, Jolly and Scott, 1985). It is worthwhile making an effort to save meniscal tissue at any opportunity.

## 18.5 Ligamentous injuries

The signs, symptoms and prognosis are such that these must be divided into acute and chronic.

In the acute ligamentous injury a clear account of its nature is most helpful in that certain types of injury are associated with a predictable pattern of ligamentous disruption. These are non-contact injuries. Contact injuries give a less predictable pattern of damage. In the course of normal activity there are two stable end point positions of the knee and when the joint is forced through one of these positions something must give. The knee finishes up in flexion with the leg and foot externally rotated and a valgus force applied at the knee or in extension with the foot internally rotated and a varus force applied to the knee. When either of these positions is exceeded there is damage to any or all of the anterior cruciate ligament, the posterior oblique ligament, the medial collateral ligament and the medial meniscus. It must be remembered that the anterior cruciate ligament has been torn to some extent in 72% of acute haemarthroses. The posterior oblique ligament is a thickening of the posteromedial capsule supported by downwards and forwards running fibres from the reflected insertion of semimembranosus. Similarly there is the injury from a rapid inwards turn on the flexed knee in which the posterolateral structures (the popliteus tendon, the arcuate ligament and fibular collateral ligament) may be torn in whole or in part.

Where the injury is the consequence of a direct blow the type of damage is less predictable but usually a varus force will tear the lateral structures first followed by the cruciates while a valgus force will tear the medial structures followed by the cruciates. However, this picture may be confused by the bone giving way rather than the soft tissues. A hyperextension force may damage the posterior capsule and cruciate while a blow to the front of the flexed knee may tear the posterior cruciate in isolation or damage the posterolateral complex. Any of the above injuries may also produce a slicing chondral or osteochondral fracture.

The management of any injury is firstly to recognize the possibility of severe damage and then to fully evaluate the knee. The knee with complete anteroposterior dislocation may be easily, frequently spontaneously, reduced but the risk of arterial occlusion at the trifurcation remains for 72 hours. The risks of missing the other injuries are not quite so dramatic but the results of operating late, when secondary changes have taken place in the articular cartilage and initially intact ligaments, are at best uncertain. Even where conservative treatment is used routinely for all such injuries a complete diagnosis of the pathological anatomy must be made so that a proper comparison between immediate operation and aggressive conservative treatment with bracing is established (Jokl et al., 1984). When a tense swelling is obviously restricting movement this can be aspirated under a local anaesthetic. It is essential to observe full sterile precautions as a haemarthrosis is an excellent culture medium. The presence of small fat globules confirms that the marrow space has been opened and that some form of intra-articular fracture has occurred. The unswollen knee with a history of major injury indicates that there is enough capsular disruption to allow the haematoma to leak into the periarticular tissues and swelling may in fact be detected in the calf. Accurate localization of tenderness is of great importance in pinpointing the pathology. The origin and insertion of each and every ligament must be palpated and it is essential to remember the low tibial attachment of the medial collateral ligament some 7.5 cm (3 in) below the joint line. Once oedema and spasm are established examination under anaesthesia is mandatory, with or without washing out the joint. An arthroscopic evaluation at this time depends on the available skills because of the risk of excessive extravasation referred to above. Routine X-rays are frequently unhelpful although small bone avulsions sometimes mark the ends of the torn ligaments. On the whole stress X-rays are most useful in the immature skeleton to distinguish separation of the epiphyseal plate from disruption of the ligaments.

Once the full diagnosis is made the choice between conservative and surgical treatment can be made. If surgery is chosen at this time it is usually possible to approximate the ends of all the torn ligaments including the cruciates (Fig. 18.9) even though the sutures may have to be run into the bones at each end. The operation is not significantly prolonged by such manoeuvres and there is no doubt that full function can be restored in many cases. There is also the opportunity to replace and fix large chondral and osteochondral fragments. Postoperative casting and bracing are usual with intensive physiotherapy and a delay in return to sport until there is full control of the knee (evidenced by running backwards in a figure of eight) and restoration of muscle bulk. The use of postoperative continuous passive motion in these cases is not yet evaluated but the preliminary reports are exciting (Salter, 1984). Conservative treatment is best reserved for isolated lesions especially of the medial ligament although Jokl et al. (1984) claim good results when the anterior cruciate ligament is torn as well. The keystone of conservative

384

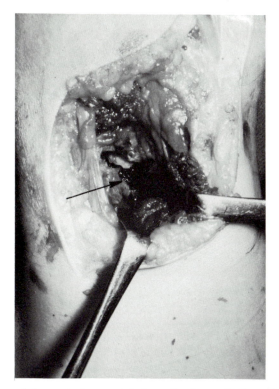

*Fig. 18.9*   Tear of the posterior cruciate from the bone; the bone bed is arrowed with the detached fragment just above.

treatment is early elevation, ice and compression to reduce the swelling followed by progressive mobilization and weightbearing within a protective brace.

A pivotal issue about immediate repair is the performance of the knee without a specific ligament and the most controversial of these is the anterior cruciate. The function of this structure in the uninjured knee remains to an extent debatable and the consequences of its deficiency vary enormously. At present an indicator of the likely future performance of the knee is lacking. It is needed because traumatic haemarthrosis of the knee is one of the commonest problems in sports medicine today and 72% are associated with complete or partial tears of the anterior cruciate (Holden and Jackson, 1985; Dehaven, 1980; Noyes, Matthews and Mooar, 1980). It is possible that the disability may be linked to the degree of the downwards and backwards slope of the lateral femoral condyle which produces an anteriorly directed resultant force under axial load (Scotland and Weir, 1984).

# Knee injuries

## 18.5.1 CHRONIC LIGAMENTOUS INJURY

This is a very complex subject and it is impossible to give other than guidelines in a chapter such as this. The classification of the various types of laxity is still evolving (Andrews and Axe, 1985). The whole field has been bedevilled by the variation in the terminology but in fact there are only three modes of failure that can occur, namely angulation, translation and rotation, which may be present individually or in combination. It would seem logical to attempt to use a classification based solely on the abnormal movement. The dispute arises when particular tissues are blamed for the presence of specific abnormalities of motion. In clinical practice it is therefore reasonable to take a wholly pragmatic view and attempt to identify the component of abnormal motion that is producing symptoms and direct surgery to the control of that abnormal motion without implying that a specific tissue defect is responsible. This is not to say that an understanding of the function of the tissues about the knee is not essential and in some cases well understood but its debate rather clouds the clinical issues at present. The reader is referred to *Orthopaedic Clinics of North America*, **16,** 1, for an introduction to this field.

The pragmatic approach referred to above is very dependent on the physical examination. In the chronically injured knee this must be done with the patient awake. The knee may exhibit a significant range of abnormal motion (laxity) but there will be one or two components that duplicate the patient's complaint (instability) and the patient must recognize this. A lax knee may allow secondary changes such as a torn meniscus or articular cartilage degeneration to occur and these must also be identified in the course of the examination. Meniscectomy may be all that is needed to cure the instability. Even major reconstruction will not produce significant improvement in the face of osteoarthritis. X-rays may be helpful in these cases in showing the degeneration and may even show the consequence of the original injury which is new bone formation under the periosteum next to the attachment of the ligament, the Pelligrini-Steida lesion (Fig. 18.10). The history must include an account of the initiating injury in terms of contact/non-contact, a tearing or popping sensation, swelling, when and where, and duration of disability. An account of the current problem must include precisely when giving occurs, most commonly on turning outwards on the loaded slightly flexed knee; does locking take place and is there swelling of the knee. Pain is not a feature of instability with the exception of a posterolateral problem and usually suggests some other, possibly additional intra-articular pathology. The following paragraphs describe physical signs and the tests commonly used to elicit them.

*Abnormal anteroposterior translation* in the flexed knee is tested in a

386

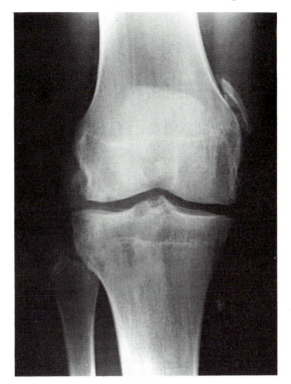

*Fig. 18.10*   Shows the new bone of the Pelligrini–Steida lesion.

variety of ways. The anterior drawer sign is performed with the patient supine, the knee flexed and the foot stabilized by the examiner's haunch. The proximal tibia is grasped with both hands, the index fingers being left free to palpate the hamstring muscles throughout the action of pulling the tibia forwards. Spasm in these muscles at any time may block the abnormal anterior motion. The posterior drawer sign is done in the same position with a backwards push on the tibia. If the tibia does come forward with the anterior drawer it is essential to look across both knees flexed the same amount, and in the relaxed position, to exclude the knee starting in the position of a positive posterior drawer sign, which will have been produced in this position by gravity. It may be very difficult to define the neutral point in some cases of abnormal anteroposterior translation. The Slocum–Larsen test (1968a) is performed in the same way as the anterior drawer but three times, firstly with the foot in neutral rotation then internal and finally external rotation. When positive, the amount of abnormal anterior motion increases with the external rotation of the tibia as the stabilizing posterior structures becomes progressively

# Knee injuries

more relaxed. Abnormal posterior motion can be detected if the whole of the tibia is moving back or if only the lateral plateau does so. This is a matter of fine judgement to distinguish between the two and may be made easier by performing dynamic radiographs. A lateral view of the knee in flexion is taken with the tibia pulled forward and free to rotate and then pushed backwards and free to rotate. The femur must stay in the same position. The lateral side is identified by the fibular styloid and the medial by a paper clip taped to the skin and the relative excursions of the two sides can be compared (King and Sudlow, 1982; Fig. 18.11). Abnormal anterior motion may be sought in the slightly flexed knee if the leg is small or the examiner's hands big. The distal femur and proximal tibia are grasped and anteroposterior translation attempted. The degree of motion is difficult to assess and the quality of the end point is important, a soft

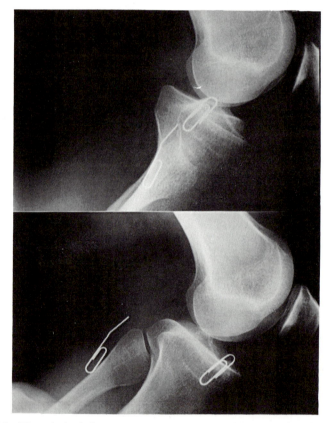

*Fig. 18.11*   The relatively larger posterior excursion of the lateral side of the knee, in this case also marked with a paper clip.

388

stop being pathological. The test is attributed to Lachman in the USA (Torg, Conrad and Kalen, 1976) and to Trillat in Europe.

*Abnormal angulation* is sought with the knee flexed to about 15 to 20° to relax the posterior capsular structures and a valgus or varus force is applied. It is essential to hold the limb in such a way that rotation which can mimic abnormal angulation is eliminated or recognized. Methods of doing this depend on the examiner and vary from holding the lower tibia in the armpit and putting both hands on the knee to dropping the leg over the edge of the examining couch so that the thigh is stabilized by contact with its surface and the limb below the knee can be moved from side to side. Abnormal motion is graded subjectively into very little (one plus), a lot (three pluses) and intermediate (two pluses).

Tests for *abnormal rotation* tend to be the most complex. Part of the assessment of rotational laxity has been mentioned in the description of the Slocum–Larsen test in which the medial tibial plateau is coming forwards, and the rotational component of the posterior drawer sign in which the lateral tibial plateau is moving backwards. A variety of tests are described to identify abnormal anterior motion of the lateral tibial plateau. The affected limb is held in extension. The foot is internally rotated and a valgus force applied to the knee. In this position the knee is flexed and if the test is positive there is a sudden posterior movement of the lateral tibial plateau at about 30° at it relocates from its anteriorly subluxed position. This sensation is immediately recognized by the patient if it is the cause of their problem and they may allow it only once because of apprehension. This can be overcome if the thumb of the hand applying the valgus force is placed under the head of the fibula. This allows control of the backwards motion and its easier recognition in mild cases. The test is associated with the name of MacIntosh (Galway, Beaupre and MacIntosh, 1972), and is called the 'pivot shift' test. The modification is described by Casey (personal communication).

A similar test is performed with internal rotation and valgus but with the knee starting in the flexed position and going to extension. A little short of extension there is a sudden movement as the lateral plateau goes to the position of anterior subluxation and this test is usually attributed to Losee, Johnson and Southwick (1978). Hughston *et al.* (1976) describe a similar test from flexion to full extension, the 'jerk' being produced by the rapid dislocation of the subluxed plateau in the last few degrees of extension. These two are thus signs of dislocation rather than relocation, although as extension is completed the plateau again relocates which occasionally gives a second jump. A further test is used to distinguish dynamically abnormal posterior subluxation of the lateral plateau. The leg is held in about 40° of flexion with the foot externally rotated and extended from this position with a valgus force on the knee. As the knee

389

approaches full extension there is a sudden movement as the posteriorly subluxed plateau goes back into place. This is called the reverse pivot shift. If this is combined with anterior subluxation the disability is great as there is no position of rotation in which the patient can put the knee to make it stable.

## 18.6 Surgical guidelines based on the physical signs

The indication for operation on any chronically injured knee is failure of conservative treatment. This is a full rehabilitation programme under the control of an experienced physiotherapist. In the majority of the cases some part of the tibia moves forward to produce the instability and it is sad to see the main emphasis still on the quadriceps power. The only muscles capable of holding back the tibia or allowing controlled forward motion are the hamstrings and it is essential that exercises are given to increase the strength and improve the co-ordination of these muscles. Even if the abnormal motion remains on clinical testing it may no longer produce instability because it is controlled. Braces and strapping are used to control the instability far more in North America than in Europe. There is no doubt that in some cases of minor instability they are all that is needed.

Acceptable results can be obtained in the majority of patients by the correction of the main component of the laxity which produces the instability. In some cases there is a need to correct abnormal motion on both the medial and lateral sides and there is some evidence now to suggest that even this is not enough in the very active professional athlete. It has been suggested that they routinely have surgery to both sides and the centre of the joint. This view awaits validation outside the realms of Australian rules football. The commonest complaint is anterior subluxation of the lateral tibial plateau, or perhaps the sudden movement as it relocates, recognized by giving on twisting on the partially flexed knee. In isolation this is demonstrated by the pivot shift test or variants described above. If there is not a significant anterior excursion of the medial plateau at the same time (a three plus anterior drawer sign or three plus Slocum–Larsen) then surgery is directed to control this abnormal excursion alone. This has proved satisfactory in the short term (King and Bulstrode, 1985) The technique is based on that described by MacIntosh (Galway et al., 1972), in which a distally based band of fascia lata is elevated from the tubercle of Gerdy. This is passed posteriorly to the fibular collateral ligament and anchored there above the mid-point by either transfixion or encircling the collateral ligament, while the foot is fully externally rotated. The band is then passed to the lower part of the lateral intermuscular septum and transfixed from front to back. It is then passed down to the lateral half of the lateral head of the gastrocnemius muscle, below the joint line, going through the muscle and taking a bite of the underlying junction of periosteum and capsule. The defect in the fascia is meticulously repaired. A fascial repair may stretch out in the long term. The same technique has recently been performed using carbon fibre. The short-term clinical results show an improvement but free fibre has been identified within the joint despite rigorous extra-articular technique and the long-term results await evaluation.

This type of technique is passive in that no active muscle belly is attached to the repair tissues. There are other procedures described to control this problem in which muscles are thought to play an active part which are called dynamic reconstructions. Ellison (1979) uses a fascial strip based proximally and ending with a piece of bone from Gerdy's tubercle, which is passed deep to the fibular ligament, the deep wall of the tunnel being made by the capsule being sutured deep to it. Kennedy, Stewart and Walker (1978) describe a further modification of this. The concept of dynamic reconstruction is tempting, but in no case has the dynamic component been proven and the results are better in those cases where the pivot shift has been passively obliterated at the operation. Other attempts at dynamic reconstruction are attributed to Slocum by Campbell (1980) in the use of the biceps and Torg is completing an evaluation of the results of biceps advancement.

When a medial reconstruction is necessary, usually in combination with the lateral side, there is a wide choice of procedures. Slocum, Larsen and James (1974) dissect the posteromedial structures and divide the capsule rather vertically along the front of the medial head of the gastrocnemius. The flaps are overlapped so as to give a downwards and backwards suture line and reinforced by bringing up the distal part of the semimembranosus tendon in continuity and suturing it to the repair. To some extent the line of the repair seems illogical and it is the author's habit to fashion similar flaps but with the distal ends based anteriorly so that the overlapped repair line runs downwards and forwards in a direction to resist the forward motion of the tibia on the femur. In addition the semi-membranosus is used to reinforce the repair and if the tissues are very poor a downwards and forwards running darn of carbon fibre can be added. There are of course many other operations designed to correct the medial side and the pesplasty of Slocum–Larsen (1968b) and the 'five-in-one' of Nicholas (1973) are good examples. The pesplasty basically consists of a proximal reinsertion of the distal part of the insertion of the pes anserinus by freeing it from the bone, turning it up over the proximal part and suturing the free edge to the medial edge of the patella ligament. The 'five-in-one' consists of total meniscectomy, proximal and posterior repositioning of the femoral end of the medial ligament, reefing of the posterior oblique ligament, an advancement of vastus medialis and a pesplasty. Readers are referred to the original articles for a full description of the procedures. Their use in isolation is now rare.

The instability of posterior subluxation of the lateral tibial plateau is not common but is recognized even less frequently. There is giving way on internal rotation on the flexed knee but importantly this is the only instability associated with pain, which comes on after prolonged standing and may be caused by stress of the scarred posterior capsular structures. Classically it is said that there is always a slight degree of hyperextension but this is not always present. The key test is the reverse pivot shift described above. When the knee is in valgus and there is no obvious lateral thrust during gait the following operation can be performed. The lateral side of the joint is exposed and the combined insertion of the fibular collateral ligament and popliteus tendon elevated from the femur with a block of bone. The anterior and posterior margins of the block are developed distally until the whole pedicle is based solely on the tibia. Posteriorly the incision is developed into the arcuate ligament which is usually the site of scarring. The bone block is transposed to a new bed formed proximally and anteriorly so as to pull the tibia forwards and tighten the collateral ligament and the arcuate ligament is reefed. This may be augmented with a distally based strip of the biceps tendon. This is inadequate in a varus or varus thrust knee when a valgus osteotomy will almost surely be indicated. This instability associated with loss of the posterior cruciate is one of the most complex and the reader should consult specialist texts.

All procedures so far described are peripheral reconstructions. The alternatives are the 'through the joint' procedures, the best known of which is the Trillat/Eriksson (Eriksson, 1976) modification of the Kenneth Jones (1963) operation in which the medial one-third of the patella ligament is elevated based on the tibia with a thin piece of patella bone, threaded through a tibial tunnel, through the joint in the line of the original anterior cruciate and anchored to the medial side of the lateral femoral condyle on to an area of freshened bone and held there by stitches through the condyle. There are many modifications of this and again the reader must consult the specialist texts. On the whole the indication for this is a neutral anterior drawer sign of more than two plus. In isolation, despite good early results, there is a deterioration against time and it may be that this should be done only with a medial and/or lateral repair.

Operations to repair the posterior cruciate are not so common. In fact, in an isolated tear of the posterior cruciate there may be no symptoms. This injury often occurs in association with a posterior dislocation of the hip and may be an incidental finding many years after the accident.

However, when the cause of the injury was hyperextension, symptoms often occur because the capsule has been torn as well. The direction of the laxity is posterior but it is distressing still to find the scar of a failed anterior repair on so many of these knees. It is important to distinguish between the posterolateral complex injury described above, the isolated posterior cruciate which is often symptom-free and the complex posterior capsular injury which may be disabling. Techniques for posterior cruciate repair vary. Carbon fibre has been used as has the medial meniscus, the medial one-third of the medial head of the gastrocnemius and a free patellar ligament graft at different times and in all cases there has been improvement in the symptoms but no patient has returned to the highest echelons of sporting activity. No repair in this region is complete without some reefing of the posterior capsule at the same time.

### 18.7  Management of the swollen knee

It is conventional to regard the swollen knee as the site of important pathology. It is more important to beware of the unswollen knee after a major injury. The haematoma has leaked out through the torn capsule leaving no fluid in the joint. There may be a spectacular collection of fluid in the periarticular tissues if sought for and often the extravasation extends well down into the calf. In these cases there is always some degree of detectable laxity and the tenderness may be some distance from the joint in the calf. When there is fluid in the joint it is necessary to decide if it is blood or synovial fluid. The large effusion will demonstrate cross fluctuation of the fluid between the examining hands placed above and below the patella. The small effusion can be detected by emptying the medial parapatellar gutter towards the thigh with a sweep of the hand and then pressing gently on the suprapatellar pouch with the flat of the hand, the fluid just filling the previously emptied space. Occasionally it may be possible to press the fluid from the suprapatellar pouch with the flat of the hand, and then bounce the back of the patella on the front of the femur as the two have been separated by the fluid. Blood accumulates quickly and has a rather boggy feel, whereas synovial fluid is slower to arrive and feels more liquid. In both cases if the joint is tightly distended the fluid must be aspirated with a wide bore needle inserted at the upper outer aspect of the patella and directed underneath it, using full sterile precautions. To leave a tight effusion of any cause in the joint invites distension of the capsular structures with the risk of laxity in the long term and renders diagnosis very difficult.

If clear fluid is aspirated it must be sent for estimation of the cell content and the presence of crystals. If the joint is tense and full of blood then it must be washed out and examined arthroscopically as there will probably

# Knee injuries

be a torn cruciate. In addition, there may be a treatable lesion such as a chondral fracture or marginal tear of the meniscus. Free fat globules in the aspirate indicate some form of fracture communicating with the marrow space. Lax effusions are usually synovial and motion is possible so that there is not the same urgency to relieve the pressure and get the joint moving but if it persists a diagnostic aspiration should be performed.

## 18.8  Loose bodies

Apart from the rare penetrating wounds that introduce a loose body all loose pieces are generated from within. Chondral fractures and separated meniscal lesions produce a radiolucent loose body. Osteochondral fractures and osteochondritis dissecans result in a radio-opaque loose body, usually not more than three, while synovial osteochondromatosis produces a myriad of loose bodies which may be opaque or translucent. The story is of giving way or locking with the knee getting briefly jammed without movement in either direction. X-ray must include an intercondylar view but it is important to remember that absence of the loose body on the X-ray does not exclude it. Treatment is removal.

## 18.9  The extensor apparatus

This composite of the quadriceps muscle, the quadriceps tendon, the patella and the patella ligament is subject to very great loads and any part may fail, although the site of failure varies with age. Tears of the quadriceps apparatus are described in the chapter on the thigh. In the more elderly patient the quadriceps ligament may tear just above the patella and requires repair. More common in the athletic age group is pain in the upper part of the patella ligament usually at or close to the insertion into the patella. The symptoms are of local pain on activity and well localized tenderness. There has often been a cyst present or an area of granulomatous degeneration, detectable on an ultrasound scan. This is best treated by exploration and excision of the abnormal area. Rarely the patella ligament itself tears, sometimes following surgery or injection of steroids (Ismail, Balakrishnan and Rajakumar, 1969). Treatment is by repair of the tear and some form of splintage such as a wire loop holding the patella to the upper tibia. Occasionally the patella itself gives way. There is a transverse break of the bone and a similar tear in the retinacular fibres of both sides. Some form of dynamic fixation is best for the bone (e.g. a figure of 8 wire wrapped around the ends of two parallel K wires) and the soft tissues must be meticulously repaired. In all these cases rehabilitation is essential before return to activity.

## 18.10 Other conditions affecting the knee

In any large group of athletes there will be some who have a non-sports-related condition but ascribe the symptoms to their sporting activities. It is vital to remember this fact and enquire closely into the history. In the last year two osteosarcomas had a delay in diagnosis because the pain was treated as an injury for many weeks.

Within the knee itself any of the arthritides may mimic the consequences of injury or overuse. Rheumatoid arthritis presents early in a number of patients with anterior knee pain and crystal arthropathy is not rare. Pigmented villonodular synovitis does occur in the knee but is less frequent than synovial osteochondromatosis which presents with the features of chronic synovitis plus locking and giving. Finally it must be remembered that many athletes are in the sexually active age group and both gonococcal arthritis and Reiter's disease may present with a swollen knee attributed to injury.

Overuse problems abound around the knee. Problems of the patella ligament have already been alluded to. On the medial side of the joint the insertion of the semimembranosus may become tender and is often associated with swelling around the distal part which is often erroneously called a Baker's cyst. Treatment is rest, local steroids and local physiotherapy. Operative removal is necessary if the size makes it a mechanical problem. It is common in the young and may often spontaneously resolve. The parents always need reassurance. Also on the medial side is the inflammation of the bursa under the pes anserinus which may be associated with or initiated by a strain of the lower end of the medial ligament. This is commonly seen in the breaststroker and is best treated by an alteration of the kick. If persistent, local injections may help.

On the lateral side there can be problems associated with the proximal tibiofibular joint. The main part of the biceps femoris is inserted here and there may be loosening of the joint capsule under repeated pulling with localizable pain. On examination it may be possible to move the fibula backwards and forwards and reproduce the complaints. If local injections and rest do not work then the deep part of the fibula at the joint can be resected. There does not seem to be an advantage in temporary stabilization of the joint with a screw, which also necessitates further surgery to remove it before it breaks. In much the same area is the tenderness from inflammation of the popliteus tendon which, if not considered, may cause confusion in the diagnosis of pain in this region. Slightly more proximal is the pain from the iliotibial tract (ITT syndrome) (Noble, 1980; Renne, 1975) where it rubs over the edge of the femoral condylar expansion on its way down to the tubercle of Gerdy. The presentation is

# Knee injuries

of pain in this region, often in middle distance runners. Examination reveals local tenderness with occasional crepitus during flexion/extension. It seems more common in the varus knee. Treatment is local with physiotherapy and injection until pain-free. On resumption of activity an outer wedge should be worn. In resistant cases it may be necessary to divide the fibres of the iliotibial tract as they cross this area, lengthening them slightly by a Z-plasty.

# References

Aicroth, P. (1971) Osteochondritis of the knee: a clinical survey. *J. Bone Joint Surg.*, **53B**, 440.

Andrews, J. R. and Axe, R. A. (1985) The classification of knee ligament instability. *Orthop. Clin. N. Amer.*, **16(1)**, 69.

Apley, A. G. (1947) The diagnosis of meniscal injury. Some new clinical methods. *J. Bone Joint Surg.*, **29**, 78.

Blazina, M. E. (1973) Jumper's knee. *Orthop. Clin. N. Amer.*, **4(3)**, 665.

Caffey, J., Madell, S. H. and Royer, C. (1958) Ossification of the distal femoral epiphysis. *J. Bone Joint Surg.*, **40A**, 647.

*Campbell's Operative Orthopaedics* (1980) (eds A. S. Edmonson and A. H. Crenshaw) 6th edn. C. V. Mosby, St Louis, p. 967.

Chen, C., Helal, B., King, J. and Roper, B. A. (1976) Closed lateral release for chondromalacial patellae. *Rheumatologie*, **35**.

Cox, J. S. (1976) An evaluation of the Elmslie-Trillat procedure for management of patella dislocations and subluxations: a preliminary report. *Amer. J. Sports Med.*, **4**, 72.

Dandy, D. J. (1978) Early results of closed partial meniscectomy. *Brit. Med. J.*, **1**, 1099.

Dandy, D. J. (1981) *Arthroscopic Surgery of the Knee*, Churchill Livingstone, Edinburgh and London.

Dandy, D. J. and Northmore-Ball, M. D. (1981) A comparative study of arthroscopic and open meniscectomy. *Brit. Orthop. Assoc.*

Deacon, O. (1981) A new method to fix osteochondritis dissecans. *Sicot Proc.*, **480**.

Dehaven, K. E. (1980) Diagnosis of acute knee injuries with haemarthrosis. *Amer. J. Sports Med.*, **8**, 9.

Ellison, A. E. (1979) Distal iliotibial band transfer for anterolateral instability of the knee. *J. Bone Joint Surg.*, **61A**, 330.

Eriksson, E. (1976) Reconstruction of the anterior cruciate ligament. *Orthop. Clin. N. Amer.*, **7**, 167.

Ficat, P., Arlet, J. and Mazieres, B. (1975) Osteochondritis dissecans and osteonecrosis of the lower portion of the femur; advantage of functional medurray exploration. *Sem. Hosp. Paris*, **15**, 1907.

Galeazzi, R. (1922) Nuove applicazione del trapiamato muscolare e tendineo. *Arch. Ortoped.*, p. 3.

Galway, R. D., Beaupre, A. and MacIntosh, D. L. (1972) A clinical sign of symptomatic anterior cruciate deficiency. *J. Bone Joint Surg.*, **54B**, 763.

# References

Goldthwait, J. E. (1899) Permanent dislocation of the patella. *Ann. Surg.*, **29**, 62.

Grange, W. and King, J. (1981) A seven year follow up of closed lateral release. *Sicot Proc.*, 234.

Gray, D. J. and Gardner, E. (1950) Pre-natal development of the human knee and superior tibiofibular joints. *Amer. J. Anat.*, **86**, 235.

Hauser, E. D. W. (1938) Total tendon transplant for slipping patella: a new operation for recurrent dislocation of the patella. *Surg. Gyn. Obst.*, **66**, 199.

Helfet, A. J. (1982) *Disorders of the Knee*, J. P. Lippincott, Philadelphia and Toronto.

Henning, C. E., Jolly, B. L. and Scott, G. A. (1985) Arthroscopic intra-articular meniscus repair. *Amer. Acad. Orthop. Surg.*, *Las Vegas*.

Holden, D. L. and Jackson, D. W. (1985) Treatment selection in the acute anterior cruciate ligament tears. *Orthop. Clin. N. Amer.*, **16(1)**, 99.

Hughston, J. C., Andrews, J. R., Cross, M. J. and Moschi, A. (1976) Classification of knee ligament instability: part I: the medial component and cruciate ligaments. *J. Bone Joint Surg.*, **58A**, 159.

Ireland, J., Trickey, E. L. and Stoker, D. J. (1980) Arthroscopy and arthrography of the knee, a critical review. *J. Bone Joint Surg.*, **62B**, 3.

Ismail, A. M., Balakrishnan, R. and Rajakumar, M. K. (1969) Rupture of the patella ligament after steroid infiltration: a case report. *J. Bone Joint Surg.*, **51A**, 503.

Jackson, R. W. and Dandy, D. J. (1976) *Arthroscopy of the Knee*, Grune and Stratton, New York.

Jokl, P., Kaplan, N., Stovell, P. and Keggi, K. (1984) Non-operative treatment of severe injuries to the medial and anterior cruciate ligaments of the knee. *J. Bone Joint Surg.*, **66A**, 5, 701.

Jones, K. G. (1963) Reconstruction of the anterior cruciate ligament. A technique using the mid one third of the patella ligament. *J. Bone Joint Surg.*, **45A**, 925.

Kaplan, E. B. (1955) The embryology of the menisci of the knee joint. *Bull. Hosp. Joint Dis.*, **16**, 111.

Kennedy, J. C. (1979) *The Injured Adolescent Knee*, Williams and Wilkins, Baltimore and London.

Kennedy, J. C., Stewart, R. and Walker, D. M. (1978) Anterolateral rotatory instability of the knee joint. *J. Bone Joint Surg.*, **60A**, 1031.

King, J. and Bulstrode, C. (1985) Polylactate-coated carbon fiber in extra-articular reconstruction of the unstable knee. *Clin. Orthop. Rel. Res.*, **196**, 139.

King, J. B. and Sudlow, R. (1982) *Compte Rendu* of the *Deuxième Congrès National Scientifique de la Société Française de Médecine du Sport*.

Losee, R. L., Johnson, T. R. and Southwick, W. O. (1978) Anterior subluxation of the lateral tibial plateau: a diagnostic test and operative repair. *J. Bone Joint Surg.*, **60A**, 1015.

Maquet, P. (1976) Advancement of the tibial tuberosity. *Clin. Orthop.*, **115**, 225.

McGinty, J. B., Guess, L. F. and Marvin, R. A. (1977) Partial or total meniscectomy: a comparative analysis. *J. Bone Joint Surg.*, **59A**, 763.

McMurray, T. P. (1942) The semilunar cartilages. *Brit. J. Surg.*, **29**, 407.

Meachim, G. (1971) The effect of age on the thickness of adult articular cartilage in the shoulder joint. *Ann. Rheum. Dis.*, **30**, 43.

Medlar, R. C. and Lyne, E. D. (1978) Sinding–Larsen–Johansson disease. *J. Bone Joint Surg.*, **60A**, 1113.

## Knee injuries

Nicholas, J. A. (1973) Reconstruction for antero medial instability of the knee. *J. Bone Joint Surg.*, **55a**, 899.

Nicholas, J. A. and Minkoff, J. (1978) Iliotibial band transfer through the intercondular notch but combined anterior instability. *Amer. J. Sports Med.*, **6**, 341.

Noble, C. A. (1980) Iliotibial band friction syndrome in runners. *Amer. J. Sports Med.*, **8**, 232.

Northmore-Ball, and Dandy, D. J. (1982) Long term results of partial arthroscopic meniscectomy. *Clin. Orthop. Rel. Res.*, **167**, 34.

Noyes, F. R., Matthews, D. S. and Mooar, P. A. (1983) Symptomatic anterior cruciate deficient knee. Part II: the results of rehabilitation activity modification and counselling on functional disability. *J. Bone Joint Surg.*, **65A**, 163.

Osgood, R. B. (1903) Lesions of the tibial tubercle, occurring during adolescence. *Boston Med. Surg. J.*, **148**, 114.

Peek, R. D. and Haynes, D. W. (1984) Compartmental syndrome as a complication of arthroscopy. A case report and study of interstitial pressures. *Amer. J. Sports Med.*, **12(6)**, 464.

Pickett, J. C. and Radin, E. L. (eds) (1983) *Chondromalacia of the Patella*, Williams and Wilkins, Baltimore and London.

Renne, J. W. (1975) The iliotibial band fraction syndrome. *J. Bone Joint Surg.*, **57A**, 1110.

Roux (1888) Luxation habituelle de la rotule: le traitement operatoire. *Rev. Chir. Paris*, **8**, 682.

Salter, R. B. (1984) Continuous passive motion. *Sicot Proc.*

Schlatter, C. (1903) Verletzungen des schnavelformingen Fortsatzes der oberem Tibiaepiphyse. *Bruns. Beitr. Klin. Chir.*, **38**, 874.

Scotland, J. R. and Weir, J. (1984) Assessment of prognosis of anterior cruciate deficient knees by means of tomography of the lateral tibial plateau. *Proc. British Orthopaedic Association, Aviemore.*

Seedhom, B. B., Dawson, D. and Wright, V. (1974) Functions of the menisci: a preliminary study. *J. Bone Joint Surg.*, **56B**, 381.

Slocum, D. B. and Larsen R. L. (1968a) Rotatary instability of the knee. *J. Bone Joint Surg.*, **50A**, 211.

Slocum, D. B. and Larsen R. L. (1968b) Pes anserinus transplantation: a surgical procedure for control of rotatary instability of the knee. *J. Bone Joint Surg.*, **50A**, 226.

Slocum, D. B., Larsen, R. L. and James S. L. (1974) Pes anserinus transplant: impressions after a decade of experience. *Clin. Orthop.*, **100**, 23.

Smillie, I. S. (1960) *Osteochondritis Dissecans*, Churchill Livingstone, London.

Swanson, S. A. V. (1975) in *Recent Advances in Orthopaedic Surgery*, Vol. 2, Churchill Livingstone, Edinburgh, London and New York, p. 115.

Tapper, E. and Hoover, N. (1969) Late results after meniscectomy. *J. Bone Joint Surg.*, **60A**, 436.

Torg, J. S., Conrad, W. and Kalen, V. (1976) Clinical diagnosis of anterior cruciate ligament instability in the athlete. *Amer. J. Sports Med.*, **4**, 84.

Watson-Jones, R. (1952) *Fractures and Joint Injuries*, Vol. 1, Churchill Livingstone, London, p. 97.

Weaver, J. K. (1977) Bypartite patella as a cause of disability in the athlete. *Amer. J. Sports Med.*, **5**, 137.

Williams, J. G. P. (1976) in *Proceedings of the XX World Congress of Sports Medicine*.

## A glossary of diagnostic terms about the knee

LIGAMENTOUS

To describe abnormal anterior motion of the tibia on the femur without any implication of rotation:

The *anterior drawer sign*; anterior motion in neutral rotation, with relaxed hamstrings and the knee at 90°.

The *Lachman test*; anterior motion of the tibia on the femur with the knee flexed to 20–30° and with a soft 'stop'.

To describe abnormal anterior motion of the medial tibial plateau on the femur:

The *Slocum–Larsen sign*; this is an anterior drawer sign in three positions, namely of neutral, internal and external rotation of the tibia. The amount of anterior motion varies with the rotation.

To describe abnormal anterior motion of the lateral tibial plateau on the femur:

(a) From extension

*The pivot shift test*, also often called the *MacIntosh test*; with internal rotation of the foot and a valgus force on the knee in extension, the knee is flexed and at about 30° the anteriorly subluxed lateral plateau jumps backwards.

*Casey* describes a variant in which the thumb is placed behind the top of the fibula and the same manoeuvre performed. The thumb controls the 'jump' and the test is repeatable as the abnormal motion is controlled.

(b) From flexion

*Hughston* describes the 'jerk' test in which the knee starts in flexion with a valgus force on the knee and internal rotation of the tibia. It is unclear whether he finds the anterior subluxation of the lateral plateau at 30° or its reposition at 5° to be the main feature.

*Losee* starts from flexion with a valgus force but with the leg in external rotation, changing to internal rotation as extension is approached. He stabilizes the fibula with the thumb and is clear that the anterior subluxation is the positive part of his test.

(c) From either

*Slocum* has the patient lie on the good side and rest the bad leg, extended over the flexed good leg. Gravity provides the valgus force and gentle active or passive flexion and extension produces a positive 'Losee' or 'pivot shift' according to the direction.

To describe abnormal posterior motion of the tibia on the femur in the flexed knee without rotation:

The *posterior drawer sign* demonstrates abnormal posterior motion of the tibia without rotation and is the reverse of the anterior drawer sign. In the *drop back sign* the hips and knees are flexed to 90° with the horizontal tibiae supported at the feet. The tibial tuberosity on the affected side falls back.

To describe abnormal posterior motion of the lateral tibial plateau on the femur:

399

# Knee injuries

If rotation is present the *recurvatum external rotation test* of Hughston is positive in which the lateral tibial plateau falls backwards in the slightly hyperextended knee when the extended leg is elevated by the big toe.

The *reverse pivot shift* is revealed by a valgus force on the flexed knee with the tibia externally rotated. As the leg is extended the posteriorly subluxed plateau moves back into place.

*Lateral thrust* is a dynamic observation in which the knee is noted to move into its maximal varus configuration during stance phase. Its implication for the result of posterolateral reconstruction is profound.

To test for collateral ligaments:

*Valgus/varus* stressing tests the posterior structures in full extension and the collateral ligaments in some degree of flexion. Rotation of the knee must be obliterated or recognized.

## MENISCAL

*McMurray* describes a test in which the knee is flexed and the tibia rotated from side to side. The same side is subjected to compression by the appropriate valgus/varus force. It is performed in varying degrees of flexion. The test is positive if the torn segment is trapped and relocates with pain. This test can lock the knee or cause very severe pain.

*Apley* distinguishes between meniscal and ligamentous problems by examining the patient prone with the knee flexed. Rotation under compression detects a meniscal lesion and rotation with traction a ligamentous lesion.

## PATELLA/PATELLOFEMORAL

The *apprehension* test involves attempting to sublux, or dislocate the patella. The apprehension is seen on the patient's face and should not be ignored. *Clarke's* test is compression of the structures immediately above the patella with the flat of the examiner's hand followed by active contraction of the quadriceps. It is positive if painful. It is claimed to be positive in cases of patellofemoral pathology. It is positive in a large proportion of the normal population.

It is tempting to produce a glossary of operative terms. Review of the original literature compared with the interpretations of experienced colleagues as to what they actually do when performing that operation suggests that Lewis Carroll was right. 'When I use a word it means just what I choose it to mean—neither more nor less' (Humpty Dumpty in *Alice Through the Looking Glass*, Chapter 6). The historical purist should consult the original article; the pragmatist should consult the surgeon doing the operation. Description of an operation by using the name of the man who first wrote it up is useless.

# 19 *Leg injuries*

JOHN KING

The leg contains the muscles which provide power (for ankle plantarflexion and thus push off), the muscles that control position (dorsiflexion, inversion and eversion), the two bones that provide their support and the nerves and blood vessels that supply them and the foot. The muscle groups are enclosed within clearly defined fascial compartments.

## 19.1 Contact injury

The leg acts as a flail by virtue of being a rigid segment connected to another by a hinge and deriving energy from that segment. The skin in this region is often damaged, usually anteriorly because it gets trapped between the hammer of the external force and the anvil of the underlying tibia. Cuts and abrasions are very common in this area and can go on to infection if not kept scrupulously clean. The best treatment is prevention and some form of shin guard should be worn in sports where contact with an opposing foot or equipment is frequent. Abrasions on the whole may be left exposed unless severe, when some form of occlusive plastic dressing speeds recovery by providing the best micro-environment for repair. Cuts necessitate accurate apposition of the edges which may be done with adhesive sutures rather than the traditional stitches on most occasions. The most difficult problem is usually persuading the player to desist from sport for the time taken to heal the injury. The underlying periosteum is often damaged and elevated on the anteromedial aspect by a subperiosteal haematoma which presents with local pain, well localized tenderness and obvious swelling in this area. Treatment is analgesia and mobilization. As yet there is no good objective evidence that the other remedies suggested (ultrasound, shortwave and diapulse) have any greater effect. In a player of contact sport the front of the tibia may come to resemble a mountain range but reassurance is all that is necessary.

Fracture as a direct consequence of trauma (as opposed to a stress

401

fracture) does occur. Diagnosis is usually obvious and it is essential to ensure that the neurovascular status of the limb distal to the fracture is intact. In the absence of the peripheral pulse first aid treatment is to align the limb with the other and apply traction until the pulse returns. The additional first aid management of an open fracture is simply to exclude further contamination by a clean covering. In all cases urgent transfer to hospital must be arranged, ideally with the leg in an inflatable plastic splint which should be available at any sporting event.

The lateral popliteal nerve is particularly susceptible to direct injury because of its superficial position overlying the bone of the neck of the fibula. A hard bang here may produce immediate paralysis of the ankle dorsiflexors. If the commencement of recovery is delayed beyond a week or so then the total recovery may not be complete. In all cases it is necessary to provide a lively splint to pull up the foot and prevent an equinus deformity of the ankle which must be regularly moved through its full range. It is important that the ankle is rehabilitated on the wobble board (Fig. 19.1) to improve proprioception before return to sport.

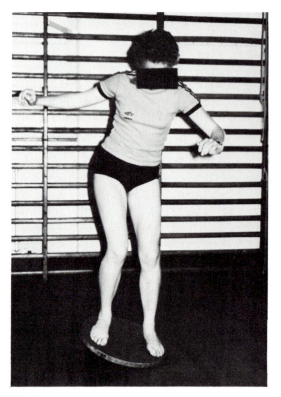

*Fig. 19.1*  Wobble board; the round type used towards the end of therapy.

The superficial peroneal nerve passes between the peronei and the extensor digitorum longus and then passes to the skin of the lower part of the outer leg through the deep fascia. It can be injured at this site leading to numbness or paraesthesiae in its distribution and rarely there may be compression as it traverses the fascia.

## 19.2   Non-contact injury

Acute non-contact injuries in the leg are rare and are usually an incomplete tear of the musculotendinous junction of the gastrocnemius/soleus complex. Tears of the plantaris are probably mythological. Ruptures of popliteal cysts may produce local pain and tenderness in the calf. Diagnosis is based on well localized pain and tenderness and an appropriate history. Treatment in all cases is elevation, rest, a heel raise and physiotherapy until full active and passive dorsiflexion is achieved. Those tears that do occur commonly are near the ankle (tear of the Achilles or posterior tibial tendons) and are dealt with in Chapter 20.

## 19.3   Overuse

Both the upper and lower joints between the tibia and the fibula may give rise to problems. The upper joint may be the site of local pain or even clinically detectable hypermobility. Rarely the symptoms come on after one identifiable acute injury. As always the first line of treatment is restriction of activity followed by a local injection of hydrocortisone. In the absence of gross laxity this may be all that is needed but some cases do fail to respond to this treatment and in these and the hypermobile cases some form of operation may be necessary. It is possible to either excise the part of the fibula deep to the insertion of biceps and produce an excision arthroplasty or to attempt to stabilize the joint by transfixion with a screw after reinforcing the capsule with a strip of biceps tendon. This latter procedure is not particularly satisfactory and it does mean a second operation to remove the screw and the current trend is to do an excision arthroplasty.

At the distal end the laxity usually follows an inversion injury of the foot with the talus spinning laterally, pushing the distal fibula backwards and tearing the anteroinferior tibiofibular ligament. The lower end of the fibula can be felt to move backwards. This is a rare injury but should not be missed because of that. The treatment is surgical and demands repair or reinforcement of the ligament and a temporary syndesmosis screw. Even if the ligament is not torn fully by the original injury there may be enough damage to some of the fibres to lead to a cyst forming within the ligament (Fig. 19.2) with well localized pain as the foot twists and as the ankle dorsiflexes and puts the ligament under tension. It must be distinguished from the lateral osteochondral talar dome fracture by radiographs and/or a radionuclide scan. Treatment is exploration and obliteration of the cyst by curetting it and closing the space with a stitch. The ankle must be immobilized in full dorsiflexion to keep the ligament on the stretch.

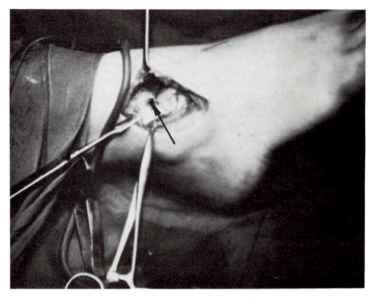

*Fig. 19.2*   Cyst in anterior inferior tibio-fibular ligament.

More commonly associated with overuse is the stress fracture which comes about from fatigue failure. Devas (1975) has demonstrated that the tibia and fibula bend towards one another when the ankle is powerfully plantarflexed and if this movement is repeated too often, before the bones can strengthen, one or other will give way. The actual pattern of failure varies from a longitudinal split to a transverse lesion. The story is of increasing pain felt in the shin and coming on during and after activity at shorter and shorter intervals from commencement. This crescendo of pain is typical during early training or after a spell of sustained activity and there may be an unpleasant aching pain after the cessation of the exercise.

Physical examination may reveal local tenderness or nothing. There may be local pain on the application of ultrasound at maximum intensity. X-rays at this early stage usually show nothing. The typical changes of a

404

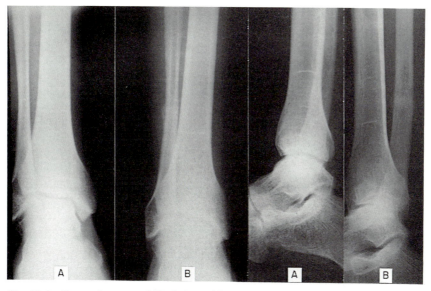

*Fig. 19.3* Stress fracture of fibula invisible on presentation (A) and visible at two weeks (B).

healing fracture may be seen with the passage of time (Fig. 19.3). To make an early confirmation of the diagnosis it is necessary to do a technetium scan which shows a well localized increase in uptake in the same region as the pain. Treatment is reduction of activity to a pain-free level with a gradual increase in the amount essayed. To advise the patient to run through the pain is dangerous. If almost complete reduction of activity does not relieve the pain, some form of removable plastic external support must be provided. The idea of treatment is to allow the bones to hypertrophy under the influence of stress while reducing the loads enough to stop them breaking. The differential diagnosis is discussed under shin splints. Some stress fractures do take a long time to heal and in these it is justifiable to elevate the periosteum overlying the lesion. The rapid subperiosteal new bone deposition speeds up the healing by increasing the girth and hence the strength of the bone. This should be done only when the normal process is slow or the fracture is recurrent. As in any other site in this age group, if the pain persists and there is not a rapid radiological evolution of a healing fracture be suspicious of a sarcoma. Sometimes a parosteal sarcoma may look exactly like a stress fracture on X-ray (Fig. 19.4) but does not settle in a reasonable time. It needs a biopsy but this must be done by whoever may undertake definitive treatment and the specimen reviewed by a very experienced bone pathologist.

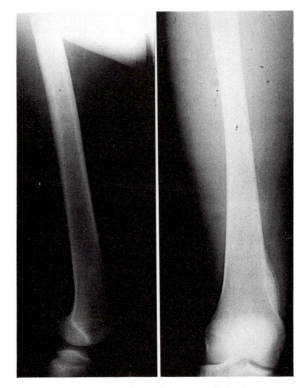

*Fig. 19.4*  Parosteal sarcoma of distal femur mimicking a stress fracture.

## 19.4  Other conditions

The superficial peroneal nerve may be compressed as it exits through the deep fascia, the symptoms usually being unpleasant paraesthesiae in its distribution. Such cases usually follow unusual activity. Most resolve without decompression of the tunnel in the fascia. The lateral popliteal nerve may be compressed by a ganglion arising from the proximal tibio-fibular joint. This may press upon the nerve or even extend within its substance. The symptoms are of progressive loss of power of ankle dorsiflexion. The loss of sensation at the base of the big toe is usually not noticed by the patient and the diagnosis is made by careful palpation of the nerve at the neck of the fibula. Removal of the ganglion removes the symptoms.

All the other conditions can be discussed under the differential diagnosis of shin splints. This is not a diagnosis but a descriptive term for exertional shin pain in an athlete (Bates, 1985) the American Medical

Association Standard Definition (1968) notwithstanding. In addition to compartmental syndromes, stress syndromes and periostitis, Sperryn (1984) lists stress fractures, vascular disease especially in the older jogger, spinal stenosis, fascial hernias, tenosynovitis, cellulitis, deep vein thrombosis, infective or varicose periostitis and tumour as potential causes, although this rather leaves no stone unturned. The syndrome is important, accounting for 10–15% of all running injuries (Gudas, 1980; James, Bates and Osternis, 1978). It is responsible for 60% of painful lesions in athletes' legs (Orava and Puranen, 1979). Andrish, Bergfield and Walheim (1974) reported an incidence of 4.07% in 2000 previously fit recruits commencing physical training.

### 19.4.1 COMPARTMENTAL SYNDROME

This condition is often called 'anterior tibial syndrome' but a review of the terms suggest that all the syndromes in this section have been called that at some time.

There are four compartments defined by the junctions of the fascia and bones of the leg (Fig. 19.5), the anterolateral, the lateral, the deep posterior and the superficial posterior, each circumscribed by inelastic tissue. They have one structure in common which is the fibula. The compartment most frequently affected is the anterolateral and the following descriptions apply to that. The other compartments have a more rare but similar story with the signs transposed appropriately.

The syndrome of raised intracompartmental pressure with ischaemia of the muscle has been described as an acute problem following trauma or an isolated episode of overuse such as a forced march, with dramatic

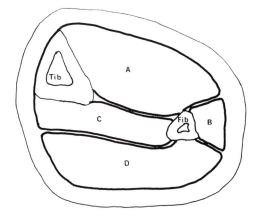

*Fig. 19.5* The fascial compartments: A: the anterior, B: the anterolateral, C: the deep posterior, and D: the superficial posterior.

changes leading to muscle death. More commonly a less dramatic sequence of events takes place in the calf muscles as a consequence of overactivity. After a certain amount of exercise the front of the leg becomes the site of a cramp-like pain and activity has to stop. There may be loss of active dorsiflexion in the severe case. With rest the pain gradually diminishes but returns on resumption of the exercise. On examination at the time of pain the front of the leg is tense and tender and passive stretching of the muscles gives rise to pain. The peripheral pulses are usually present. If the leg is seen at rest there is no abnormality to be defined.

To confirm the diagnosis it is necessary to show that there is an increase of pressure within the compartment above that which is normally expected. This is done by direct compartmental pressure measurements using a needle or wick catheter (Murbarak and Hargens, 1981). In a clinic it is most simple to use the needle technique in which an 18 gauge needle is inserted into the compartment and connected to a tube containing saline in the half connected to the needle (Fig. 19.6). The meniscus of this column of fluid provides a reference point. The tube connects to a three-way tap with the other arms to a syringe and a manometer. As the syringe is compressed the meniscus begins to move smoothly but slowly towards the leg as the saline flows in. At the same time the pressure necessary to do this is read directly off the manometer. It is necessary to compare both sides before and after activity and to put the needle in the compartments thought to be affected. This technique gives different results in different hands so that absolute values are useless. With this technique the result is regarded as positive if the rise in pressure on the abnormal side is more than twice that on the normal side, although Puranen and Alavaikko (1981) found a factor of three for pressure differences between the normal

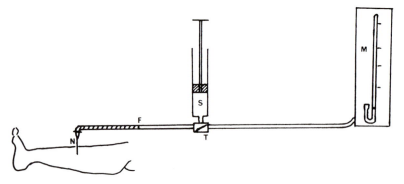

*Fig. 19.6* Diagram of the system to measure compartmental pressure. N is an 18 gauge needle, F the fluid meniscus, S the syringe, T the three-way tap and M the mercury manometer.

and symptomatic side in medial tibial pain and four in anterolateral pain. Murbarak *et al.* (1982) dispute this result for medial pain which they claim is due to periostitis but it is generally accepted that elevated anterior compartmental pressures can cause shin splint pain (Rorabeck, Bourne and Fowler, 1983).

Treatment is surgical and involves opening the fascia of the affected compartment. The extensive procedures such as extraperiosteal excision of the fibula, used in the acute lesions, are not applicable. There is usually a long scar and always a muscle hernia afterwards, but the scar can be reduced by passing an insulated wire through a small hole up inside the fascia and threading it down again outside through a second small incision at the top. The insulation at the bend is removed, the diathermy connected to the bottom ends and the wire pulled out thus cutting the fascia and securing haemostasis (Fig. 19.7). Recurrence of this problem is rare and demands rigorous assessment of the compartments and careful re-exploration under direct vision.

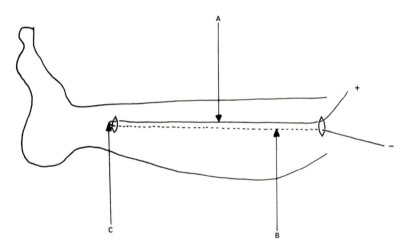

*Fig. 19.7* Diagram of closed method of fascial strip. A is an insulated wire subcutaneous and deep to fascia, B an insulated wire subcutaneous and superficial to fascia, C the point at which the insulation is removed; + or − are connected to the diathermy.

### 19.4.2 PERIOSTITIS

Shin pain associated with activity may not show any of the characteristics outlined above and may be medial. Examination may show a pronating foot in stance phase and a little tenderness on the medial rim of the tibia where the muscles insert, giving rise to the name medial tibial syndrome.

# Leg injuries

This seems to be an inflammation or irritation of the periosteum at the insertion of the fascia or at the origin of the muscles. A technetium scan may show a little diffuse increase in activity in this region. Treatment is difficult. It is best to start with a good medial arch support and provide a shock absorber such as sorbothane as a heel pad. If that simple measure fails a custom built orthosis may succeed.

## 19.4.3 TENOSYNOVITIS

Occasionally confused with the above, but simple to distinguish, is the anterior shin pain from inflammation of the tendons as they pass under the Y-shaped extensor retinaculum. The pain is present on motion, localized to the lowest part of the front of the shin, and there is local tenderness on palpation or even crepitus as the ankle is actively moved. Local injection is usually enough but release may occasionally be necessary with some consequent bowstringing of the tendons.

The three conditions—stress fracture, compartmental syndrome and periostitis—are often difficult to distinguish and represent the main differential diagnosis of shin splints. Usually one of these three causes can be separated out after use of the investigations described, but a small number of cases defy diagnosis despite consideration of the list above.

## References

AMA Subcommittee on the Classification of Sports Injuries (1966) *Standard Nomenclature of Athletic Injuries*, Chicago.
Andrish, J. T., Bergfield, J. A. and Walheim, J. (1974) A prospective study on the management of shin splints. *J. Bone Joint Surg.*, **56A**, 1697.
Bates, P. (1985) Dissertation for the Diploma in Sports Medicine, The London Hospital Medical College.
Devas, M. (1975) *Stress Fractures*, Churchill Livingstone, Edinburgh, London and New York.
Gudas, C. J. (1980) Patterns of lower extremity injury in 224 runners. *Comprehensive Ther.*, **6**, 50.
James, S. L., Bates, B. T. and Osternis, L. R. (1978) Injuries to runners. *Amer. J. Sports Med.*, **6**, 40.
Murbarak, S. J. and Hargens, A. R. (1981) *Compartment Syndromes and Volkmann's Contracture*, W. B. Saunders, Philadelphia, London, Toronto and Sydney.
Murbarak, S. J., Gould, R. N., Yu, F. L., Schmidt, D. A. and Hargens, A. R. (1982) The medial tibial stress syndrome. *Amer. J. Sports Med.*, **10**, 201.
Orava, S. and Puranen, J. (1979) Athletes' leg pain. *Brit. J. Sports Med.*, **13**, 92.
Puranen, J. and Alavaikko, A. (1981) Intracompartmental pressure increase on

exertion in patients with chronic compartmental syndrome in the leg. *J. Bone Joint Surg.*, **63A**, 1304.

Rorabeck, C. H., Bourne, R. B. and Fowler, P. J. (1983) The surgical treatment of exertional compartment syndrome in athletes. *J. Bone Joint Surg.*, **65A**, 1245.

Sperryn, P. (1984) Succouring the shin sore. *Med. News*, **October**.

# 20 *Ankle injuries*

S. C. CHEN

Injuries of the ankle are very common, yet they are usually treated rather casually in the busy Accident and Emergency Department of a hospital. This cavalier treatment may not matter very much in the sedentary individual where the end result may be surprisingly good. However, what may be regarded as moderate injuries of the ankle in the sedentary individual may have disastrous consequences in the sportsman. Tendons, ligaments, capsule and articular cartilage may be injured.

## 20.1  Tendon injuries

Although tendon injuries are less common than ligament or bony injuries, they give rise to the same degree of disability as these latter injuries, if improperly treated. A tendon can be damaged if a sudden strain is applied to it. This can occur in a very vigorous push-off as in a sudden lurch forwards in an athletic sprint, and when trying to retrieve a ball at squash or a shuttlecock at badminton, or it could occur in a sudden reflex contraction to stabilize the ankle or subtalar joints, as in landing after jumping up to hit or catch a ball.

In normal walking the anterior tibial muscle contracts and stabilizes the ankle at heel strike. During the toe-off phase the calf muscles contract and force the ball of the foot against the ground, whilst the peroneal and posterior tibial muscles act as guy ropes stabilizing the foot and preventing it from inverting or everting, and at the same time helping the calf muscles in the push-off phase.

Tendons are largely composed of collagen fibres. Collagen is a heterogeneous structural protein of which there are different types. Five types are recognized, each with tissue-specific functions and distribution. The normal Achilles tendon contains 85% collagen almost entirely of Type I. In ruptured Achilles tendons there are Type I and III collagen fibres and it is postulated that the presence of Type III collagen might account for

# Ankle injuries

decreased resistance to tensile forces and to spontaneous rupture (Coombs *et al.*, 1980).

## 20.1.1 ACHILLES TENDON RUPTURE

The Achilles tendon can be injured either at the musculotendinous junction or near its insertion to the calcaneum (Fig. 20.1).

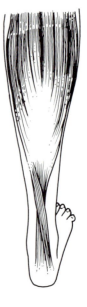

*Fig. 20.1* Posterior view of the tendo achillis to show the rotation of the fibres from medial to lateral.

### (a) Tears at the musculotendinous junction

One still hears mention of a plantaris tendon rupture. This, as everyone should know, is a myth. The plantaris tendon never ruptures. What is usually mistaken for this non-existent condition is a rupture of a few muscle fibres of the gastrocnemius and/or soleus at the musculotendinous junction, the Achilles tendon itself being intact. Treatment consists of rest from sports for about three to four weeks, oral analgesics and a supportive bandage.

### (b) Tendon rupture

The classical story is that whilst playing tennis or any other ball game, the patient feels as if he is kicked or struck at the heel, and if anyone is unfortunate enough to be nearby, he may be accused of kicking him and be the recipient of a retaliatory assault. Such a patient is usually middle-aged, plays occasionally and has a rather aggressive nature.

414

The fibres of the Achilles tendon pursue a spiral course from its musculotendinous junction to its bony insertion and two muscles, the gastrocnemius and soleus, are attached to this one tendon. The fibres which are attached to the gastrocnemius and those which are attached to the soleus cross each other. During the act of jumping, the gastroncnemius and soleus contract to plantarflex the ankle and at the same time the quadriceps muscles contract strongly to extend the knee and further lengthen the already contracted gastrocnemius which is attached across the knee to the back of the femoral condyles. Christensen (1953) proposed a mechanical cause, having noted that the tendon fibres of the gastrocnemius and soleus intersect each other in a rotating manner, and a saw-like action between these fibres can occur. On the other hand De Stefano (1975) suggested that an asymptomatic degeneration of the Achilles tendon preceded a rupture after studying biopsy specimens of acute ruptures. The site of rupture is usually about 4 cm proximal to its insertion as this is the most avascular part (Lagergren and Lindholm, 1958).

The diagnosis of a ruptured Achilles tendon is surprisingly difficult. The tendon may be only partially torn, when there is disruption of the individual fibres at various levels but no visible or palpable gap in the tendon. Partial rupture was thought to be uncommon until Ljunqvist (1968) reported twenty-four cases, thus establishing its relative frequency. Even when the tear is complete, haematoma formation can mask the gap in the tendon. Approximately 25% of ruptured Achilles tendons are missed at initial examination by a doctor (Inglis *et al.*, 1970). Flexion of the foot can still occur due to action of the posterior tibial, peroneal and toe flexor muscles. There are two tests which are very reliable:

(1) Simmonds' test, which is performed on the prone patient whose feet extend beyond the examination couch. The relaxed calf muscles are gently squeezed with one hand. If the Achilles tendon is intact there is passive plantarflexion of the foot. If it is ruptured, this does not occur.
(2) The patient is unable to stand on tiptoe, as the muscles mentioned above are not strong enough by themselves for this action.

Treatment can be conservative or surgical. There are several methods, but the principle is the same, that is to approximate the ends. If conservative treatment does not do so then surgery is necessary. It is very important to immobilize the ankle for eight weeks, the first four weeks in equinus and the second four weeks in as much dorsiflexion of the ankle as possible. This change of plaster is carried out at four weeks on a conscious patient so as not to strain the repair.

The main problem with surgical repair of a ruptured Achilles tendon is delayed wound healing and skin necrosis. This is due to the relatively poor vascular supply of the skin in this region. One method of surgical repair which overcomes this is to carry out the repair percutaneously (Ma and Griffith, 1977).

Conservative treatment of Achilles tendon rupture in a below knee plaster cast with the foot in equinus as popularized by Lea and Smith (1968) is not favoured as there is a high incidence of re-rupture (Inglis *et al.*, 1970; Coombs, 1981). Even in Lea and Smith's series there is a 25% re-rupture rate. Although Nistor (1981) favoured non-surgical treatment because of a shorter morbidity and no hospital stay, his series included five re-ruptures in the non-surgical group compared to two re-ruptures in the surgical group.

In middle-aged people who participate in vigorous exercises, an exquisitely tender lump about three inches above the insertion of the Achilles tendon may develop. This lump may not be painful at rest but becomes painful when doing active sports. It is due to an intratendinous rupture giving rise to an area of softening and fibrosis. This lesion does not respond to conservative measures such as rest, heel raise, shortwave diathermy or cortisone injections, and should be removed and the defect sutured (Bromberger, 1982).

### 20.1.2 CHRONIC ACHILLES TENDINITIS AND BURSITIS

Athletes who participate in endurance events may develop Achilles tendinitis and/or bursitis. The main symptom is pain in the back of the ankle, which is aggravated by activity, especially walking or running on slopes. Clinically there is tenderness when the Achilles tendon is palpated. When bursitis is present, tenderness in front of the tendon can be elicited also.

The Achilles tendon is surrounded by a fine paratenon which becomes inflamed due to repetitive friction (Lipscomb, 1950). The Achilles bursa which lies in front of the tendon can be similarly affected. Treatment in the early stages is rest with an elastic strapping for support. Ultrasound therapy may be helpful. In the chronic condition which does not respond to conservative treatment within two to three months, surgical stripping of the paratenon surrounding the tendon should be carried out (Kvist and Kvist, 1980). Following stripping of the paratenon, immediate post-operative mobilization is essential. This operation should not be performed in acute paratendonitis. If the bursa is thickened by chronic inflammation, it may also have to be excised.

### 20.1.3 CALCANEAL EXOSTOSIS OR 'PUMP BUMP'

This is a condition due to ill-fitting footwear, such as jogging shoes, which may give rise to a painful swelling just above the insertion of the Achilles tendon. This swelling may be medial or lateral to the tendon and is due to reactive bone formation from constant friction and pressure. This condition is called 'pump bump' in the USA because it is commonly seen in teenage and young adult females who wear high-heeled shoes.

Treatment is non-surgical in the early stages and consists of rest till symptoms settle and wearing low-heeled and well fitting laced up shoes. In late cases the bony calcaneal prominence may have to be excised.

### 20.1.4 POSTERIOR TIBIAL TENDON INJURY

*(a) Tenosynovitis*

The posterior tibial tendon lies in a tendon sheath and runs behind the medial malleolus, curving forwards and downwards to be inserted into the navicular bone (Fig. 20.2). This confined space and curved direction of pull predispose to tenosynovitis and tendinitis following strenuous sporting activities of the endurance type, for example long distance running.

Usually a middle-aged patient presents with pain behind the medial aspect of the ankle. On examination there is tenderness and sometimes swelling behind the medial malleolus. The patient has difficulty in standing on tiptoe, although the Achilles tendon is intact. There is pain on forced inversion of the foot. The patient is usually flat-footed (Williams, 1963).

Treatment consists of rest from sporting activities for three to four weeks, oral anti-inflammatory drugs, a supportive ankle strap and valgus insoles. Local steroid injections should be avoided as this may precipitate

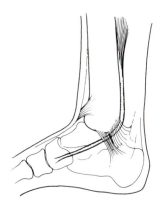

*Fig. 20.2* Medial view of the ankle to show the posterior tibial tendon being inserted to the navicular bone.

417

Ankle injuries

a tendon rupture. In chronic cases there may be an associated teno-vaginitis similar to de Quervain's disease at the wrist, and surgical release may have to be carried out.

*(b)   Tendinitis and tendon rupture*

It is very difficult to distinguish between tenosynovitis and tendinitis but the latter condition is more severe with more pain and restriction of ankle and subtalar movement. It is very important to anticipate a tendon rupture in a severe case of tendinitis. A history of the patient feeling a sudden snap in his ankle must be taken very seriously. If a tendon rupture is suspected a tenogram must be done and early surgical repair undertaken. If this is not carried out the patient will suffer a progressive pes plano-valgus deformity and will have difficulty in standing on tiptoe. In the late stages he will complain of tiredness and ache in his affected foot after a few holes of golf or after walking a short distance.

In the severe case of tendinitis it is advisable to decompress the tendon surgically. In a recent tendon rupture it is possible to suture the ruptured ends together followed by a four week period of plaster immobilization. In a late tendon rupture it is not possible to bring the ruptured ends together and in such a situation, the proximal and distal ends of the ruptured posterior tibial tendon can be sutured to the flexor digitorum longus tendon.

*(c)   Avulsion fracture of the navicular bone at the posterior tibial tendon insertion*

If an athlete decelerates suddenly, the tendon insertion to the navicular can be avulsed together with a piece of bone. If it is undisplaced, treatment consists of a below knee plaster cast for four weeks. If it is displaced (Fig. 20.3) the piece of bone must be fixed back into place with a screw followed by plaster immobilization for four weeks. One must differentiate this from an accessory ossicle of the navicular which is usually present in both feet. This accessory ossicle or os naviculare can sometimes cause pressure symptoms when wearing shoes, and in severe cases has to be excised followed by careful repair of the tendinous attachments.

20.1.5   PERONEAL TENDON INJURY

The peroneal longus and brevis muscles are strong everters of the foot and primary lateral stabilizers of the ankle. The peroneal tendons lie behind the lateral malleolus, held in place by the superior and inferior peroneal retinacula and pursue a downward and forward course (Fig. 20.4). The tendon of brevis is inserted into the tip of the styloid process of the base of the fifth metatarsal and the tendon of longus enters the sole of

418

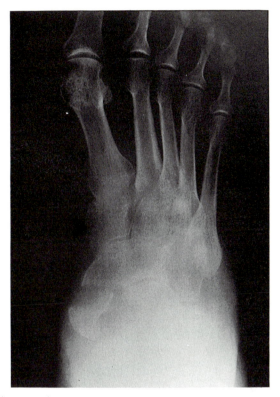

*Fig. 20.3* Radiograph of the foot to show avulsion fracture of the navicular bone.

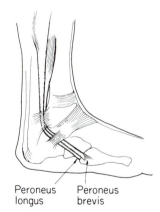

Peroneus   Peroneus
longus     brevis

*Fig. 20.4* Lateral view of the ankle to show the peroneus brevis tendon being inserted to the tip of the styloid process of the fifth metatarsal bone, and the peroneus longus tendon entering the sole of the foot. Both tendons lie behind the lateral malleolus and curve forwards predisposing to tendon injuries.

the foot and is inserted into the base of the first metatarsal and medial cuneiform.

### (a)   Tendinitis

Due to the curved direction of pull, like the posterior tibial tendon on the medial aspect of the ankle, the peroneal tendon can become inflamed. The patient presents with pain on the lateral side of the ankle. On examination there is tenderness and sometimes a swelling along the direction of the peroneal tendons. Forced eversion of the foot produces pain.

Treatment consists of rest from sporting activities for three to four weeks, using a supportive ankle strap and occasionally a below knee plaster cast in the severe case during this period. In severe cases, a tenovaginitis, similar to a de Quervain's disease at the wrist, may have to be released surgically, but care must be taken to preserve a pulley to prevent subsequent subluxation or dislocation of the peroneal tendons.

### (b)   Tendon rupture

Peroneal tendon rupture is extremely rare as it is not within a tendon sheath. It occurs only if the tendon is degenerated or subject to injudicious local steroid injections. If it ruptures the patient has a foot drop and is unable to evert his foot. This is a very disabling injury and should be treated surgically, approximating the ruptured ends together with sutures followed by a four week period of plaster immobilization.

### (c)   Subluxing peroneal tendons

The peroneal tendons disrupt the superior peroneal retinaculum and sublux when the muscles contract violently, whilst the foot is dorsiflexed and everted, as in skiing (Escalas, Figueras and Merino, 1980), or in a stumble when playing football or any other sport. This injury is predisposed by a shallow peroneal groove behind the lateral malleolus.

In the acute injury, it is important to immobilize the ankle and foot in a below knee plaster cast for four weeks. Any less rigid immobilization than a plaster cast is ineffective. In the late case, the subluxing peroneal tendons must be stabilized in the peroneal groove of the lateral malleolus by one of several reconstructive procedures such as a periosteal flap, bone block or deepening the groove.

### 20.1.6   ANTERIOR TIBIAL TENDON INJURY

### (a)   Tendinitis

This injury is very rare and occurs sometimes in skiers, long distance runners or hikers, particularly when travelling downhill for long distances. They can experience pain in the anterior tibial compartment and in the anterior tibial tendon at the level of the ankle. This condition usually settles down very quickly. Treatment consists of rest for a couple of weeks and oral analgesics.

*(b)  Rupture*

This tendon is rarely ruptured as it has a direct and straight attachment to the medial cuneiform and first metatarsal (Fig. 20.5). It has a good vascular supply. The few cases of anterior tibial tendon rupture reported in the literature have been due to degeneration of the tendon in the middle-aged athlete. These present with a mild foot drop as the anterior tibial tendon contributes 80% of the muscle power in dorsiflexion. Surgical repair gives excellent results.

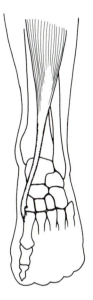

*Fig. 20.5*  Drawing of the front of the ankle to show the tibialis anterior tendon being inserted into the medial cuneiform and first metatarsal bones.

## 20.2  Ligament and capsular injuries

These injuries are usually referred to as a 'sprained' ankle, which is a totally inadequate diagnosis. The injury must be pinpointed, not only to a particular ligament but if possible to a particular part of a ligament. Furthermore it is necessary to distinguish between a complete rupture and a partial rupture of a ligament.

The ankle joint could be considered a closed unit with bony, ligamentous and capsular elements (Fig. 20.6). The ligaments and bone depend

# Ankle injuries

on one another for normal function and damage to one group can involve the other, and it is important to appreciate that damage to both groups can occur. Of the bony elements the lower end of the tibia and the medial malleolus are weightbearing, and constitute more than three-quarters of the bony part of the ankle, while the fibula and the lateral malleolus, besides some weightbearing (Lambert, 1971) are important lateral stabilizers of the ankle.

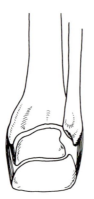

*Fig. 20.6*  Cut section of the ankle to illustrate the 'closed unit' concept.

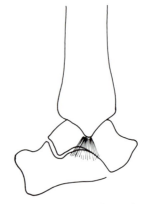

*Fig. 20.7*  Drawing to show the medial ligament consisting of a deep part and a larger fan-shaped superficial part.

The medial ligament is the most important structure in preventing the talus from moving laterally even if the inferior tibiofibular ligament is ruptured (Fig. 20.7). It consists of a deep part which is fused with the joint capsule and a superficial part which fans out in a triangular shape from the medial malleolus to the talus, the sustentaculum tali, the spring ligament and base of the tuberosity of the navicular.

The next most important ligament in the ankle joint is the inferior tibiofibular ligament which holds the tibia and fibula together. It consists of a very thick and strong interosseus part and relatively weak anterior and posterior parts. The inferior tibiofibular ligament varies very much in its anatomy which may explain variations in the injuries found in this area from similar forces (Monk, 1969).

The lateral ligament consists of a strong calcaneofibular part which runs posteriorly and downwards from the tip of the lateral malleolus to the calcaneum and is taut in adduction of the ankle, a weak talofibular part which becomes taut in plantarflexion and an equally weak posterior talofibular part which becomes taut in dorsiflexion (Fig. 20.8).

The capsule of the ankle joint is a discrete structure anteriorly and

422

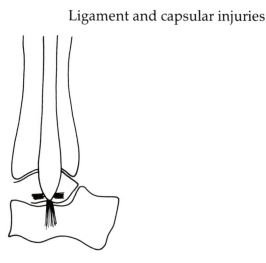

*Fig. 20.8* The lateral ligament consisting of the strong calcaneofibular part and the weaker anterior talofibular and posterior talofibular parts.

posteriorly, merging with the medial and lateral ligaments on either side of the ankle and contributing to its stability.

In any sport, where the athlete has to swerve to stop and turn suddenly, or land heavily on his feet, the ankle joint can be 'twisted'. The usual mechanism is an inversion strain, but forced plantarflexion or eversion strains can cause ligamentous and/or capsular damage.

Ligamentous injuries of the foot and ankle frequently produce a proprioceptive deficit affecting the muscles of the injured leg, and this is probably responsible for the symptom of 'giving way' of the injured leg. Many articular nerve fibres terminate in mechanoreceptors in the capsule and ligaments of joints (Freeman and Wyke, 1964) and these subserve reflexes which stabilize the joints by provoking appropriate muscle activity. In the foot and ankle, instantaneous and qualitatively precise contractions of the calf muscles must occur if the foot is to remain stable on uneven ground. When a ligament or capsule ruptures these fine and delicate nerve fibres are also ruptured and lead to partial joint de-afferentiation. This defect may be permanent. Proprioceptive defects can be elicited by asking the patient to stand on one leg in a modification of Romberg's sign. However, this test is invalid if the subtalar joint is stiff (Hicks, 1961) or if there is pain when standing on that leg, or if the calf muscle power is weak. Early mobilization with co-ordination exercises following a foot or ankle sprain can often prevent this proprioceptive deficit.

Clinically the ankle is swollen and painful. Movements are restricted. Careful examination will pinpoint the area of maximum tenderness and

423

this is a very reliable method of diagnosing the parts of a ligament which are damaged. X-rays may show no evidence of any bony injuries. On the other hand, flakes of bone may be avulsed at the ligamentous or capsular attachments and these may be important clues to the presence of such damage. Do not dismiss these flakes of bone as minor fractures. They may be minor as regards the size of the bony fragments, but they represent very severe ligamentous or capsular injuries.

To distinguish between a complete and a partial rupture of the ligament it is necessary to carry out stress films under general or regional anaesthesia. The normal ankle should be similarly examined for comparison. In a complete rupture there will be tilting of the talus in the ankle mortice. A completely torn inferior tibiofibular ligament may not be evident in X-rays, and the ankle may look deceptively normal, as the tibia and fibula lie close together in the non-weightbearing state. However, a stress film will show abnormal widening of the ankle mortice. Arthrograms of the ankle can be useful and will show a complete leak of radio-opaque dye into the soft tissues if there is a complete ligament rupture.

### 20.3 Partial ligamentous or capsular injuries

#### 20.3.1 MEDIAL LIGAMENT INJURY

This is caused by eversion, internal rotation forces with the foot in plantargrade position, or external rotation forces with the foot in dorsiflexion. Treatment consists of a figure of eight strapping relaxing the medial ligament and kept on for three weeks.

#### 20.3.2 INFERIOR TIBIOFIBULAR LIGAMENT INJURY

This is usually part of a fracture complex and is caused by a violent external rotation force of the ankle with the foot in dorsiflexion. In the isolated tears of the weak anterior inferior tibiofibular ligament, a supportive ankle strapping for three weeks should suffice.

A severe abduction injury can tear the strong inferior tibiofibular ligament, giving rise to diastasis of the inferior tibiofibular ligament. Either the medial ligament is torn or the medial malleolus is avulsed and a fracture of the shaft of the fibula above the inferior tibiofibular joint usually accompanies this injury. The talus is also displaced laterally.

It is important to stabilize the ankle joint adequately and this is done by reducing the diastasis and holding it with a screw across the inferior tibiofibular joint. The medial malleolar and the fibular fractures must be accurately reduced and held with screws with or without a small plate

424

across the fibular fracture. Early non-weightbearing mobilization can be started soon after the operation to prevent ankle stiffness.

## 20.4   Lateral ligament injury

### 20.4.1   RUPTURE OF THE ANTERIOR TALOFIBULAR PART

This injury is caused when the foot twists whilst in plantarflexion. It can cause prolonged disability if not adequately treated. A lateral X-ray of the ankle in slight plantarflexion will show the talus is slightly subluxed forwards and the congruity of the ankle joint is lost. If this is the only injury, the ankle is strapped using elastic adhesive bandage with dorsiflexion of the ankle, the strapping being a supportive U, and figure of eight.

### 20.4.2   RUPTURE OF THE POSTERIOR TALOFIBULAR AND CALCANEOFIBULAR PARTS

The posterior talofibular part is rarely injured and, if it is, it is usually in combination with the calcaneofibular part.

In severe twisting injuries of the plantarflexed foot a complete rupture of the calcaneofibular part occurs. It may be advisable in some instances where gross instability is demonstrated in stress radiographs to operate on these complete ruptures to prevent late instability of the ankle. The ruptured fibres are brought together and held with absorbable sutures. A period of four weeks in a below knee plaster cast is necessary. However, in patients where instability cannot be demonstrated, or there is only slight instability, early mobilization with a supportive strapping will give the best results (Freeman, 1965a and b).

## 20.5   Capsular injuries

### 20.5.1   ANTERIOR CAPSULAR STRAIN

The anterior capsule of the ankle joint can be strained or partially ruptured in forced plantarflexion injuries. Pain and tenderness are most marked along the front of the ankle. X-rays may show tiny flakes of bone separated from the dorsum of the talus. Test for forward subluxation of the talus in the ankle mortice in lateral stress films. As always, compare any shift in position with the normal side.

Treatment is strapping of the ankle in slight dorsiflexion for three weeks so as to relax the damaged capsule. It is very important to appreciate that ligamentous and capsular injuries usually occur together, although one element of the injury may predominate. Furthermore, more than one ligament may be damaged. When there is obvious medial ligament damage one may have to exclude a more serious injury, particularly of the inferior tibiofibular ligament complex, which may not be obvious unless specifically looked for.

## 20.6   Rehabilitation in ligamentous and capsular injuries

The rehabilitation period for a ligamentous or capsular injury is much longer than following a fracture. The athlete can expect to experience varying degrees of pain for periods up to several months. This is the reason why, as a general rule, plaster immobilization is not used unless extremely necessary (e.g. following a surgical repair of a completely ruptured ligament) for this lengthens the rehabilitation period because of periarticular adhesions.

Following the period of rest in a supportive strapping or in a plaster cast, physiotherapy consisting of gentle mobilization exercises is carried out routinely. At the same time proprioceptive toning exercises such as 'wobble board' exercises are instituted (Freeman, 1965a). After about three weeks of this regime the patient is allowed to train in graduated stages for another fortnight and then allowed to participate in sports. Further strapping may then be necessary when returning to sport. This is not so much to 'support' the ankle, which this clearly cannot do, but to increase the proprioceptive 'feedback' from the skin. In severe cases an ankle orthosis may be required.

## 20.7   Tarsal tunnel syndromes

There are two rare conditions connected with entrapment of the posterior tibial and deep peroneal nerves.

### 20.7.1   POSTERIOR TARSAL TUNNEL SYNDROME

The posterior tibial nerve is trapped at the medial malleolus, where it gives sensory fibres to the sole of the foot and motor branches to the intrinsic muscles of the foot. The posterior tibial nerve divides at this level into three divisions: the medial plantar, the lateral plantar and the calcaneal branches. Any or all of these may be affected, and hence there may be symptoms related to the entire sole or to only a part of it. The syndrome is due to trauma such as fracture or dislocation at the ankle.

Tendinitis of the posterior tibial or toe flexors may lead to swelling and compression of the posterior tibial nerve. The usual symptoms are pain in the sole of the foot, which resembles that of carpal tunnel syndrome in that it is of a burning quality. Pain during the night is characteristic, and is made worse following activity. Diagnosis is sometimes difficult as there are many causes of foot pain. Gentle percussion over the tarsal tunnel, which is behind and below the medial malleolus, produces tingling. Sensory loss in the distribution of the affected nerve may be present, and intrinsic muscle weakness may occur.

Treatment consists of anti-inflammatory drugs and a valgus insole. In resistant cases surgical decompression of the posterior tibial nerve may be necessary.

## 20.7.2 ANTERIOR TARSAL TUNNEL SYNDROME

The terminal branches of the deep peroneal nerve may be trapped beneath the dense superficial fascia of the ankle. The syndrome is also due to trauma to the dorsum of the foot. The nerve lies on bone and may be injured. Violent plantarflexion of the foot can also injure it. Symptoms are mainly numbness and paraesthesia on the dorsum of the foot, mainly in the first dorsal web space. The pain is made worse in certain positions of the foot such as plantarflexion and inversion, and may be relieved by dorsiflexion or eversion. Night pain and paraesthesia may be present as in the carpal tunnel syndrome.

Clinically there may be sensory loss in the first dorsal web space but the tips of the toes are usually not affected. Gentle tapping of the affected nerve may produce tingling. The extensor digitorum brevis muscle may be wasted and weak. Treatment consists of a local steroid injection and active prevention of excessive plantarflexion and inversion by the patient. In resistant cases extensive surgical release of the affected nerve from under the extensor retinaculum of the ankle to the dorsum of the mid-foot may have to be carried out.

## 20.8  Fractures of the ankle

The ankle and the subtalar joints are two hinge joints acting together as one unit. The ankle hinge has a transverse axis in the coronal plane and the subtalar hinge has an axis of 45° to the ground and 15° to the sagittal plane (Fig. 20.9). A hinge joining two segments at an angle functions as a torque converter and rotation of one segment causes rotation of the other segment (Rose, 1958). Hence supination of the foot causes external rotation of the tibia and pronation of the foot causes internal rotation of the tibia. This is a very important concept, because in walking a torque

427

Ankle injuries

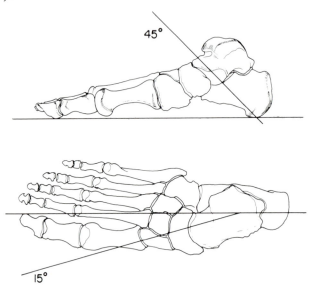

*Fig. 20.9* Diagrams to show the subtalar joint axis at 45° to the ground and 15° to the longitudinal axis of the foot.

force is applied to the ankle joint and in running this torque force can not only be great but also rapidly cyclic in nature and any accidental twisting of the foot during running, such as stepping into a pot hole or stumbling over high ground, can cause rotational injuries to the ankle.

The ankle joint can be injured by inversion, eversion, external rotation, internal rotation, plantarflexion, dorsiflexion or compression forces. Usually a combination of these forces (the commonest being inversion and external rotation) act resulting in a wide variety of fracture complexes. Basically the fractures can be stable or unstable in relation to the talus within the ankle mortice. The fractures are stable if there is no shift or no danger of shift of the talus within the ankle mortice. The fractures are unstable if the talus has shifted or is in danger of shifting within the ankle mortice. This talar shift is usually in a lateral direction but could also be posterolateral, anterolateral or medial.

The medial, lateral or posterior malleolus (the posterior lip of the lower end of tibia) can be fractured in combination with other fractures or ligamentous injuries.

A medial malleolar fracture may appear to be undisplaced but if there is a fracture gap then it has to be internally fixed, as there is usually some periosteal tissue interposed in the gap preventing bony union (Fig. 20.10).

The level of fracture of the lateral malleolus in a twisting injury of the

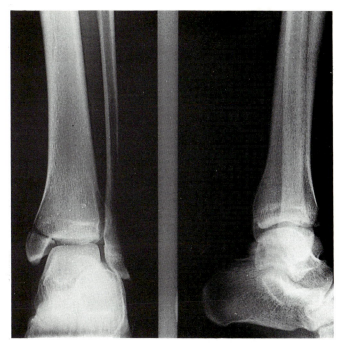

*Fig. 20.10*   Medial malleolar fracture with a gap.

ankle is important because it gives an indication of whether the inferior tibiofibular ligament is ruptured or not (Fig. 20.11(a) and (b)). The most common lateral malleolar fracture is an oblique fracture directed backwards and upwards from the level of the anterior inferior tibio-fibular ligament. In this fracture only part of the inferior tibiofibular ligament is ruptured and therefore there is no tibiofibular diastasis. If this fracture is below the inferior tibiofibular joint then this ligament has been spared. If it is above the joint then the ligament must have ruptured. The maissoneuve fracture is an extreme example of this where the spiral fracture is at the neck of the fibula (Fig. 20.12). It is very important to restore the length of the lateral malleolus when reducing the fracture or normal function of the ankle cannot be regained especially for the exacting demands of sporting activities.

A fracture of the posterior malleolus involving less than one-quarter of the articular surface can be treated conservatively by dorsiflexing the ankle joint to a plantargrade position as this would reduce the posterior malleolus since the posterior capsule is attached to it (Fig. 20.13). A fracture of the posterior malleolus involving more than one-quarter of the articular surface must be reduced accurately and internally fixed.

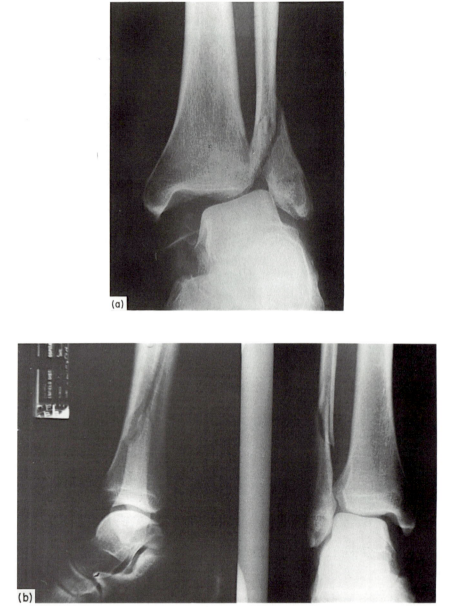

*Fig. 20.11* (a) The lateral malleolar fracture is at the level of the inferior tibiofibular joint but the ankle joint is unstable because of a complete medial ligament rupture. Note the flakes of bone detached with the medial ligament. (b) Fracture of the fibular above the inferior tibiofibular joint showing instability of the ankle joint due to disruption of the inferior tibiofibular joint.

430

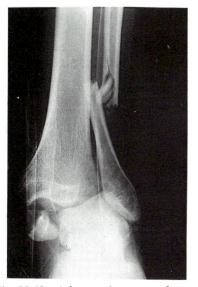

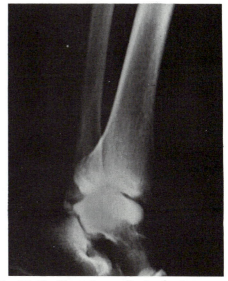

*Fig. 20.12*  A low maissoneuve fracture with a medial malleolar fracture.
The ankle is unstable due to disruption of the inferior tibiofibular joint.
The fibula can be fractured as high as
the neck and this could be missed if a
careful clinical examination is not
carried out.

*Fig. 20.13*  Posterior malleolar fracture.

A special type of fracture called the Tillaux fracture can be missed
unless one is aware of this entity and appreciates the gravity of this injury
(Fig. 20.14(a) and (b)). In a pronation external rotation injury a small
fragment of the anterior tibial lip of the inferior tibio-fibular joint is
avulsed by the anterior inferior tibiofibular ligament. This has to be
reduced and internally fixed.

Because an ankle injury is usually due to a twisting strain, the talus can
be crushed against the ankle mortice, causing damage to the articular
cartilage and subchondral bone. Unfortunately these intra-articular
injuries are very difficult to treat. If a large fragment of bone is sheared off
as in the 'dome' fracture (Nisbet, 1954) this has to be removed (Fig.
20.15(a)–(c)). The worst example of articular cartilage damage occurs
when the ankle joint is injured by a compression force combined with
rotational or other forces – the articular surface of the talus can be severely
damaged and as well gross comminution of the lower end of the tibia and
fibula can occur.

Accurate reduction of the lateral malleolus is very important, especially

431

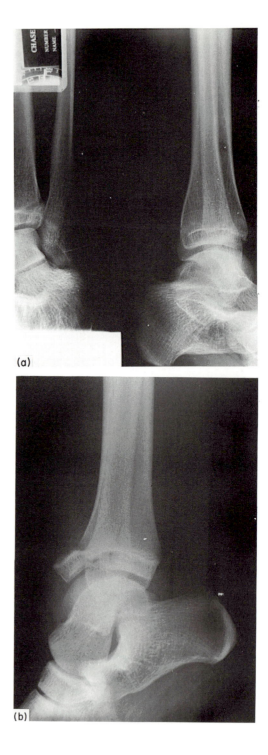

*Fig. 20.14* (a) Fracture of the anterior tibial lip of the inferior tibiofibular joint – Tillaux fracture. (b) An adolescent type of Tillaux fracture where a much larger fragment of the anterior tibial lip including a portion of the inferior tibial epiphysis is avulsed.

432

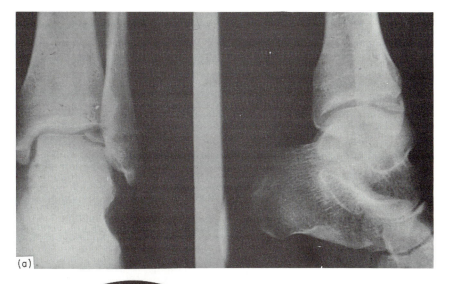

*Fig. 20.15* (a) A dome fracture of the talus, usually at the lateral corner of the dome. (b), (c) Arthroscopic appearances of a dome fracture showing the osteochondral fragment. (Courtesy of David Dandy.)

(a)

(b)

(c)

433

# Ankle injuries

in the athlete, otherwise residual pain will persist due to impingement of the tip of the lateral malleolus on the talus. A slight lateral shift of the talus may occur with a displaced lateral malleolar fracture, and if this displacement is not reduced by accurately reducing the fracture, pain, swelling and stiffness of the ankle will occur, preventing the patient from participating in active sports.

In football, the foot can be violently plantarflexed if it strikes an immovable object such as the ground, as in a miskick when tackled, and this can cause a fracture of the posterior malleolus of the tibia due to posterior subluxation of the talus as well as damage to either or both of the medial and lateral ligaments. Needless to say, if the patient is to return to his sport, accurate reduction of the fracture is important.

Osteochondral fractures of the dome of the talus can occur either in isolation or in combination with other fractures around the ankle. They are caused by impingement of the talus in the ankle mortice shearing off a small osteochondral fragment. When undisplaced they are treated with plaster immobilization for three weeks followed by intensive physiotherapy. When displaced they should be removed. Fortunately the fragment is usually a small one, and its removal does not appear to cause any functional problems, although from a long-term point of view post-traumatic osteoarthritis may occur due to damage to the articular surface.

## 20.9   Diagnosis

In an ankle 'sprain', always suspect a serious injury, either a ligamentous rupture or a fracture, till proved otherwise. The ankle is usually swollen and painful by the time the patient attends for examination. A careful history will elicit the mechanism of injury and also the magnitude of force applied to the ankle. A previous history of a 'weak' ankle or previous trauma may lead one to suspect a severe ligamentous injury if there is no bony injury.

Careful clinical examination should elicit points of maximum tenderness which give an indication of the ligaments injured. A tender anterior inferior tibiofibular ligament usually indicates a rotational injury. The degree of bruising gives the extent of damage. A large haematoma or boggy feel over the major ligaments may be an indication of a complete ligament rupture. The fibula should be gently palpated from top to bottom to exclude a high spiral fracture. X-rays of the ankle, not only the standard anteroposterior and lateral views, but also oblique views and dome views of the talus are important. Tiny flakes of bone within the ankle joint and the presence of loose fragments in the joint may be the only clue to intra-articular fractures.

434

Examinations using an image intensifier, and stress films of the ankle preferably under a general anaesthetic, will unmask a complete rupture of the inferior tibiofibular ligament in an apparently normal looking ankle. Tilting of the talus when an eversion stress is applied indicates a ruptured medial ligament. Anteroposterior subluxation can be demonstrated if the anterior talofibular ligament is ruptured. A trial reduction of a posterior malleolar fragment can be carried out by dorsiflexing the ankle to see whether it would reduce completely or whether it would require open reduction and internal fixation.

## 20.10   Treatment

In order to ensure that an individual returns to sporting activities it is very important to obtain perfect reduction and adequate fixation of the fractures. It would be far worse to fix surgically a fracture imperfectly than to accept a slight displacement by conservative management. All unstable ankle fractures must be surgically treated. At the same time the soft tissues around the ankle joint should not be unnecessarily interfered with or damaged. Therefore careful planning of the various skin incisions must be done beforehand.

In addition to dealing with the fractures it is necessary to repair any complete ruptures of the medial or lateral ligaments. If the inferior tibiofibular ligament is ruptured the fibula is internally fixed, usually with a plate and screws, and the stability of the inferior tibiofibular joint is tested using an image intensifier. If there is widening of this joint when stressed then a diastasis screw must be used, which should then be removed after eight weeks.

Following surgery it is important to rest the leg on two pillows and to elevate the foot of the bed for forty-eight hours till any oedema settles. At the same time the ankle is gently mobilized but only dorsiflexion and plantarflexion exercises are permitted. If ruptured ligaments have been repaired a hinged ankle cast brace is applied to prevent accidental inversion and eversion. The patient can be mobilized non-weightbearing using crutches after a week and gentle flexion/extension ankle exercises are continued. At the end of six weeks the cast brace is removed and partial weightbearing with crutches started. At the end of eight weeks the patient may fully weightbear with crutches or sticks. At the end of twelve weeks full weightbearing and gradual return to normal activities with sports training are permitted, leading progressively to full sporting activities at four months.

# Ankle injuries

## References

Bromberger, A. (1982) The pathology and treatment of lumps in the tendo Achillis. *J. Bone Joint Surg.*, **64B**, 118.

Christensen, I. B. (1953) Rupture of the Achilles tendon. Analysis of 57 cases. *Acta Chir. Scand.*, **106**, 50.

Coombs, R. R. H. (1981) Prospective trial of conservative and surgical treatment of Achilles tendon rupture. *J. Bone Joint Surg.*, **63B**, 288.

Coombs, R. R. H., Klenerman, L., Narcisi, P., *et al.* (1980) Collagen typing in Achilles tendon rupture. *J. Bone Joint Surg.*, **62B**, 258.

De Stefano, V. (1975) Pathogenesis and diagnosis of ruptured Achilles tendon. *Orthop. Rev.*, **4**, 17.

Escalas, F., Figueras, J. M. and Merino, J. A. (1980) Dislocation of the peroneal tendons. *J. Bone Joint Surg.*, **62A**, 451.

Freeman, M. A. R. (1965a) Treatment of ruptures of the lateral ligament of the ankle. *J. Bone Joint Surg.*, **47B**, 661.

Freeman, M. A. R. (1965b) Instability of the foot after injuries to the lateral ligament of the ankle. *J. Bone Joint Surg.*, **47B**, 669.

Freeman, M. A. R. and Wyke, B. D. (1964) The innervation of the cat's knee joint. *J. Anat.*, **98**, 299.

Hicks, J. H. (1961) The three weight-bearing mechanisms of the foot, in *Studies of the Musculo-Skeletal System* (ed. F. Gaynor Evans), Charles C. Thomas, Springfield, Illinois, p. 172.

Inglis, A. E., Scott, W. N., Sculco, T. P. and Ponterson, A. H. (1970) Ruptures of the tendo Achillis. An objective assessment of surgical and non-surgical treatment. *J. Bone Joint Surg.*, **58A**, 990.

Kvist, H. and Kvist, M. (1980) The operative treatment of chronic calcaneal paratenonitis. *J. Bone Joint Surg.*, **62B**, 353.

Lagergren, C. and Lindholm, A. (1958) Vascular distribution in the Achilles tendon. *Acta Chir. Scand.*, **116**, 491.

Lambert, K. L. (1971) The weight bearing function of the fibula. *J. Bone Joint Surg.*, **53A**, 507.

Lea, R. B. and Smith, L. (1968) Rupture of the Achilles tendon, non-surgical treatment. *Clin. Orthop.*, **60**, 115.

Lipscomb, P. R. (1950) Non-suppurative tenosynovitis and paratendinitis. Instructional Course Lectures, Vol. 7, American Academy of Orthopaedic Surgeons.

Ljunqvist, R. (1968) Subcutaneous partial rupture of the Achilles tendon. *Acta Orthop. Scand.*, Supplement, 113.

Ma, G. W. C. and Griffith, T. G. (1977) Percutaneous repair of acute closed ruptured Achilles tendon. *Clin. Orthop.*, **128**, 247.

Monk, C. J. E. (1969) Injuries of the tibio-fibular ligaments. *J. Bone Joint Surg.*, **51B**, 330.

Nisbet, N. W. (1954) Dome fracture of the talus. *J. Bone Joint Surg.*, **36B**, 244.

Nistor, L. (1981) Surgical and non-surgical treatment of Achilles tendon rupture. *J. Bone Joint Surg.*, **63A**, 394.

Rose, G. K. (1958) Correction of the pronated foot. *J. Bone Joint Surg.*, **40B**, 674.

Williams, R. (1963) Chronic nonspecific tendosynovitis of the tibialis posterior. *J. Bone Joint Surg.*, **45B**, 542.

# 21 *Foot problems*

BASIL HELAL

The foot is in use in virtually every sport and even in those sports where it plays little part, such as shooting, a foot problem giving rise to pain can distract the sportsman and produce a poor performance. Indeed Hippocrates said 'He who has pain in the foot has pain everywhere'. The foot ranks in functional importance with the hip and knee, for equivalent weight and stress is taken by it.

Analysis of the reasons for consultations during the Olympic Games (1980) reveals that foot problems were responsible for some 18% of the visits. Of these 70% of the problems were avoidable, 50% were due to deficient footwear and 20% avoidable by foot hygiene and nail care. Of the remainder 28% arose because of intrinsic disorders of shape and alignment and other pathology and only 2% were due to direct injury in the course of the sport.

## 21.1  Foot deformities

These are often compatible with high performance sporting activity. It is common to encounter minor degrees of cavus or valgus feet or metatarsus varus and these can be symptomless and do not inhibit performance. A patient seen in Zurich five years ago had a forefoot that was so severely supinated that he walked on the dorsum of the foot. He proved to be a successful inside forward of a good class local amateur football team and was totally free from symptoms!

## 21.2  Referred pain

It must always be borne in mind that pain, particularly on the outer border of the foot can be produced by lumbar disc lesions and peroneal nerve entrapment in the peroneal canal round the neck of the fibula or superficial peroneal nerve entrapment as it emerges from the deep fascia, some 10 cm above the external malleolus. This gives rise to pain and numbness on the dorsum of the foot (Henry, 1945; Kernohan, Levack and Wilson, 1985). Symptoms can be relieved by surgical decompression at the appropriate site. Pain may also arise because of vascular insufficiency and pulses should always be felt. Ischaemia of the intrinsic muscles or an impending Volkmann contracture of the intrinsics can produce severe plantar pain.

## 21.3   Muscle cramp

This is usually circulatory in nature and can be due to vascular insufficiency, either proximal in the limb or due to arteriolar spasm secondary to cold. Occasionally it is due to insufficiency of venous return or overuse and fatigue of the intrinsic muscles. Stretching of the toes into extension usually produces relief. It is important to check the calcium level to exclude a tetanic cause.

## 21.4   The skin

In snorkelling and scuba diving, stepping on sea urchin spines requires individual removal of barbs or application of papaya paste to dissolve them. Coral cuts, particularly fire coral, can produce blisters and itching. Blisters from chafing by ill-fitting shoes should be treated by evacuation leaving the overlying dead epidermal layer as a dressing. Swimmers or users of communal showers can pick up fungal infections and infective viral warts. Prophylaxis by careful washing and application of antifungal powders will avoid this hazard. Chronic fungal infections may be caused to persist especially in the fourth web space where the toes are 'tight packed', producing a lack of drainage and constant moist environment. An osteotomy of the base of the proximal phalanx producing some abduction of the little toe will solve this problem if all conservative measures, including systemic antifungal drugs, fail. Viral warts should be treated with podophyllum and kept isolated by dressings. If the wart is not responding then curettage under local anaesthetic is indicated.

## 21.5   Callosities

These can be pared down but if examination reveals a footwear or underlying cause such as foot deformity or 'dropped' metatarsal head then a suitable orthosis or, if necessary, corrective surgery is indicated.

## 21.6 Nails

A common injury to the nail is the subungual haematoma produced by a shoe with too much 'recoil' (Fig. 21.1(a) and (b)) due to too springy a sole. Whitlows due to ingrowing nails can be a great nuisance to the sportsman. Initially wedge resection or simple avulsion of the nail to allow drainage will relieve pain and may allow participation in the sport almost immediately.

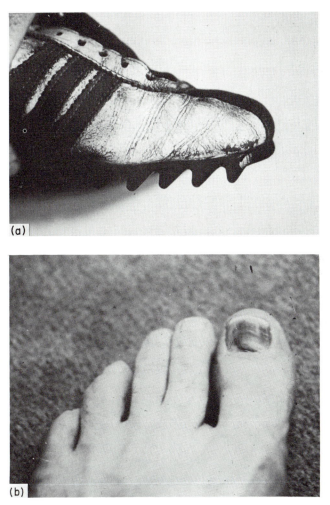

(a)

(b)

*Fig. 21.1* This type of springy sole (a) can produce the great toe nail lesion shown by excessive 'recoil' (b).

439

## Foot problems

Recurrent problems with the nail are best treated by radical ablation of the nail bed. I like to use the chiropodial technique of phenolization of the collateral margins of the nail bed to ensure destruction of the matrix at these sites.

Prolonged immersion of the foot in water in sailing and rowing can produce blisters and cooling of the wet foot in ill-fitting skiboots can produce frostbite. It is important to note that frostbite can produce premature fusion of the epiphysis in the growing child and this can result in serious growth disturbances. Frostbitten areas are now treated by rapid warming by immersion in a warm bath.

### 21.7 Tendons

Tenosynovitis of the peronei or of the tendons in the tarsal tunnel may occur due to abnormal pressure on these sites due to footwear or to malalignment of the foot associated with excessive use. Ice, rest and steroid injections can be of help. Persistent synovitis should lead one to think of disease of the synovium as in connective tissue disease or villonodular synovitis. Occasionally, synovitis of one of the toe flexors or extensors can occur.

### 21.8 Cystic lumps

These cysts frequently arise from adjacent joints or may be enlargements of existing bursae. They are usually annoying because they take up space in the shoe. They may respond to needling and evacuation of the contents but may need excision to effect a permanent cure. If they are removed they should always be sent for histology – particularly the intermetatarsal bursa which causes adjacent toes to divaricate on weightbearing – for they may be the harbinger of rheumatoid disease.

### 21.9 Fractures and dislocations

Any of the foot bones may be fractured. Sports such as parachuting, gliding, motor cycle and car racing and sometimes pole vaulting have produced some very serious fractures. In karate the foot is used as a weapon and the front kick can produce fractured sesamoids of the great toe. The 'knife edge' kick can fracture the fifth metatarsal base. Inversion sprains can cause avulsion fracture of the fifth metatarsal which occasionally gives rise to non-union if the fragments are separated and it often saves time and trouble to fix (by a screw) those that are separated.

440

Fractures of the talus, especially those involving the body or neck, can result in avascular necrosis as can talar dislocation. Fractures of the os calcis involving the subtalar joint and with loss of the talar angle give rise to controversy with regards to their management but it is thought are best managed by elevation and grafting and early mobilization. Tarsal fractures involving joints should be kept non-weightbearing, compressed and mobilized early.

## 21.10   Stress fractures

The os calcis can be involved, especially in dancers, and stress fractures of both the os calcis and talus have been described. Otherwise these mostly occur in the metatarsals, most commonly the second or third. In the early stages when there are no X-ray changes a technetium scan will show an area of activity. The treatment consists of support and rest followed by progressive activity (see also Section 21.25).

## 21.11   Heel pain

This may occur behind the heel at the insertion of the tendo achillis and can be due to a pulling osteochondritis, damaging the apophysis of the os calcis, usually before the age of sixteen years when it fuses. This is called Severs osteochondritis and is treated by rest and raising the heel. This is preferably done with an impact absorbing polymer (sorbothane) and will always resolve without more active measures.

There are two bursae related to the insertion of the Achilles tendon, one deep to the tendon and one superficial, one or both of which may inflame and give rise to symptoms (Fig. 21.2). If they do not respond to conserva-

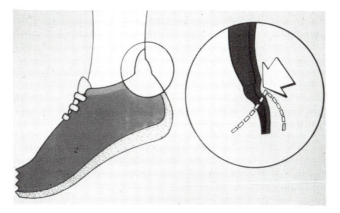

*Fig. 21.2*   The heel tab can be a source of injury to the Achilles tendon.

tive measures such as heel inserts and rest or steroid infiltration they may need excision.

## 21.12   The posterior heel exostosis

This may be accompanied by an overlying bursitis. Removing the stiffener from the shoe and inserting a soft back may solve this problem, as may a change in the height of the shoe back. Occasionally, removal of the exostosis is necessary. If it is centrally placed and cannot be removed without damage to the insertion of the Achilles tendon, then a dorsally based closing wedge osteotomy of the os calcis just anterior to the Achilles tendon will produce an effective cure.

## 21.13   Bony heel spurs

These occur at the heel attachment of the plantar ligament. They are common and are of no significance. I have never found an indication to excise them and where they have been excised elsewhere, more often than not, no benefit accrues.

## 21.14   Jogger's foot

Pain in the heel and medial plantar aspect of the foot can be the result of medial calcaneal neuritis. The medial calcaneal and plantar branches of the posterior tibial nerve give off medial calcaneal and plantar branches which can be damaged by the overlying fascia when the foot is pronated. If correction of pronation by orthosis does not help then a steroid injection into the area just below the tarsal tunnel is carried out. Occasionally surgical release of the fascia is necessary (Rask, 1978).

## 21.15   Plantar fascia

Acute tears of the plantar fascia or fatigue of intrinsic muscles with subsequent microtears of the fascia of the foot can produce pain. Because the plantar fascia is mobile anteriorly and fixed at the heel it tends to tear posteriorly giving rise to heel pad pain. Treatment should be directed to supporting the longitudinal arch with a well built up valgus support and intrinsic exercises. An injection of local anaesthetic and steroid helps produce a rapid relief of symptoms and anti-inflammatory medicines such as Brufen are useful.

Chronic problems can sometimes be relieved by local radiotherapy or, as a last resort, a release of the plantar fascia at the heel (Steindler operation) may be indicated. It is important in persistent plantar fasciitis to exclude conditions such as rheumatoid arthritis, gout and ankylosing spondylitis and Reiter's disease, all of which may present in this manner.

## 21.16 Tarsal tunnel syndrome

The tarsal tunnel is a compartment lying behind and beneath the internal malleolus which is bounded by fascial and ligamentous walls and contains the tibialis posterior and toe flexor tendons and the vessels and nerves passing to the sole of the foot.

Rarely entrapment of the posterior tibial nerve may occur, usually secondary to a tenosynovitis here, giving rise to paraesthesia, pain and burning sensation in the sole of the foot and medial three toes. Compression of this compartment will reproduce the symptoms and this can be confirmed by electrical conduction tests. If local steroid injections and an inner side heel wedge do not restore normality then decompression of the tarsal tunnel is carried out.

## 21.17 Anterior tarsal syndrome

The anterior tarsal syndrome (Edwards *et al.*, 1969; Gessini, Jandolo and Pietrangel, 1984) consists of aching and paraesthesiae felt on the dorsum of the foot. The physical signs are numbness of the first web space between the great and second toes, a positive Tinel sign on percussion over the anterior tibial (deep peroneal) nerve in front of the ankle and electrical evidence of denervation of extensor digitorum brevis. It is due to an entrapment of the anterior tibial (deep peroneal) nerve beneath the inferior extensor retinaculum of the ankle. Local steroid injection will settle the majority of cases but if there are persistent symptoms then a decompression by surgical division of the retinaculum may be necessary.

## 21.18 Midtarsal problems

Pain in the midtarsal area may be due to an osteochondritis of the navicular bone (Kohler's disease) in the growing child – this results in a 'crush' of the bone which then gradually returns to normal. Pain is the feature and it is diagnosed by X-ray. No active measure other than rest is necessary. A similar condition with avascular necrosis may rarely occur in the adult. This condition is not so benign and destruction of the adjacent midtarsal joint and the joint between this and the cuneiform bones may occur and require subsequent fusion. Both these conditions have been seen in sports people diagnosed and treated as sprains by trainers, including one in a Sussex fast bowler.

### 21.19 Sinus tarsi syndrome

The sinus tarsi syndrome (Taillard *et al.*, 1981) consists of pain and tenderness over the lateral side of the sinus tarsi and a feeling of ankle instability on uneven ground. Symptoms are decreased by infiltration with local anaesthetic. The syndrome is associated with one or more ankle sprains and it is not certain whether these precipitate or follow upon disturbance of the subtalar joint. Arthrography reveals rupture of the subtalar joint capsule and disappearance of the recesses along the inter-osseous ligament. Electromyography reveals no tone in the peroneus longus and brevis. Conservative management involves rest, sometimes for two to three weeks in plaster, followed by rehabilitation particularly of proprioception with exercises on a balancing board. Surgical treatment consists of excision of the tissue filling the lateral portion of the sinus tarsi for 1–1.5 cm. Resistant cases have been subjected to fusion of the subtalar joint.

### 21.20 Osteochondritis dissecans of the talar head

Two long distance runners have presented with midtarsal pain and have proved to have this problem. One of them required removal of a loose osteochondral fragment.

### 21.21 The 'overbone'

This is an osteophyte overlying the dorsum of the medial cuneiform and first metatarsal joint. In longstanding cases there is an overlying bursa. Usually sponge padding of the tongue of the shoe suffices. Occasionally these osteophytes need to be excised.

### 21.22 Cuboid instability syndrome

The cuboid instability syndrome (Newell and Woodle, 1981) is said to comprise 4% of 'athletic' foot conditions and most of those with this problem in Newell's series had pronated feet. Pain is felt vaguely on the outer border of the foot or over the fourth and fifth metatarsals, especially when walking or running on uneven ground. The condition is often mistaken for peroneal tendinitis or stress fracture of the cuboid. A calcaneo navicular bar should be excluded by appropriate radiographs.

The theory is that with the foot pronated, the midtarsal joint is lax and the peroneus longus has a strong mechanical advantage which moves the lateral margin of the cuboid dorsally and the medial side tilts down 'locking' the cuboid. A manipulation is carried out which reverses this, that is the cuboid is pushed upwards and laterally from its medial and plantar aspect.

### 21.23   Short leg syndrome

Leg length discrepancy is said to occur in some 40% of the athletes examined by Subotnick (1981). Some have real skeletal shortening and others are due to abnormal joint positioning. These patients tend to externally rotate the leg on the short side dropping excessive weight onto the medial aspect of the foot and forcing this into pronation, resulting in pain. Correction of length by an appropriate raise and a correct orthosis for the foot until symptoms abate is all that is necessary.

### 21.24   Pronated foot problems

Excessive pronation (eversion) results in aching feet, particularly along the medial border, and pain in the dorsiflexor and everter muscles. Secondarily shin splints and backache may occur. On examination hallux valgus, an enlarged abductor hallucis muscle and claw toes are all supportive signs. Corrective exercises to the inverters are very important and orthoses to tilt the foot into supination are helpful.

### 21.25   The great toe metatarsophalangeal joint

#### 21.25.1   HALLUX VALGUS

This can be a serious problem, especially to the ballet dancer who has to dance on points. This often means the end of a dancing career unless a careful realignment is carried out. It is important to align the joint horizontal to the ground when the dancer is on points and this is best achieved by a double osteotomy at the base of the proximal phalanx and at the neck of the first metatarsal. Alignment is adjusted and the ray

445

transfixed by a fine Kirchner wire to stabilize the position for four weeks.

Other forms of hallux valgus can be managed by osteotomy if the metatarsophalangeal joint is mobile (Helal, 1977, 1981b).

## 21.25.2 HALLUX RIGIDUS

There are two causes for this condition: an osteochondritis dissecans of the first metatarsal head and, more rarely, a chondromalacia of the sesamoids of the great toe leading on to degenerative changes (Fig. 21.3).

Any form of arthroplasty of the joint will end a top class athletic career. Usually pain is experienced because of a block to extension of this joint. If the arc of movement is shifted dorsally then very often comfortable running can be continued (Fig. 21.4). This is achieved by a dorsally based wedge osteotomy of the neck of the proximal phalanx or the neck of the first metatarsal if there is a request to correct a concomitant valgus deformity of the joint. This procedure frequently produces an additional benefit in some regression of the osteoarthrosis of the joint due to the biological effects of the osteotomy (Brooks and Helal, 1968).

## 21.26  Lateral metatarsalgia

### 21.26.1  STRESS FRACTURE

This is due to progressive trabecular failure under repeated overload. Malalignment, fatigue of muscles or stretching of ligaments which normally take some of the stress off the underlying bone or a malalignment of the foot resulting in abnormal overload is the basic cause. Pain is the presenting feature; occasionally there is swelling. No X-ray changes are visible initially but periosteal bone appears around the site two to three weeks later. A technetium scan will show a hot spot before any bone changes are visible radiologically.

Various causes for this have been seen in athletes. Fatigue or stress fractures of the second, third or fourth and, more rarely, of the fifth metatarsal have all been observed. Occasionally first ray problems have been the initiating cause by forcing the athlete to supinate the forefoot and so place added stress on the lateral metatarsals.

### 21.26.2  'DROPPED' METATARSAL HEADS

This perhaps is a misnomer as Martorell (1971) and others have shown that what seems to happen is that the metatarsal involved in fact loses its mobility at the tarsometatarsal joint and so does not rise under load. If orthoses cannot solve the problem then a telescoping metatarsal

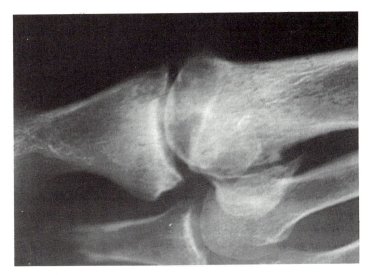

*Fig. 21.3* The sesamo-metatarsal degeneration preceded the general arthrosis of this great toe metatarsophalangeal joint.

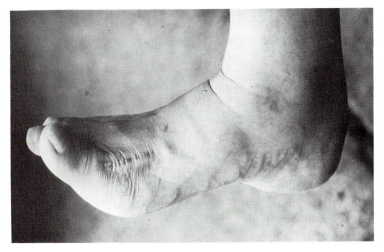

*Fig. 21.4* A dorsally based wedge osteotomy in this, a cross country runner, with hallux rigidus enabled this degree of great toe metatarsophalangeal extension with relief of symptoms.

osteotomy relieves the symptoms and can be carried out on high performance athletes with success (Fig. 21.5(a)–(d); Helal, 1975).

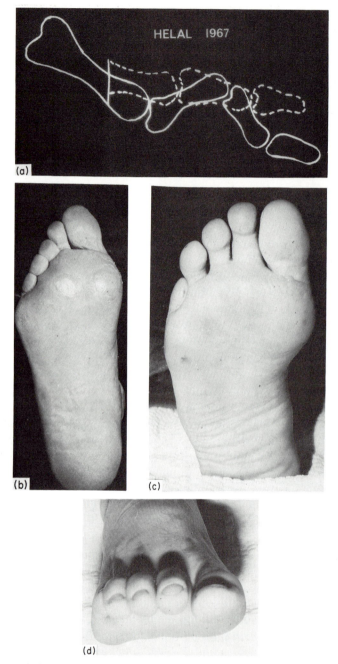

*Fig. 21.5* (a) This type of osteotomy has converted this foot (b) with callosities to (c) without. Note the restoration of metatarsal alignment in (d).

### 21.26.3 OSTEOCHONDRITIS OF THE METATARSAL HEADS (FRIEBERG, PANNER, KOHLER'S SECOND DISEASE)

This is a condition encountered in sports people before maturity. It is due in fact to a dorsal crush of the epiphysis. If encountered in the early stages it should be treated by a dorsal cancellous bone graft which will restore the shape of the metatarsal head and restore the integrity of the joint affected permanently. In the later stages, when there has been distortion of the metatarsophalangeal joint, an osteotomy allowing the head to telescope is sometimes very effective in relieving discomfort. Alternatively, if the joint has to be excised then it is best to carry the excision out on the base of the proximal phalanx inserting a small silicone elastomer spacer.

### 21.26.4 BUNIONETTE OF THE FIFTH METATARSAL HEAD

This is usually secondary to a valgus fifth metatarsal. Excision of the prominent portion of the metatarsal head gives poor results. The condition is best treated by an osteotomy of the neck of the fifth metatarsal to displace the head medially (Fig. 21.6).

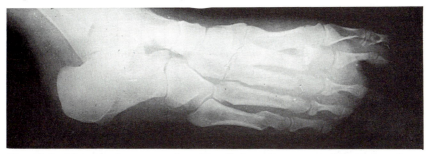

*Fig. 21.6* Metatarsal osteotomies. The little toe metatarsal head has been displaced medially for a bunionette deformity.

### 21.26.5 MORTON'S NEUROMA

The nerve is compressed either by the intermetatarsal ligament or by an intermetatarsal bursa. The typical symptoms are present in both, namely, burning pain in a cleft usually between the third and fourth toes, but it can occur in the others. In the case of a bursa, weightbearing causes the affected pair of toes to divaricate. Excision of the bursa or the neuroma or division of the intermetatarsal ligament alone will effect a cure if supports and intrinsic exercises should fail. The excised bursal tissue should always be sent for histology as it has been shown that the bursitis may have a rheumatoid origin (Shepherd and Vernon Roberts, 1975).

Foot problems

## 21.27 Toe deformities

Congenital overlap of little toes, clawed toes and hammered toes are not infrequently seen in sports people who perform to a high standard. If correction is required then this is usually by surgery. The overlapped little toe is best treated by V–Y plasty of the skin combined with flexor to extensor tendon transfer (Helal and Chen, 1978).

Similar management is recommended for mobile claw toes (Fig. 21.7). It is not recommended for the sprinter, who is best left untreated until his career is interrupted. Stiff claw toes require digital joint fusions in the corrected position. Hammer toes can be treated by excision of the proximal interphalangeal joint. Fusion is generally unnecessary unless correction is not held, in which case Kirchner wire fixation for six weeks is recommended.

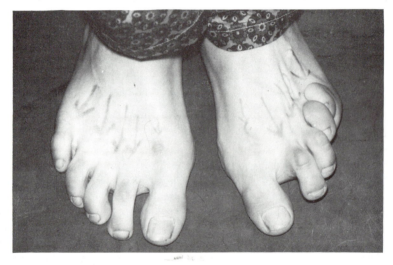

*Fig. 21.7*   The toes of a well known marathon runner. Callosities and sores over the dorsae of the proximal phalanges required corrective surgery in the form of realignment and fusions. He went on to win a race six months later.

## 21.28 The ossicles of the foot

There are numerous accessory bones in the foot. They divide into two categories: sesamoid bones which are laid down in cartilage and are a regular and typical part of the skeleton, and true ossicles formed from embryonic elements which, instead of disappearing, sometimes persist.

450

Some of them, occasionally in man, are atavistic but are always present in certain animals. It is important to be aware of the likely sites for ossicles as they may be mistaken for fractures. Generally speaking the true ossicles are applied to an adjacent major bone by fibrous tissue, whereas sesamoids are closely applied to a tendon and very frequently have one surface forming part of a synovial joint.

### 21.28.1 OS TRIGONUM

It is said (Quirk, 1982) that this is sometimes a source of symptoms, especially in activities which require a good deal of ankle flexion as in ballet dancers on points, and may sometimes have to be removed if giving rise to persistent pain. The author's experience as advisor to a ballet school suggests that the condition is very uncommon. One dancer who presented with symptoms in this area that were not due to a stress fracture of the os calcis or an Achilles or deep bursal problem had had the os trigonum removed and was suffering discomfort from local scarring and adhesions (Table 21.1).

*Table 21.1* Athletes with foot sesamoid problems

| | |
|---|---|
| Great toe sesamoids | 16 |
| Tibiale externum (accessory navicular) | 2 |
| Peroneal sesamoid | 1 |

Two other ossicles, the tibiale externum (Fig. 21.8(a), (b) and (c)) and the peroneal ossicle have presented as persistent problems in athletes. In two patients, both male cross country runners, seventeen and twenty-two, the tibiale externum was the site of pain and in one patient, a professional cyclist at twenty-six, the peroneal sesamoid was at fault. All three patients had had a considerable number of conservative treatments, including supports, rest in plaster and steroid injections. All three lost their symptoms after excision of these bones and were able to return to perform their sport at their former standards. Macroscopically and histologically the excised ossicles show classical chondromalacic changes (Fig. 21.8(c)).

### 21.28.2 SESAMOIDS

The sesamoids under the head of the great toe metatarsal are constant and problems associated with these are not excessively rare (Fig. 21.9; Helal, 1981a).

451

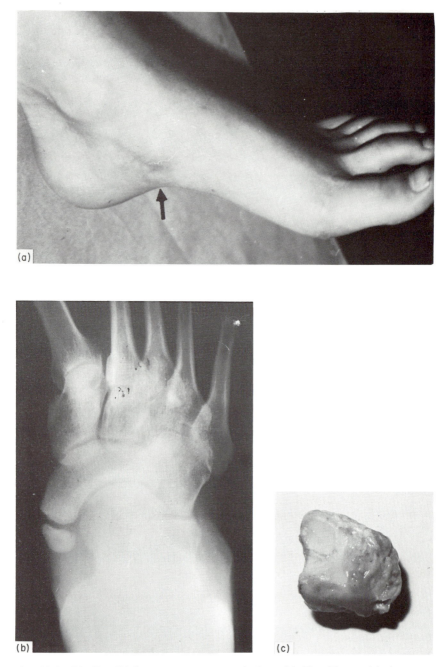

*Fig. 21.8* (a) Os tibiale or accessory navicular. (b) The X-ray. (c) Appearance of excised os tibiale showing malacic changes in the lining cartilage.

452

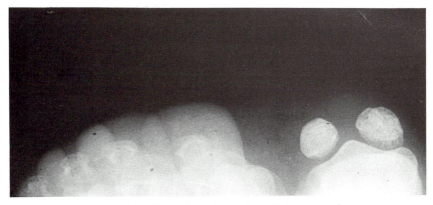

*Fig. 21.9* 'Crush' fracture of medial sesamoid.

The great toe sesamoids have an interesting background in mythology. Named 'Albadaran' by the ancient Arabs they were considered to have magical properties. The Rabbi Ushaia in 400 AD sought the seat of the soul and inspected the old graves in his quest. He noted that the best preserved bones were the sesamoid bones (probably because they are compact and not too riddled with vascular channels). He therefore decided that these were the repository for the soul and on the day of judgement they would be watered with celestial dew, whereupon the body would be reconstituted around them. He stated this with such conviction that 1000 years later in Caspar Bauhinus' textbook of anatomy it was noted that 'the sesamoids are the seat of the soul'.

Experimentation and clinical studies have confirmed the close similarities between the patella and the great toe sesamoids, indeed they suffer many of the same injuries and pathological processes.

In the author's practice forty-four patients with pathology confined to the great toe sesamoids have been presented over a decade and of these sixteen were athletes: four women and twelve men, with age ranges from twelve to twenty-eight years (Table 21.2). All were in sports involving

*Table 21.2* Great toe sesamoid problems in the athlete's foot

| 12 Men<br>4 Women } 16 | Age<br>12–28 |
|---|---|

Fractures 8 (avulsion 6, crush 2)
Presesamoid bursitis 3
Infection 1
Chondromalacia 4

Foot problems

running or jumping; eight were fractures, six of the avulsion type, and two were crush fractures and diagnosed as so called 'osteochondritis'. Cadaver experiments producing crush fractures will result in identical X-ray appearances and indeed histology demonstrates healing fractures. Three had presesamoid bursitis; one had infection with a sinus leading to the sesamoid; four had typical chondromalacia (Fig. 21.10). All but two had excision of a sesamoid – generally the medial. One had a lateral sesamoid excised and two had both sesamoids excised.

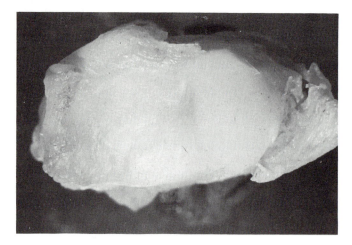

*Fig. 21.10*   Typical chondromalacia in an excised bipartite medial sesamoid.

The first patient with excision of both sesamoids developed a lateral metatarsalgia which was relieved by wearing a small rubber pad under the metatarsal head and the other had artificial sesamoids implanted. This patient was a jogger who slipped off a step on a bridge and hyperextended his great toe. He suffered a fractured lateral sesamoid and distraction of the two elements of a bipartite medial sesamoid. After much conservative treatment both were excised and in order to prevent lowering of the metatarsal head silicone rubber sesamoids were fashioned and implanted. It is now two years since his operation. He has been running painlessly for over a year (Fig. 21.11(a), (b) and (c)).

Eleven of the sixteen returned to their sport within three to six months. Eight achieved an athletic prowess of a standard equivalent to that before their troubles commenced. Two retired from competitive sport but played games such as tennis and squash and one, who had a degree of hallux rigidus, decided to give up sport entirely.

Conservative management consists of protecting the sesamoid from weightbearing for at least a six week period. Persistent pain suggests that

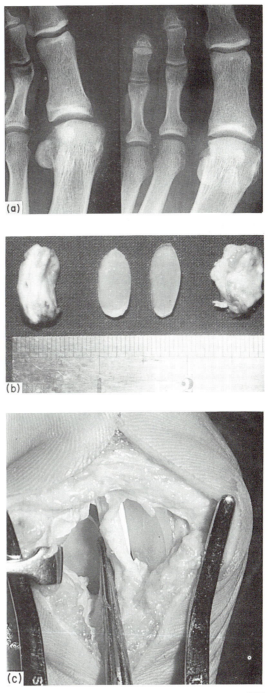

*Fig. 21.11* (a) The injury to the sesamoids. (b) The appearance of the damaged excised sesamoids and their silicone rubber replacements. (c) The silicone rubber sesamoids in place.

a surgical solution is necessary. If possible, avoid excision of both sesamoids. If this is necessary then silicone elastomer replacements may help to avoid the complication of lateral weight shift due to loss of height of the first metatarsal head. Awareness of the possibility of problems arising in the great toe sesamoids will uncover many more patients with similar problems.

The foot has been the 'Cinderella' of orthopaedic surgery. Fortunately a realization of its importance and complexity has dawned. The foot is a shock absorbing mechanism and a torque converter and its many intrinsic problems and its influence on the rest of the lower limb have aroused much interest. Foot societies have stimulated much research and discovery. Our understanding of foot problems and their solution is growing rapidly.

## A note on terminology

The term for tilting the sole to face outwards is eversion or pronation (following the same line as the ipsilateral forearm). Tilting the sole to face the midline is called inversion or supination. Pointing the foot downwards as in standing on tiptoe is equinus. Drawing the foot back so that the heel is the lowest point is called calcaneus.

## References

Brooks, M. and Helal, B. (1968) Primary osteoarthritis venous engorgement and osteogenesis. *J. Bone Joint Surg.*, **50B**, 493.

Edwards, W. G., Lincoln, C. R., Bassett, F. H. III and Goldner, L. J. (1969) The tarsal tunnel syndrome, diagnosis and treatment. *J. Amer. Med. Assoc.*, **207**, 716.

Gessini, L., Jandolo, G. and Pietrangel, A. (1984) Anterior tarsal syndrome. *J. Bone Joint Surg.*, **66A**, 786.

Helal, B. (1975) Metatarsal osteotomy for metatarsalgia. *J. Bone Joint Surg.*, **57B**, 187.

Helal, B. (1977) Surgery of the forefoot. *Brit. Med. J.*, **29 January**, 276.

Helal, B. (1981a) The great toe sesamoid bones. *Clin. Orthop. Rel. Res.*, **175**, 82.

Helal, B. (1981b) Surgery for adolescent hallux valgus. *Clin. Orthop. Rel. Res.*, June, 50.

Helal, B. and Chen, S. C. (1978) Flexor to extensor transfer for clawing of the lateral four toes, *Operative Surgery*, eds C. Rob and R. Smith, 3rd edn, Orthopaedics p. 917. Butterworths, London.

Henry, A. K. (1945) *Extensile Exposure*, E. and J. Livingstone, Edinburgh and London, p. 296.

456

# References

Kernohan, J., Levack, B. and Wilson, J. N. (1985) Entrapment of the superficial peroneal nerve. *J. Bone Joint Surg.*, **67B**, 60.

Martorell, J. (1971) Algunas aspectos de la metatarsalgia. *Podologie*, **6**, 159.

Newell, G. S. and Woodle, A. (1981) Cuboid instability syndrome. *Phys. Sportsmed.*, **9**, 71.

Quirk, R. (1982) Talar compression syndrome in dancers. *Foot and Ankle*, **3**, 65.

Rask, M. R. (1978) Medial plantar neuropraxia (jogger's foot). *Clin. Orthop.*, **134**, 193.

Shepherd, E. and Vernon Roberts, B. (1975) Paper read to the British Orthopaedic Foot Surgery Society.

Subotnick, S. K. (1981) Short leg syndrome. *J. Orthop. Sports*, **3**, 11, 16.

Taillard, W., Meyer, J. M., Garcia, J. and Blanc, Y. (1981) Sinus tarsi syndrome. *Int. Orthop.*, **5**, 117.

# 22 *Sports footwear*

MARGARET ELLIS

## 22.1 Introduction

A recent exhibition in the British Museum illustrated the evolution of sportswear (Fig. 22.1). There is now a vast range of sports footwear available. Many, almost identical, types of shoe are produced by different manufacturers. Despite recent changes and developments defects in design still remain in the final product. Many members of the public who find difficulties with ordinary shoes can find comfort in sports shoes. Some sports shoes are comparatively cheap, so that for an individual needing two different sized shoes for their right and left feet, the purchase of two pairs of running shoes may be cheaper than buying ordinary shoes. It is clear that the requirements necessary for walking every day in such shoes differ from those for running one or two hours each day since many sportsmen find problems in their sports footwear.

The foot needs to be flexible to adapt to its external environment and to be rigid to provide an effective thrust on push-off. During walking there is a rotation of the leg which starts at the pelvis and increases in magnitude in the distal segments of the lower limb. Thus it is 6° at the pelvis, 13° in the femur and 18° in the tibia. This rotation is internal in the swing phase and at the beginning of the stance phase, and external during the start of the walking cycle (Mann, 1975; Fig. 22.2).

The foot obtains its stability at push-off as a result of the external rotation that occurs when it is weightbearing. The subtalar joint is an oblique hinge so that when the talus is rotated the calcaneum rotates along an axis at right angles to the talar movement. Thus, when the foot is on the ground external rotation of the leg will produce inversion of the heel and internal rotation will produce eversion of the heel. This, combined with the windlass effect of the plantar fascia which tightens as the toes are extended for push-off, stabilizes the joints of the foot giving it the necessary rigidity for an efficient propulsion thrust. Some people

459

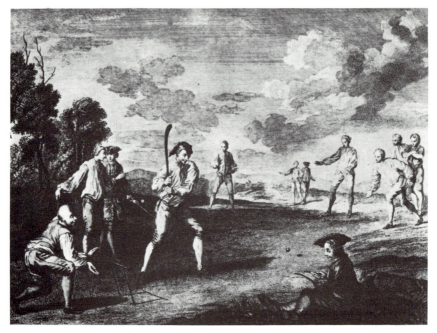

*Fig. 22.1* Examples of early English sports: cricket (a) and tennis (b) (courtesy of the British Museum).

have a greater or lesser tendency to internal or external rotation in the leg with resulting 'in' or 'out' toed gait.

Any abnormality of rotation in any section of the lower limb will be reflected in an abnormal gait. This will lead to an alteration in the wear pattern of the shoes. The pressures involved in walking are increased when running. The constant positioning of the foot inside the shoe is accentuated. Thrust and heel strike over prolonged periods will markedly increase potential areas of pressure. Abnormal distal pressures can of course be translated proximally and damage proximal joints. The knee is especially vulnerable to injury from unsuitable types of shoe and length of cleat (Torg and Quendenfeld, 1971). The repetitive actions involved in running and jumping will lead to abnormal pressure inside the shoe and explain some of the difficulties experienced by sportspeople with their sports footwear. The position of the foot on landing is therefore important (Fig. 22.3). Depending on whether the foot is in a neutral, inverted or everted position on landing, the pressure on the sole of the foot will be 'normal' or disturbed. An abnormal foot pressure distribution will result in abnormal wear on the sole of the shoe. There are recognized patterns of 'normal' shoe sole wear (Fig. 22.4).

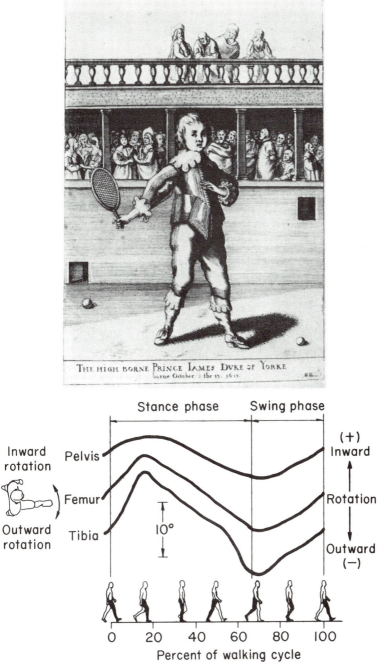

Fig. 22.2  Rotation in the lower limb during the normal walking cycle.

461

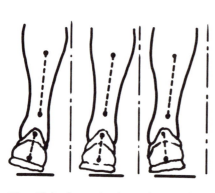

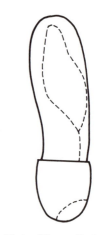

Fig. 22.3 Inversion/eversion variations on landing.

Fig. 22.4 'Normal' shoe wear.

Major deviation from normal shoe wear can be observed by inspection of the sole of the shoe, for example, in situations where the lateral border of the foot takes a majority of the body weight. The wear on the sole may also help to indicate any tendency to inversion or excessive eversion on landing. Shoes generally reduce the peak pressure areas especially at the heel and first metatarsal head when compared to barefoot walking. The inside of the shoe may show pressure patterns even more clearly and may also indicate other abnormalities such as squashed toes or abnormal sweating.

A survey of the literature on sports footwear has been undertaken from medical and sports journals, manufacturers of sports footwear and advertisements. Shoe adaptations and orthoses have also been included. A postal questionnaire has been sent to all the participants in the British Olympic field and track events to seek information on their methods of shoe selection, preference and experience. The questions also covered any foot problems thought to have been caused by faulty shoe design. A similar questionnaire was circulated among a group of patients attending The London Hospital Sports Clinic and among a number of other sports enthusiasts. Other information was sought from a large department store in London having a sizeable sports section. The author is most grateful to all those who assisted with their helpful contributions.

## 22.2 Shoe design

The range of shoes available can be rather bewildering. There are now more than two hundred types of road running shoes available in the

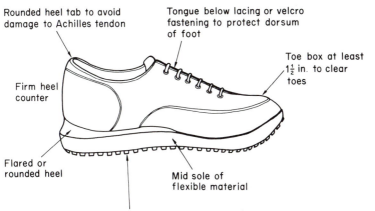

Rounded heel tab to avoid damage to Achilles tendon

Tongue below lacing or velcro fastening to protect dorsum of foot

Firm heel counter

Toe box at least $1\frac{1}{2}$ in. to clear toes

Flared or rounded heel

Mid sole of flexible material

Studded sole to absorb shock and help grip

*Fig. 22.5* Components of a shoe.

United Kingdom alone (Linton, 1983). With such a wide range of possibilities it is important to consider various aspects of shoe design (Fig. 22.5). Sperryn (1980) has made a notable contribution to the study of sports footwear and has drawn the attention of sportspeople and their advisers as well as manufacturers to many design faults and many of the features described derive from his publications.

Unless there is a foot deformity present the design of the shoe last should be straight so as not to push the foot into an angulated gait (Fig. 22.6). The last should be deep enough to accommodate the foot, leaving plenty of room for movement during function. This is particularly

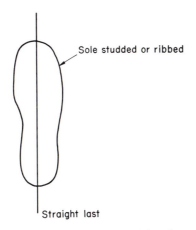

Sole studded or ribbed

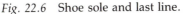

Straight last

*Fig. 22.6* Shoe sole and last line.

important over the area of the toe box, so as to avoid unnecessary bruising. If there are any 'overbones' (as referred to in Chapter 21) the depth of the shoe is also important. In many shoes there is not enough space for either insoles or padding on the dorsum of the foot to be added.

The sole of the shoe needs to have some form of patterning to help grip the ground surface. Often the pattern is not deep enough. Studding of the sole may help shock absorption and help improve grip but must not be too long as excessive grip may predispose to ankle injury. The studs have to be short enough to penetrate and allow sole contact in the ground. This especially applies to rugby and soccer shoes (Williams, 1976). The mid-sole area should be flexible so as not to hinder normal function. The choice of materials available for the sole is wide. Durability is important, but must not override the basic requirements of flexibility. If the sole is too springy there will be a recoil effect which can result in subungual haematomata of the great toe. The outer border of the soles of shoes can be built up to accommodate inversion or eversion gait patterns. A thicker sole may be provided in the case of leg shortening. The toe section of the sole should be rounded to avoid snags and potential 'catching' edges. The heel section of the sole may also be rounded to avoid point impact, that is to spread the impact load. There is a more recent tendency to flared designs which bend into the heel itself, though too much flare is unsuitable for court games such as squash where frequent slewing of the shoe occurs.

The inner sole provides additional padding between the foot and the ground. Some shoes have removable insoles which are heated and shaped to the individual foot. It is surprising that more sports footwear manufacturers do not incorporate such an insole, such as that produced by the 'Thermofit' process used for skiboots. Presumably the cost of this has been prohibitive, but it seems a pity that a similar process is not more readily available for other sports footwear.

The area under the heel may have an additional heel wedge. This is most frequently made of some soft resilient material. In designs where the heel is flared this wedge will also be flared to conform to the shape of the heel.

Many materials are available for the upper section of sports shoes. Lightweight shoes may be of cotton or canvas, heavier ones of leather or manmade fibres. The actual design details themselves sometimes cause problems for the sportsman. Stitching and stripes have been known to cause chafing. In some cases, where the design of the upper does not contour the anatomy of the foot, there may be creases and folds in the material which will cause similar damage. In some instances where the upper is too tightly stretched across the foot, blisters may result. If such shoes are worn frequently, permanent damage to the foot may result.

Moulded uppers might remove the need for seaming across the foot and eliminate this problem.

The heel counter should be quite firm to provide good hindfoot stability. The upper rim by the heel part of the shoe should not be too high. If the heel counter is too high in any part, rubbing will result around the ankle joint. In recent times we have seen examples of 'Achilles tabs' which were supposed to support and avoid irritation of the Achilles tendon. Unfortunately, the opposite has been experienced in models with high heel tabs. It is surprising that even in some of the most expensive products this practice still persists. Designs with high heel tabs should be avoided or cut down to avoid damage. Responses to the postal questionnaire on sports footwear showed that 12% thought such heel tabs should be reduced.

The tongue should be wide enough to protect the dorsum of the foot from the fastening or lacing. The tongue should be shaped to keep the shoe well positioned so as not to allow rotation over the foot. The method of fastening is commonly with laces, although more sports shoes are gradually being introduced with 'Velcro' fastenings. Whichever method is used the fastening usually controls the last variable to width. 'Velcro' straps allow a range of positions for the wearer to use and are quickly placed and removed. Some people prefer laces as they feel more secure. The design with variable lacing has introduced more possibilities for width adaptions. Short lacing is desirable in a training shoe to allow free mobility of the toe end of the shoe. A good fit must not rely on slack being taken up by laces. Rucking can be reduced by double lacing which is particularly useful when the shoe throat is very long (Sperryn, 1980).

## 22.3   Materials for sports shoes

As has already been mentioned a wide range of materials is used for producing sports shoes. Some are natural products, but many manmade fibres are used, some of which have been shown to be very strong and resilient. This has enabled cheaper and more standard production of sports shoes. Ventilation difficulties have been overcome by a patterning of holes in the material. Many of the manmade fibres are easy to wash and therefore may be kept clean more simply than natural materials. 'Vinyls', 'urethane' and 'poromerics' are the main groups of manmade fibres used for shoe production (Rossie, 1983a). Any sports shoes produced with manmade fibre uppers, except for some 'poromerics' will act like closed containers, trapping moisture around the feet. As tests in the United States Tanners Council Research Laboratories have shown, the average

465

pair of adult feet gives off about half a pint of moisture daily. It is therefore not surprising that athletes wearing such closed shoes will suffer from macerated skin and rashes. Natural fibres such as leather have more 'breathability'. The most satisfactory combination is that of manmade soles and natural material uppers.

Suggestions were made in replies to our questionnaire that seamless shoes might be advantageous and of necessity this would require manmade fibres to be used. Many would like a lighter shoe. We are aware that some successful athletes, such as Zola Budd, resort to running without shoes because of their weight and the resulting slowing effect on performance. In addition some sportsmen were concerned about the wear shown inside the shoe on the heel counter liner. This may be improved in the future by using more resilient materials.

## 22.4 Shoe sizes and widths

The major difficulty is that there is not one accepted method of shoe sizing. The English, American, Canadian and French all use different systems. Rossie (1983b) explains that an American 7 is equal to an English $6\frac{1}{2}$, a French 40 or 41 and a metric size 27. Many attempts have been made to devise an internationally accepted system, but without success. There are also different sizes for men and women; for example a lady's English 8 is much smaller than a man's 8.

Many sports shoes are found to be too narrow for the wearer's foot (Fig. 22.7). Constant wearing of such shoes will lead to bruising, blisters and cramping of toes. Shoes which are too shallow will lead to bruised toes and rubbing of the foot. Shoes which are too long will allow a pumping action in the shoe and may cause redness and blisters around the heel and on the toes.

Some shops have small track surfaces where shoes can be tried out more realistically. Serious sportsmen will obviously tend to go to shops catering for their needs. When the sportsman is purchasing sports shoes, he must remember to wear the type of socks, liners and insoles he would normally wear. These make a great difference to an efficient fit. Alternatively, some sportsmen do not wear any interface and in this case must remember to remove socks when trying on shoes.

Most shoes are selected personally. Of the Olympic sportsmen who replied to our questionnaire 88% said they chose their own footwear, whereas *all* the hobby sportsmen chose their shoes. Despite this 16% of the total were not satisfied with their shoes, 26% had made some complaint to the manufacturer about some aspect of the product, but only 16% felt satisfied with the response from the manufacturer, 38% of the

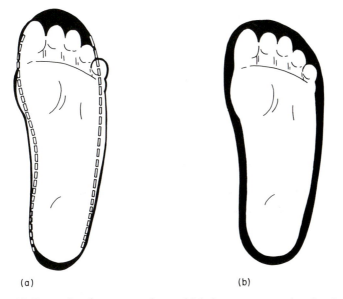

*Fig. 22.7* (a) Example of a sports shoe which is too narrow for the foot. (b) Example of shoe allowing space for the foot.

respondents had made some alterations to their sports shoes, 17% had either added inner soles or changed the inner sole, 12% had removed the heel tabs, 6% had added heel pads, and 6% had raised the heels. Some of the changes were quite radical but perhaps this is not surprising when 57% of the replies said they had sustained damage to their feet because of their sports footwear. One-third had undergone some form of treatment for this damage. The greatest number of cases included damage to the metatarsal and heel areas.

## 22.5  Types of orthoses and adaptations

The International Society for Prosthetics and Orthotics defines an orthosis as a support around a weakened body segment. The range of orthoses most frequently used fall into two main categories, those which are mass produced and those which are custom made for the individual. Some of these custom made orthoses will be produced by the sportsmen themselves, often in an attempt to overcome a new pressure area or blister. At the other extreme, podiatrists, orthotists and others will specially design orthoses from a range of thermoplastic materials. Some of these may be far more expensive than the shoes themselves. However, this may be the only solution to a chronic problem or disability. It is essential that the person producing the orthosis has adequate training in the field as an inappropriate orthosis may create more damage. Mass produced orthoses may be bought in shoe shops or chemists. Products such as those made by Scholl may be a simple solution to the existing problem. Whichever device is chosen, whether self-selected or that obtained through a special orthotic clinic, it is important to make regular checks to ensure that the orthosis is solving the problem. Careful assessment of each case is advisable. Footprints or pedobarographic assessments may be of assistance in this and the latter may be repeated with the orthosis in place (Fig. 22.8).

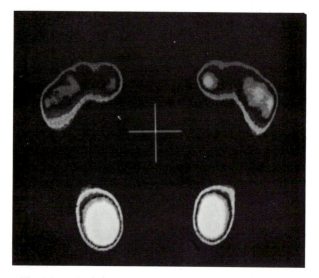

*Fig. 22.8*  Pedobaric assessment showing zonal pressure.

Some orthoses are static without any moving parts; dynamic orthoses allow, or actively encourage, movement. Most orthoses provided by the sportsmen themselves seem to be static. Padding to tongues, heel counters and soles are the most common. Insoles frequently correct medial or lateral border positioning (Fig. 22.9). Others change the angulation of metatarsal heads. Shock absorbing materials have been incorporated into the inner soles of some sportswear to help overcome heel strike thrust. High thrust at heel strike will increase the amount of stress, not only through the subtalar joint, but through the whole of the lower limb (Hlavac, 1979). Severe pain in the hip, knee and spine may be encountered as a result. If the sportsman cannot be trained to correct such action serious damage may result. Heel pads of material such as sor-

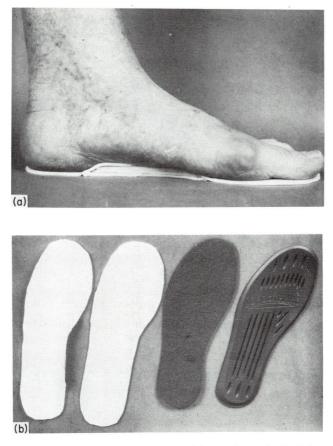

*Fig. 22.9* (a) Insoles to correct the position of the medial arch. (b) Other examples of insoles to correct lateral or medial borders of the foot and absorb shock.

bothane may also be used (Fig. 22.10). In cases of heel spurs, pressure relieving orthoses may help (Fig. 22.11). Heels or ankles may be supported by flexible strapping or anklets (Fig. 22.12) or by a rigid heel cup of 'orthoplast' or 'polypropylene' (Fig. 22.13). Some clinicians believe that protection of the ankle joint places greater pressure on the knee and can increase the number of injuries of the knee (Reid and Healion, 1959).

Dynamic orthoses are mainly prescribed for specific acute or chronic disabilities. Examples include ankle foot orthoses and fracture braces (Fig. 22.14). Any orthosis or adaptation to be put inside the sports shoe must be worn for periods of time to accustom the wearer to the change. It is important not to allow a long training period immediately after fitting. The wearer should follow any instructions carefully and make regular

469

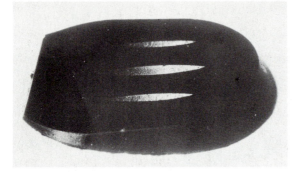

Fig. 22.10   Sorbothane heel pad.

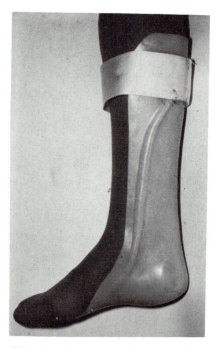

Fig. 22.11   Orthosis for heel spurs.

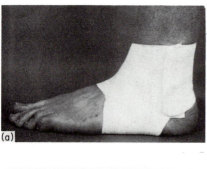

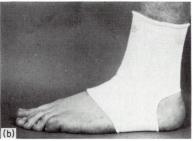

Fig. 22.12   (a) and (b) Ankle and heel supports.

Fig. 22.13   Example of rigid polypropylene ankle foot orthosis.

470

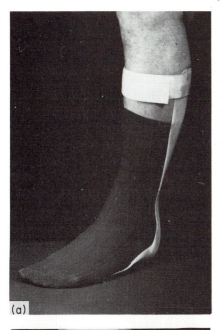

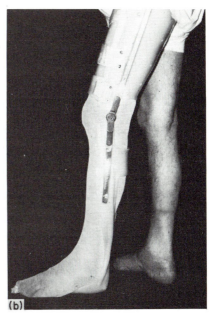

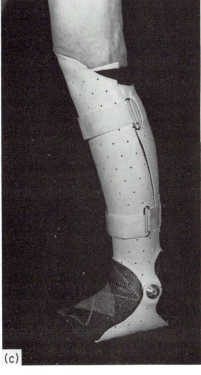

*Fig. 22.14* (a) Dynamic ankle foot orthosis made of polypropylene. (b) Dynamic knee ankle orthosis for femoral shaft fracture. (c) Dynamic tibial fracture brace made of orthoplast.

471

# Sports footwear

checks for abnormal skin colour or pressure problems caused by the orthosis.

## References

Hlavac, H. (1979) *The Foot Book. Advice for Athletes*, World Publications, Mountain View, California.

Linton, I. (1983) Running with the pack. Marketing sales promotion supplement, 8 September, 27.

Mann, R. A. (1975) *Atlas of Orthotics: Biomechanical Principles and Applications* (Ed. American Academy of Orthopaedic Surgeons). C.V. Mosby, St Louis, pp. 257.

Reid, S. E. and Healion, T. E. (1959) Knee and ankle injuries. *Wisc. Med. J.*, **58**, 561.

Rossie, W. A. (1983a) Manmade shoe materials and foot health. *J. Amer. Pod. Assoc.*, **73(6)**, 320.

Rossie, W. A. (1983b) The enigma of shoe sizes. *J. Amer. Pod. Assoc.*, **73(5)**, 272.

Sperryn, P. N. (1980) Running and training shoes. *Medisport*, **2(2)**, 42.

Torg, J. S. and Quendenfeld, T. (1971) Effect of the shoe type and cleat length on incidence and severity of knee injuries among high school football players. *Res. Q. Am. Assoc. Health Phys. Ed.*, **42**, 203.

Williams, J. G. P. (1976) The problem of football boots. Proceedings of the Centenary Medical Congress, Dublin, of the Irish Rugby Football Union.

# 23  *Medicine, sport and the law*

J. M. CAMERON

## 23.1  Introduction

Sports medicine is a specialty that concerns not only ill athletes but healthy ones as well. In it the medical profession can be confronted with a new array of situations, some of them demanding an intervention in fields outside the common experience of many physicians.

As in other specialties in medicine, medical negligence in sports medicine may result in damage, by negligence in diagnosis, treatment or rehabilitation of the 'alleged' injured athlete. One must remember, however, that medical intervention to improve artificially athletic performance is a common practice and in itself can cause iatrogenic disease which could be considered as medical negligence. This occurs as a result of the use of methods which may not be in general accord with professional ethics or which may be harmful to the sportsman/woman or athlete.

As a result of the concern expressed by this major medical association in the world regarding the unethical and illicit use of certain medical practices in sports, the World Medical Association in September 1981 met in Lisbon. They approved the Declaration of Principles of Health Care for Sports Medicine and within the thirteen articles of the Declaration an attempt was made to establish a set of rules to which medical intervention should comply worldwide.

The medicolegal aspects of sport are usually associated with death or injuries caused by physical activity. Medical intervention to improve artificially athletic performance, however, represents a relatively new field where specialists in sports medicine and team doctors are confronted with new ethical issues (Reys, 1982). The World Medical Association in its Declaration produced in Lisbon (1981) can be assumed to have prepared a Code of Ethics for Sports Medicine (Reys, 1982). Amongst its recommendations many are particularly concerned with the prevention of iatrogenic damage to athletes and sportsmen.

# Medicine, sport and the law

One of the great myths in which Britain as a sports-crazed nation fondly believes is an increasing age of sporting leisure time (Grayson, 1978). Two High Court awards in the 1970s in England confirmed what the criminal courts in England had established in 1878, namely that a foul tackle could be a civil as well as a common assault. This contradicted the idea that the great god sport transcends the country's laws.

Nowadays more and more people are becoming involved and concerned with the vast sporting complex of the nation which gave sport its concept of fair play to the world. This (Grayson, 1978) creates an overriding entanglement with the country's legal system spanning the internal administration of any particular game or pastime. 'Sport is fun, politics often is not. The two cannot mix; politics can only destroy sport' (Grayson, 1983).

Medical professional practice is not all a bed of roses. The best intentions of doctors sometimes go awry. Mistakes mar the handling of patients, create errors in diagnosis, and spoil the chances of successful treatment. It is only when these arise from a lack of ease, failure to ensure accuracy in records or communications, or from a more serious disregard of ethical standards, that trouble is bound to follow.

As more and more leisure time is created, more and more people become seduced by the joys of sport: playing, watching or administering. Therefore there is a great need to know the rights and privileges which sport provides both economically and socially; the duties and obligations that exist not only under the laws of each particular sport but also under the laws of the land which is supreme.

## (a) Spectators

Spectators constitute the greatest section of the sports loving public. Today in Britain the Safety of Sports Ground Act 1975 has created headaches all round. A spectator generally has no protection against a promoter who regulates his affairs safely, or the player who performs within the rules of a particular game.

## (b) Player athletes

The playing area creates the greatest scope for errors, ignorance and misunderstanding relating sport to law and law to sport.

The sporting scene in Britain has traditionally been well served and guided at national levels from the legal profession. This is reflected in the high standards throughout the administration of all sports. For example, the British Boxing Board of Control has been and still is served by a successive generation of practising King's and Queen's Counsel who see that the Queensbury Rules are maintained. The Football League Management Committee has frequently been chaired by practising solicitors, the

474

Lawn Tennis Association has in recent years been presided over by a former Old Bailey Judge (Sir Carl Aarvold), and the current president of the International Lawn Tennis Association is a Chancery Queen's Counsel (Grayson, 1978).

## 23.2 Medical aspects

The Declaration of Principles of Health Care for Sports Medicine is particularly concerned with the prevention of iatrogenic damage to athletes as sportsmen and women.

Modification of blood constituents and biochemistry, use of drugs, psychological manipulation, pain suppression and alterations of sex and age features are all condemned by ethical standards. The risks of iatrogenesis inherent to each of these medical interventions are of different magnitude, and not all of these are prevented by law. On the other hand prohibition laws without satisfactory methods to enforce them are not effective. In some cases, as in psychological manipulation, no reliable control is available. Laboratory methods to detect auto- or hetero-transfusions, use of corticosteroids and of some other hormones are currently being investigated. Analytical control of doping has advanced and nowadays it requires a very high level of technology and expertise.

It is known that physical activity has some risks when practised without medical supervision. Unfortunately it has to be recognized that certain medical practices to improve artificially the athlete's performance are not only unfair and unethical but represent a potential source of iatrogenic disease. They have to be discouraged by legislative measures supported by appropriate methods of enforcement.

Doping may be defined as the administration of drugs to increase artificially an athlete's performance. The main group of drugs are psychomotor stimulant drugs, sympathomimetic drugs, other central nervous stimulants, narcotic analgesics and anabolic steroids. Adverse reaction to these drugs may include acute health hazard or chronic disability, either of them potentially fatal. Laboratory control of drug abuse is feasible by analytical methods such as thin layer chromatography, gas liquid chromatography and mass spectrometry.

Some controversial practices such as hypnosis or extreme psychological pressure have no legal grounds to control them. As a matter of fact hypnosis was considered a forbidden practice in one of the former Regulations for Anti-Doping Control at the Olympic Games, but it had to be withdrawn for lack of practical ways to prove it.

Narcotic analgesics and local anaesthetics are the main drugs used to mask pain. This happens not only in contact sports such as boxing and wrestling but also in football, soccer and other games where serious lesions may occur. Corticotherapy is frequently used for its anti-inflammatory actions and also because it is credited with anti-stress properties. The long-term use of corticosteroids in athletes and sportsmen may induce chronic disabilities and even death. The resource to analgesics is forbidden if they are intended to keep an injured athlete or sportsman in competition. However, while detection of major analgesics offers no difficulty with current laboratory methods, the control of corticosteroids is much more difficult.

Certain sport activities benefit from small complexion and weight of athletes. Such is the case with gymnastics, for example, where smaller and lighter female gymnasts have distinct advantages over their heavier and older rivals. Slowing of puberty and development is perfectly within the realm of medical possibilities. From 1978 on, medical authorities have been suspicious that some participants have been treated with drugs acting probably on the pituitary gland. So far this has not been confirmed, but growing concern with this matter is expressed in the second article of the Declaration:

> When the sports participant is a child or an adolescent the physician must give first consideration to the growth and stage of development.

On the other hand, anabolic steroids have deserved much more attention. The use of steroids by healthy sportsmen is condemned but the onus of discovery and elimination rests on the sports medical authorities. Laboratory tests for anabolic steroids are available, but they are expensive and require considerable expertise.

In cases of doubtful sex, mainly in feminine contests, the necessity to confirm the sex of the participant may arise. Karyotype study has replaced the gynaecological examination or sex chromatin determination for this purpose.

With regard to training and taking part in events in conditions compatible with the preservation of the athlete's fitness, health and safety, it should be a matter of common sense to prohibit strenuous physical activity when the athlete's health or other conditions make it inadvisable. However, fatal accidents do occur and, for example, heat stroke can be a cause of death in sportsmen.

Medicolegal aspects of sports are usually associated with death or injuries caused by physical activity. However, medical intervention to improve artificially athletic performance represents a relatively new field where sports doctors are confronted with new ethical issues. This World Medical Association has stated in its Declaration of Principles of Health Care for Sport Medicine the main ethical guidelines for physicians in order to meet the needs of athletes. This Declaration can be assumed as a code of ethics for sports medicine and amongst its recommendations are some concerned particularly with the prevention of iatrogenic damage to athletes and sportsmen (see Appendix 2).

## References

Reys, L. L. (1982) Iatrogenic disease in sports medicine. *Acta Med. Leg. Social.*, **32**, 283.
Grayson, E. (1978) *Sport and the Law, Sunday Telegraph* Publications.
Grayson, E. (1983) Forget politics and play the game. *Sunday Telegraph* magazine.

# Appendix 1 *Articles of association and rules of the Amateur Boxing Association of England. 2nd edition 1984*

## Procedure following K.Os

It is advisable to send every boxer who has suffered from concussion or amnesia during a boxing contest to hospital for examination.

*Procedure after knockouts and when the referee has stopped the fight*

(1) A boxer who has been knocked out as a result of a head blow, or if the referee has stopped the contest due to a boxer having received hard blows to the head, making him defenceless or incapable of continuing, shall be examined by a doctor immediately afterwards; he should be accompanied to his home or suitable accommodation by one of the officials on duty at the tournament.

(2) A boxer who has been knocked out during a contest, or if the referee has stopped the contest due to a boxer having received hard blows to the head, making him defenceless or incapable of continuing, shall not be permitted to take part in competitive boxing or sparring for a period of at least twenty-eight days after he has been knocked out.

(3) A boxer who has been knocked out during a contest, or if the referee has stopped the contest due to a boxer having received hard blows to the head, making him defenceless or incapable of continuing twice in a period of 84 days, shall not be permitted to take part in competitive boxing or sparring during a period of 84 days from the second knockout or fight which has been stopped by the referee.

(4) A boxer who has been knocked out during a contest, or if the referee has stopped the contest due to a boxer having received hard blows to the head, making him defenceless or incapable of continuing three times in a period of 12 months, shall not be allowed to take part in competitive boxing or sparring for a period of one year from the third knockout or fight which has been stopped.

(5) The referee will indicate to the officer in charge and judges to endorse the score card 'R.S.C.(H)' when he has stopped the contest as a result of a boxer being unable to continue as a result of blows to the head.

# Appendix 2 *Prohibited drugs recommended by the Medical Commission of the Olympic Association*

## (a) Psychomotor stimulant drugs

Amphetamine
Benzphetamine
Chlophentermine
Cocaine
Diethylpropion
Dimethylamphetamine
Ethylamphetamine
Fencamfamin
Meclofenoxate
Methylamphetamine

Methylphenidate
Norpseudoephedrine
Pemoline
Phendimetrazine
Phenmetrazine
Phentermine
Pipradrol
Prolintane
and related compounds

## (b) Sympathomimetic amines

Chlorprenaline
Ephedrine
Etafedrine
Isoetharine

Isoprenaline
Methoxyphenamine
Methylephedrine
and related compounds

## (c) Miscellaneous central nervous system stimulants

Amiphenazole
Bemigride
Caffeine (if the urine concentration exceeds 15 µg ml$^{-1}$)
Cropropamide
Crotethamide
Doxapram

Ethamivan
Leptazol
Nikethamide
Picrotoxine
Strychnine
and related compounds

## Appendix 2

### (d) Narcotic analgesics

Anileridine
Codeine
Dextromoramide
Dihydrocodeine
Dipipanone
Ethylmorphine
Heroin
Hydrocodone
Hydromorphone
Levorphanol
Methadone

Morphine
Oxocodone
Oxomorphone
Pentazocine
Pethidine
Phenazocine
Piminodine
Thebacon
Trimeperidine
and related compounds

### (e) Anabolic steroids

Clostebol
Dehydrochlormethyltestosterone
Fluoxymesterone
Mesterolone
Metenolone
Methandienone
Methyltestosterone
Nandrolone
Norethandrolone

Oxymesterone
Oxymetholone
Stanozolol
Testosterone (if the ratio of the total concentration of testosterone to that of epi-testosterone in the urine exceeds 6)
and related compounds

### (f) Beta-adrenoceptor blocking drugs

Acebutolol
Atenolol
Labetalol
Metoprolol
Nadolol
Propranolol

Oxprenolol
Penbutolol
Pindolol
Sotalol
Timolol
and related compounds

The technique of blood enhancement when a sportsman receives a transfusion of his own blood taken previously is now prohibited.

# Index

# Index

484

# Index

486

# Index

# Index

490

# Index

# Index

494

# Index

# Index

knee injuries, 367
  posterior elbow pain, 273
Whitlow due to ingrowing nail, 439
Wilson's sign, 376
Winding of abdomen, 168
Wire fixation of upper vertebrae, 137
Wobble board, 402
World Medical Association, Lisbon, 1981,
  473
Wrestling, ulnar nerve damage, 308
Wrist
  bursitis, 283
  fractures, 289
  injuries, 281–317
  level problems, 282–3
  median entrapment, 283–4
  pain causes on radial side, 282–3
  pain causes on ulnar side, 282
  sprains, 292
  tendinitis, 283
  tenosynovitis, 283

ulnar collateral ligament sprains, 286
ulnar head subluxation and styloid fracture, 286

X-ray
  in abdominal injuries, 166–7
  of elbow and forearm injuries, 248–9
  of elbow, gravity stress, 260
  of sacro-iliac joints, 334

Yachtsmen
  foot problems, 440
  severed finger flexors, 307
  tenosynovitis, 304–5

'Z'-plasties for finger wounds, 294–5
  for knee injury, 396
Ziehl–Neelsen's stain, 200
Zygomatic bone complex fractures, 72, 74
  summary of signs, 77
  treatment, 86–7